BUILT
TO THE
HILT

BUILT TO THE HILT

Creating A Muscularly Strong And Superbly Conditioned Body
That Will Last A Lifetime

BY
Josh Bryant

Special thanks from the publisher and author to
Michael Neveux, Kevin Jordan, Dr. Sal Arria, Betty Abrantes, and Lynette Smith

PUBLISHED BY
The Creative Syndicate
10400 Overland Road, Suite 143
Boise, Idaho, USA 83709

BOOK INFORMATION:
www.BuiltToTheHilt.com
http://JoshStrength.com

PHOTOGRAPHY BY Michael Neveux

MODEL: Kevin Jordan

LAYOUT & DESIGN: Betty Abrantes

COPYEDITING: Lynette Smith

ISBN (PRINT): 978-1-937939-34-2
ISBN (EBOOK): 978-1-937939-35-9
First Printing 2014
Library of Congress Control Number 2013956589

BUILT
TO THE
HILT

**CREATING A MUSCULARLY
STRONG AND SUPERBLY
CONDITIONED BODY THAT
WILL LAST A LIFETIME**

By

JOSH BRYANT

To Dr. Fred Hatfield

For his tremendous help with this book
and for serving as my first inspiration
to investigate the scientific side
of lifting

CONTENTS

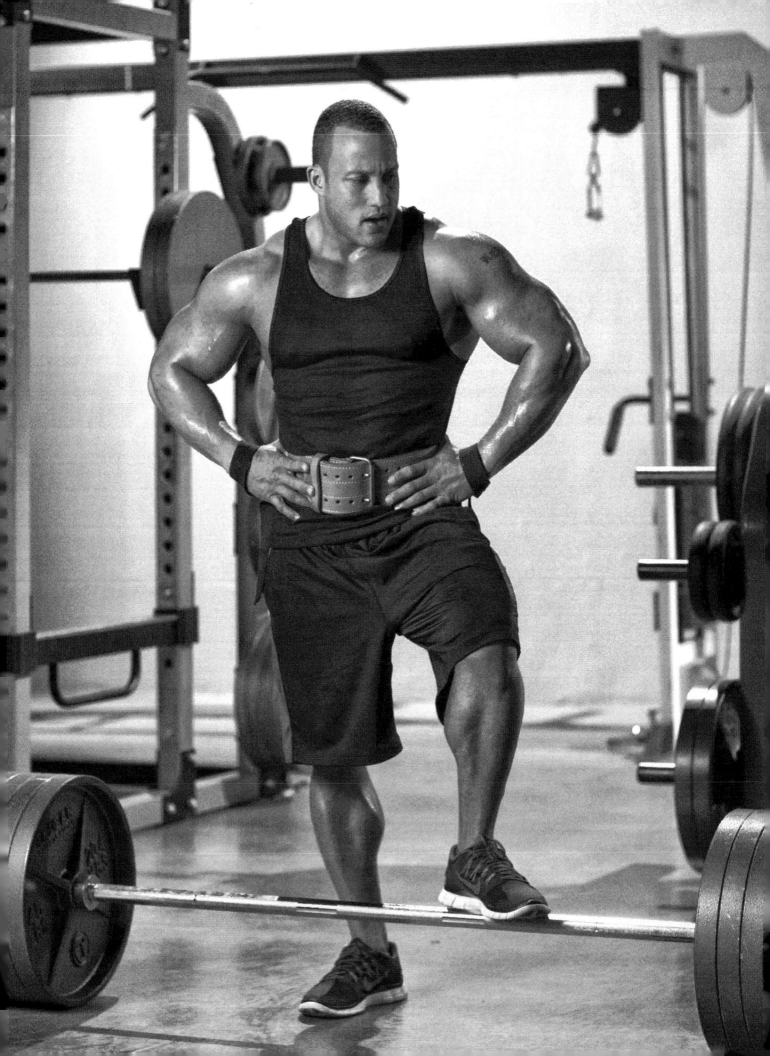

CHAPTER 1.

Bodybuilding Methods and Traditions

"Bro science" is an anecdotal creed emanating from bodybuilding circles. It has driven training methodologies for generations of iron disciples. Some of these methods are validated by scientific studies, while others need to be eradicated from the body-builder's regimen.

Let's take a look at a number of popular methodologies commonly used by bodybuilders.

SPLIT SYSTEM TRAINING

For beginners, entire body training sessions are sufficient as they provide an ample stimulus for neural adaptation and trigger muscle growth. In fact, effective full body sessions may consist of only one set per body part. However, the gains from full body sessions taper off rather quickly, necessitating more advanced protocols.

Super Sets, Giant Sets, Rest Pause Sets, Drop Sets, Pyramiding, High Volume Training and sets consisting of multiple movements, or triple sets, are used by bodybuilders to prompt more muscle growth.

Keep in mind that using these advanced tactics while engaging in full body training sessions may be difficult, due to the extreme neural, mechanical, and metabolic demands placed on the body.

As such, a good idea is to shift your full body training to Split System Training, which will allow for maximal muscle stimulation while permitting time for your body to recover. This division of training is known as the Split System.

If you decide to train the same exercises repeatedly throughout the week with a goal of accelerating neural adaptations, you could find yourself sacrificing intensity, and working within percentages well below your one-rep maximum, thus shortchanging any gains in hypertrophy or strength.

One classic program is the 5 x 5, which calls for performing five sets of five repetitions of the squat, bench press and power clean, done three days per week.

Obviously you could choose to train each lift at full tilt during each session, but that would quickly lead to physical and mental burnout. Alternatively, you could fluctuate the training stresses throughout the week while still ingraining movement patterns, necessary to expedite neural adaptations, by alternating heavy (H), medium (M) and light (L) days for each movement.

That would look like this:

Monday
Power Clean (H)
Squat (M)
Bench Press (L)

Wednesday
Power Clean (M)
Squat (L)
Bench Press (H)

Friday
Power Clean (L)
Squat (H)
Bench Press (M)

Because of neural adaptations, you can improve at the movement without running the risk of overtraining. The split may not be divided by body part; however, intensity is cycled, or waved, breaking up the training stimulus in a sensible manner. You can easily adapt the aforementioned outline to any series of lifts on a three-day-per-week training split.

Training splits can be arranged in a seemingly infinite number of combinations. Another popular split, adapted from old school college football strength and conditioning programs, is the push/pull system, broken down by training pressing and squatting movements one day and training pulling movements, which would include chin-ups, rows, and deadlifts, on the other day.

A time-efficient twist to the push/pull system is to combine the movements in the same session and perform them as supersets throughout the workout. A pushing movement would be paired with a pulling movement.

Examples are:

- Vertical Push Movement (Military Press) superset with Vertical Pulling Movement (Chin-up)
- Horizontal Pushing Movement (Bench Press) superset with Horizontal Pulling Movement (T-Bar Row)

Seemingly infinite combinations of training splits can be designed. Commonly employed splits include body-part training splits, where only one or two muscle groups are targeted each workout; antagonist body-part splits, where muscles that oppose one another are trained in the same workout; and movement-based splits, in which one compound movement, such as a squat, bench, or deadlift, is performed each workout.

Splits may also consist of training to failure, such as High Intensity Training, or they may emphasize phases of muscular contractions to induce more muscle growth. The realm of possibilities is practically endless.

Regardless of what split you choose to follow, it is imperative that you adhere to proven training principles. You must maximize energy levels for individual workouts and know that the results of a training program are the sum of individual workouts. When things are done right, the outcome is greater than the sum. In other words, synergy takes place and puts you on the road to building a championship physique.

SUPERSET

A superset is when two exercises are performed consecutively without a break. Originally, supersets were defined as combing two exercises of antagonist (opposing) muscle groups. An example would be a biceps curl immediately followed by a triceps extension.

A very popular method of supersetting, because of the emphasis on proper postural alignment and the elimination of muscle imbalances, is the push/pull superset system. This could be a horizontal or vertical pressing movement followed by a horizontal or vertical pull movement. An example would be a bench press paired with bent over row or a military press paired with a chin-up. The obvious benefit is that symmetrical development of opposition muscle groups is enhanced. This system is more intense than the traditional set system.

Arnold Schwarzenegger popularized supersets with the idea, "More work could get done in less time."

Here are some practical examples of traditional supersets:

Legs
Leg Extensions / Stiff Leg Deadlifts
Sissy Squats / Leg Curls

Chest, Shoulders and Back
Flat Benches / T-Bar Rows
Military Press / Chin-ups
Front Raises / Face Pulls

Arms
Close Grip Bench Press / One-Armed Eccentric Barbell Curls
Tricep Push-downs / Scott Curls

In today's world of bodybuilding, the term superset is sometimes used differently than its original intent. Frequently, it is used to describe a single-joint (isolation) movement paired with a multi-joint (compound movement) for the same muscle group.

A popular chest superset would be a pec deck and a bench press. Some of our more artistically inclined bodybuilding brethren perform two movements for the same muscle group with different emphasis. An example of this would be the incline press supersetted with a weighted dip. The incline press would be for the clavicular portion of the pectoralis muscle group (upper chest) and the dips for the sternal aspect of the same muscle group (lower chest).

Examples of within group supersets:

Quadriceps from Different Angles
Leg Extensions and Hack Squats
Upper Back from Different Angles
Chin-ups and Seated Rows
Shoulders from Different Angles
Lateral Raises and Overhead Presses

GIANT SETS

As we climb our way up the mountain of intensity, we step into the land of Giant Sets. A Giant Set consists of combining three exercises and sometimes even more without resting between exercises.

A Giant/Tri Set, in its original intention, would be used to develop individual muscles within groups consisting of three or more muscles. An example would be lateral raises, inverted flyes, and front raises. These three exercises would work the three heads of the deltoids (lateral "side," posterior "rear," and anterior "front") as independently as possible.

Here are some examples of giant sets:

Quadriceps at Different Angles
Leg Extension, Sissy Squats, Front Squats
Chest at Different Angles
Chain Flyes, Chain Bench Press, Bench Presses
Triceps at Different Angles
Triceps Push-downs, Upright Bar Dips, Barbell Triceps Extension, Triceps Extension
Back at Different Angles
Chin-ups, Dumbbell Rows, Reverse Hyper Extensions

REST-PAUSE METHOD

Rest-pause training breaks down one set into several mini-sets with a brief rest between each. Depending on the intensity level and what you hope to accomplish, several different methods can be used.

For strength, this involves taking a single at 85%–95% of your one-repetition max, then waiting 15–30 seconds and then performing another single with the same weight and repeating this process until failure. Typically, 6–8 singles can be done. This method is extremely taxing on the central nervous system and can be dangerous. Generally, the adaptations are more neurologically driven for strength than for increases in muscle size.

Many old-time strength aficionados swear by this method and it has certainly worked for some; but with everything we do in training, we must weigh the risks and benefits. Proceed with caution when experimenting with this method.

An example of this type of training on the bench press, for someone with a one-repetition max of 300 pounds, would be to use 275 pounds, rest 15 seconds, then keep repeating and stop after failure.

A more effective variation of this method can be used for the bodybuilder seeking muscle hypertrophy. Select your chosen exercise and select a weight you can perform for 6–10 repetitions, lift the weight to failure, stop and rest for 15 seconds, and do the same weight again to failure; this will probably be 2–3 repetitions. Repeat this process once or twice; it is very tough to go beyond three sets.

If you select the bench press as your exercise, a rest-pause series with an emphasis on hypertrophy might look something like this:

Set 1: 225 x 8 reps
Rest 15 seconds
Set 2: 225 x 3 reps
Rest 15 seconds
Set 3: 225 x 2 reps

This method is a great way to bust through a plateau and teach you to grind out reps. Your muscle fibers will be very fatigued and, because of the short repetitive bout, you will build a fantastic mind-muscle connection and experience a mind-blowing pump.

This is also very taxing on the central nervous system (CNS); do not use this method every workout or for multiple sets of the same exercises or movements. Because of the strain on the CNS, avoid doing this method for highly technical movements.

Recent research provides some interesting findings on the rest-pause method's effectiveness.

A study was published in *Journal of Science & Medicine of Sport* that consisted of 14 subjects who performed three different resistance training protocols involving 20 repetitions in the squat with 80% of their current one-rep max. The first training protocol consisted of five sets of four reps with a 3-minute rest interval; the second program consisted of five sets of four reps with 20-second rest intervals; and finally the rest-pause method consisted of the initial set to failure, then subsequent sets were completed after a 20-second rest interval.

All training methods had similar decreases in maximal force and rate of force development post workout; however, increased motor-unit recruitment was observed following the rest-pause protocol.

DROP SETS

Drops sets are an effective method for packing on slabs of muscle. However, they too place a tremendous strain on the Central Nervous System.

Drop sets should be used sparingly because it is easy to overtrain with this method. If you decide to utilize drop sets in your training program, one to two per workout won't hurt; but if used week in and week out in a training cycle, central and peripheral fatigue will quickly accumulate. Residual fatigue from prior sessions will inhibit your body's ability to recover and will severely impact CNS functioning.

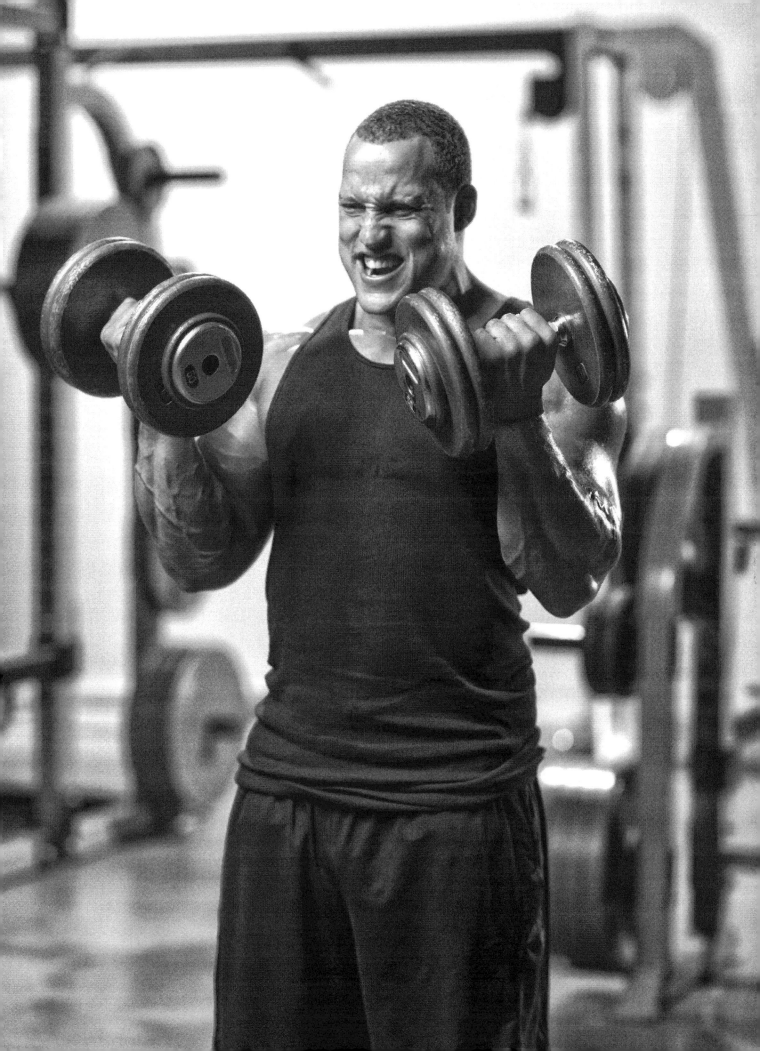

The purpose of drop setting is to provide a "shock" stimulus to the muscles by placing much more additional stress on a muscle than would be true for a traditional set, inducing a higher degree of muscle hypertrophy.

Drop sets work simply because they recruit the entire spectrum of muscle fibers, ranging from the powerful fast-twitch fibers down to the slow-twitch oxidative fibers.

Fast-twitch fibers are worked from the initial heavy weight, and the slow-twitch muscle fibers are worked from the final high repetitions. Because of the overall volume of blood that moves to the muscle group being trained, bodybuilders will experience an amazing pump, filling the area being worked with oxygenated, protein-enriched blood, setting the stage for newfound muscle growth.

Traditionally, drop sets have been used as a way to continue exercise with a lower intensity once muscular failure has been achieved at a higher intensity.

Muscular failure is key to making muscles grow, because it stimulates the release of growth hormone (GH) and insulin-like growth factor-1 (IGF-1). Many bodybuilders opt to perform their drop sets on plate-loaded or selectorized machines, as it's relatively safer and because it allows bodybuilders or workout partners to quickly reduce the load, either by shedding plates or by adjusting the pin along the weight stack. Some ambitious bodybuilders use drop sets with barbell and even dumbbell exercises.

I have taken this a step further and included some optimal leverage (mechanical advantage drop sets) and accommodating resistance drop-set techniques.

An example of a dumbbell drop set would be the rack and run technique. Let's use lateral raises as an example.

If your top set of lateral raises with dumbbells is 30 pounds, you would perform this weight until failure. Next, you would do the same thing with 25 pounds, then 20 pounds, then 15 pounds, then 10 pounds, and finally 5 pounds; you run down the dumbbell rack from your top set to the lightest weight on the rack.

Barbell drop sets are usually associated with the strip set, meaning you have small plates on the barbell and, once muscular failure is reached, you strip one of the plates off and continue.

An example would be doing biceps curls with 105 pounds, which would be a 45-pound bar with three 10s on each side; curl this weight until failure. Then, your partners immediately strip a 10-pound plate off each side; then you do 85 pounds until muscle failure. Repeat the process, then it is 65 pounds until failure. You could continue this all the way down to the 45-pound Olympic bar.

Accommodated resistance drop sets are simply performing a traditional exercise with the addition of bands or chains.

Let's use the bench press as an example, with 200 pounds of weight on the bar with an additional 100 pounds of chains (two 25-pound chains on each side). Complete the maximum repetitions with the two chains on the bar, racking the bar upon failure, and have a partner pull one chain off each side of the bar. Next, complete the maximum amount of repetitions with 200 pounds on the barbell and 50 pounds of chains; upon failure, remove the last pair of chains. Finally, complete the 200-pound bench press with straight bar weight.

Mechanical advantage or optimal leverage drop sets, unlike traditional drop sets, do not include a reduction in weight after each set; instead, the drop is an improvement of leverage.

Let's use the incline dumbbell press as an example. Start with the incline at 60 degrees and perform the exercise to failure. Next set, drop the adjustable incline bench to a 40-degree angle and perform the incline dumbbell press to failure. Finally, drop the incline to 20 degrees and perform the exercise to failure.

Unlike traditional drop setting where weight is reduced, this method improves leverage, so as you get tired your leverage improves. It is a different way of manipulating intensity than just reducing weight. Generally, drop sets are reduced in weight/intensity 10%–30% per drop, and 2–3 drops are performed. Again, remember to use these methods with caution!

This is just the tip of the iceberg. Be creative, experiment, and learn.

STAGGERED SETS

This type of training is when you stagger your smaller and slower developing body parts between sets for larger muscle groups, like doing a set of wrist curls or concentration curls between sets of leg presses or squats. This will allow you to train the bigger muscle group (legs, in this example) with plenty of energy and power, while also working the smaller muscle (either forearms or biceps, in this example).

Many times bodybuilders need to bring up a lagging muscle group, which may require as many as 40 sets per week for that particular muscle group. This cannot be done effectively in one workout, so increased frequency is needed. Staggered sets provide an ample opportunity to increase frequency and get in those extra sets.

TRADITIONAL PYRAMIDING

Pyramiding involves performing sets consisting of high reps at the beginning of the workout (base of pyramid), working towards the top of the pyramid by decreasing reps and increasing weight.

Because you start with lighter weights, it gives your muscles and connective tissues a chance to warm up for the heavier weight later in the workout. As you increase weight, you overload your muscle fibers, and that induces muscle hypertrophy.

Pyramid training has the advantage of many variables that can be manipulated to increase intensity; and, after all, increased intensity will increase muscle mass.

Let's look at this example of a pyramid squat workout.

Set 1: 225 x 12, rest interval 3 minutes
Set 2: 245 x 9, rest interval 3 minutes
Set 3: 260 x 7, rest interval 3 minutes
Set 4: 275 x 5, rest interval 3 minutes
Set 5: 290 x 3

With all of these different sets for a different number of repetitions, there are countless possibilities of ways to increase intensity.

If we reduce the rest interval by just 10 seconds, we have increased intensity.

If we add just one repetition to one of the sets, we have increased intensity.

If we add an extra set, we have an increased intensity, and of course we could just pile more pig iron on the bar.

Pyramids offer a plethora of ways to increase intensity, our ultimate goal, and this is something many haphazard training bodybuilders fail to track.

Many strength athletes have used pyramids for decades with success; and as bodybuilders, we must remember that our base is our limit strength!

The above example is a traditional ascending pyramid. Here are some variations of the traditional pyramid:

Triangle Pyramid ("Egyptian Pyramid")
In this technique, you work your way up (ascending) the pyramid, then back down (descending). Here is an example in the deadlift for someone with a max of 350 pounds:

Set 1: 255 pounds x 8 reps
Set 2: 285 pounds x 6reps
Set 3: 315 pounds x 4 reps
Set 4: 285 pounds x 6 reps
Set 5: 255 pounds x 8 reps

Double Wave Loads

Here is an example in the bench press for someone who has a one-repetition max of 300 pounds. Using this method, you follow an ascending pyramid two times.

> Set 1: 200 pounds x 12 reps
> Set 2: 215 pounds x 10 reps
> Set 3: 235 pounds x 8 reps
> Set 4: 200 pounds x 12 reps
> Set 5: 215 pounds x 10 reps
> Set 6: 235 pounds x 8 reps

REVERSE PYRAMIDING

As you just learned, traditional pyramiding means high reps at the beginning of the workout (the base of the pyramid) and, as you build your way up the pyramid, you decrease reps and increase weight.

Reverse pyramiding is the opposite; the base is the heavy weight and you increase reps and decrease weight as you work your way up the pyramid.

If you're burning yourself out on light weights and not giving yourself a chance to make strength gains, you're shortchanging yourself. I don't want to say traditional pyramiding is flawed, but if you need to build your base and you use this approach, you need to make sure you save enough energy for your heavier sets.

One reason some people have such effective results with traditional pyramid training is that their lighter sets are essentially warm-up sets. They are not burning themselves out; they are simply warming up.

Many college strength coaches purposely assign lighter sets that are not fatiguing prior to the heavy sets because they know the athletes will not properly warm up.

With reverse pyramid training, a proper warm-up is essential. Warming up is an art, not a science; it will ultimately come down to your personal preference.

Here is a generic warm-up that would work well for reverse pyramid training if your top set is 250 on the bench.

General warm-up: 8–10 minutes walking on the treadmill or on the bike, just to get some blood flow; then do 5–10 minutes of dynamic stretching, followed by bench press.

> Set 1 bar: 2 x 10
> Set 2 bar: 95 x 6
> Set 3 bar: 135 x 6

Set 4 bar: 185 x 4
Set 5 bar: 225 x 1

Reverse pyramiding will allow you to build strength very effectively because the most important strength-building set is the first set in this rep scheme. Therefore, the athlete is 100% fresh.

Post Activation Potentiation (PAP) refers to the enhancement of muscle function following a high force activity.

Legendary Russian Sports Scientist, Yuri Verkhoshansky, explained PAP in layman's terms: "When you perform a 3–5 rep max followed by a light explosive set… to your nervous system it's like lifting a half can of water when you think it's full." The weight feels lighter and moves faster.

When training heavy on a core lift, we are generally lifting the weight, if it is a work set, with maximal force. Most studies on PAP are generally done on things like heavy squats followed by an explosive activity like a vertical jump. Many studies show the effectiveness of PAP, but the same holds true when moving from a maximal weight to a submaximal weight.

I have used this strategy with people performing a bench press for maximum reps at a football combine. If the weight is 225 for maximum reps, they will do a single with a weight in the 275–315 range. They can always do more reps this way, as opposed to warming up and making 225 the heaviest set.

Although I do not have studies to back this up, I have found you can always do more on a rep max if you lift heavier weight first. Of course, this is assuming you don't overdo it. Simply put, 300 pounds feels lighter if you have just lifted 400 pounds.

Reverse Pyramiding can be used year round. However, it would not be a good idea to do heavy singles, doubles and triples year round. There will need to be some variation in the intensity, sets, and reps schemes. However, the concept can be used as long the variables that dictate intensity are properly manipulated.

Here is an example of a legs-oriented reverse-pyramid workout:

Legs, Bodybuilding Oriented
Squats: 3 (90%), 5 (85%), 8 (78 %), 12 (70%)
Squats: 10 (bottom half), 10 (top half), 10 (full range of motion)
Walking Lunges (per side): 6, 8, 10
Dumbbell Bulgarian Split Squats (Tempo–5-0-3-0): 5, 6, 8
Leg Press: 20, 30, 40, 50
Leg Ext (Tempo 3-0-2-0): 10, 12, 14
Leg Curl/Stiff Leg Deadlift superset (decrease weight both movements each

superset as reps increase): 6/8, 9/11, 12/15, 15/20
Abs: 8 sets

PRE-EXHAUSTION TRAINING

Using a single-joint "isolation" movement to failure before performing a heavier multi-joint "compound" movement is performed is called *pre-exhaustion training*. A practical example would be leg extensions before front squats (for the quadriceps) or cable flyes before the bench press for the chest.

This technique was popularized by Arnold Schwarzenegger in the movie *Pumping Iron*. If you watched it, you'll remember Arnold performing leg extensions before squats. While a seemingly uncanny practice, the idea behind pre-exhaustion training is this: When you fatigue the prime mover muscle with an isolation exercise prior to a heavier compound movement, you will lead to greater muscle fiber recruitment because muscular fatigue will set in before neurological fatigue.

Compound movements require a far greater degree of neuromuscular activity than single joint movements do. Theoretically, you'll get the best of both worlds by inserting pre-exhaustion training in your repertoire, as you'll recruit more muscle fibers, which will ultimately lead to much greater muscle growth.

Some prominent coaches and trainers believe pre-exhaustion training is more friendly to the joints as muscular fatigue sets in prior to training heavy compound movements, which now can be trained using lighter loads yet still yield hypertrophic benefits.

All of this sounds great! So what does science have to say?

One 2003 study in the *Journal of Strength and Conditioning Research* conducted on 17 men showed the effect of pre-exhaustion training on lower-extremity muscle activation during the leg press. Prior to performing the leg press exercise, subjects performed a 10-repetition maximum in the leg extension; then a 10-repetition maximum was performed in the leg press.

Muscle activation was measured using electromyography (EMG), which showed that activity of the quadriceps, or target muscle, was significantly less when subjects were pre-exhausted. Judging the muscle-building effect of an exercise requires more than an EMG reading, but the subjects were able to complete more repetitions and use more weight on the leg press when not in a pre-exhausted state.

The conclusion of this study was contrary to most bodybuilders' belief that pre-exhaustion training has a disadvantageous effect on performance because of decreased muscular activity and reduced strength when performing core lifts, which, after all, are the core of our training.

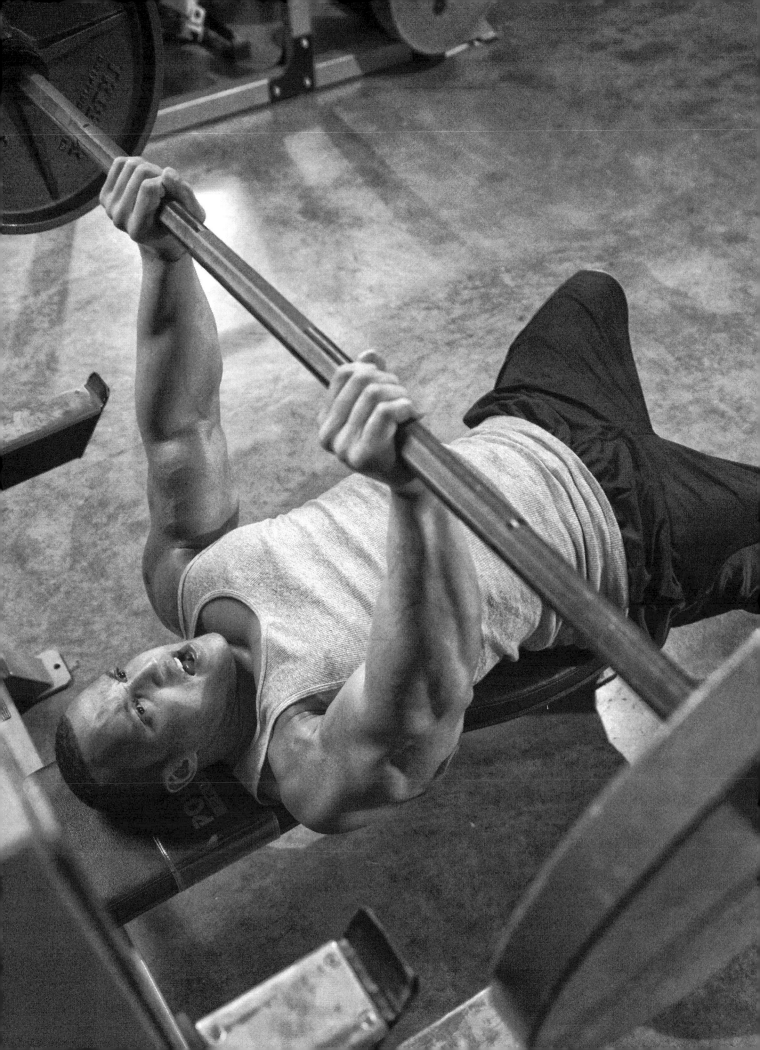

A 2007 study in Brazil titled "Effects of Exercise Order on Upper-Body Muscle Activation and Exercise Performance," produced a similar conclusion. The study, which also utilized EMG, involved performing repetitions on the machine pec deck, prior to the bench press, in a pre-exhaust style.

The study showed that the muscles of the chest were no more efficiently recruited, as EMG signals confirmed. The only muscle that had a higher EMG during the bench press was the triceps; this was simply because the chest was fatigued and motor units from the pectoralis region could not be as effectively recruited. This study concluded that if you want to get better at a particular exercise, perform it first in the training session.

Pre-exhaustion training will not lead to greater muscle fiber recruitment or even to greater joint safety, for that matter. This is due to fatigue in the muscles that are normally used as prime movers during a compound movement; that alters the motor pattern of the compound movement, resulting in less efficient and even unsafe technical execution of compound lifting movements. The majority of pre-exhaustion training benefits are simply "bro science."

Here is an example of a pre-exhaustion training for the chest:

Pec Deck: 45 seconds max reps x 3 sets
Flyes: 3 sets 12 reps, supersetted with Cable Upper Cut Flyes 3 sets 12 reps
Machine Press: 3 sets 12 (last set 3 drop sets to failure)
Bench Press: 4 sets 8 reps

POST-EXHAUSTION TRAINING

Just as you might have guessed, post-exhaustion training is the opposite of pre-exhaustion training; it is, in fact, how most powerlifters or power bodybuilders, also known as "powerbuilders," train.

Instead of pre-fatiguing the muscle with an isolation exercise prior to performing a heavy compound movement, the heavy compound movement is performed first in the workout and the isolation movements are performed later in the workout.

The advantage to this type of training is that you will be freshest for the compound movement. After all, compound movements should serve as the base of your training, as they provide the most stimulation for muscle growth and evoke a significant hormonal response to training.

Training in this manner allows the lifter to concentrate on strength for the compound movement and wrap up the workout with isolation movements for a nice pump.

Science confirms this training methodology as an effective one.

A 2012 article in the *Sports Medicine Journal* examined the sequence of resistance training exercises performed. This article examined studies from every major academic data base, including the Scielo, Science Citation Index, National Library of Medicine, MEDLINE, Scopus, SPORTDiscus~M and CINAHL®.

Acute responses were examined, as were long-term adaptations, with resistance training exercise order as the experimental variable. It was found that exercise order affects max effort strength, the ability to perform repetitions over multiple sets and total volume.

Much greater strength gains were realized when compound exercises were performed first in a session, as opposed to their being performed at the end of a session.

The research concluded that exercises should be sequenced in order of neuromuscular demand. Placing compound movements first in an exercise program is supported generally by anecdotal observations of the biggest, strongest, most muscular men on the planet, so it isn't surprising to see science back this up.

Here is an example of a post-exhaustion shoulder workout:

Overhead Press: 5 sets 5 reps
Arnold Presses: 2 sets 10 reps
Lateral Machine Raises: 3 sets 15 reps
Seated Dumbbell Lateral Raises: 1 top set to failure, 3 rest-pause sets (15 seconds rest)
Reverse Flye/Face Pull superset: 12, 12 x 3 sets
Machine Shoulder Press: 90 seconds of continuous tension (slow and light)

GERMAN VOLUME TRAINING

This method should probably be called the 10 Sets Method, but legendary strength coach Charles Poliquin has made it better known as "German Volume Training." It is believed to be originated out of German Weightlifting circles by Coach Rolf Fesser as a program to add muscle in the off season. Bill Kazmaier used this method in the bench press in the off season, as did I, the youngest person ever to bench press 600 pounds raw.

While Charles Poliquin popularized the system in North America, legendary bodybuilder and fitness trainer to the stars, Vince Gironda, used a similar method with his clients. Even Bev Francis used German Volume Training in her early bodybuilding days to pack on mass. Lots of anecdotal evidence suggests this method is highly effective.

Generally, it is recommended that a high volume protocol of multiple sets of 6–15 repetitions is the prescription for maximum muscle hypertrophy, using a moderate load between 55% and 85% of a bodybuilder's one repetition max in the movement being performed.

Volume is defined as *reps x sets x poundage lifted*. My in-the-trenches experience would agree that generally higher volume produces better muscular gains, as opposed to the same sets and repetitions using lighter weights. That's why compound movements are the method of choice for building muscle mass.

Let's look at an example where our primary emphasis is the quadriceps using the front squat and the leg extension.

If four sets of 10 repetitions are performed on the front squat with 300 pounds, the total volume is 4 x 10 x 300 = 12,000 pounds. If we did the same workout with leg extensions using 60 pounds, the total amount of volume would be 4 x 10 x 60 = 2,400 pounds. Much more work is accomplished with the front squat, and this is the premise of German Volume Training.

Even though most educated coaches and athletes correctly use compound movements as their go-to choice to add muscle mass, generally after the compound movement is performed, the goal is to hit the muscle from all different angles.

This can be accomplished via supplementary core lifts (for example, performing a dumbbell military press after a standing military press) and, of course, multiple sets and repetitions of single joint movements that more effectively isolate the muscle; this technique is known as post-exhaustion training or powerbuilding. The goal is to get the benefit of the core movement and also stimulate as many muscle fibers as possible by attacking the muscle from a variety of angles with a variety of movements.

What's the alternative? Attack the same movement with multiple sets, much higher than typically recommended.

Limited studies on German Volume Training confirm its effectiveness for building muscles.

In fact, a 2010 study published in the *Journal of Australian Strength and Conditioning* showed that German Volume Training (GVT) protocol increased muscle mass in elite kayakers after using the system for 5 weeks. Other anecdotal reports support this notion and, of course, the endorsement of the German weightlifting machine doesn't hurt!

Originally, German Volume Training (the 10-Sets Method) was a protocol of 10 sets of 10 repetitions of a compound movement, using a 20-repetition max, or approximately 60% of the athlete's one-rep max. Rest periods of 60 seconds up to 3 minutes have been advocated; however, rest depends on the movement being performed, the load used, and the anaerobic capacity of the athlete. In the event of not being able to complete all of the repetitions, reduce the load by 2.5%–5%, so if you were using 200 pounds and did not complete the final rep on the seventh set, use 190–195 pounds on the following set.

While this reduction is quite small, we want to keep the intensity as high as possible for maximum muscle growth. If you attempt to keep the weight the same and continually miss reps because of fatigue, you won't reap the intended benefits of GVT.

If you are performing only four reps on your last set, even if you had made every rep until that point, you have reduced the total volume by 60%! If you do this over multiple sets, you have significantly deviated from the protocol, which will greatly alter the adaption to the program. German Volume Training is 10 sets of 10 repetitions. If you decide to use this method, stick to it!

How Does German Volume Training Work?

Because of the high volume training load, short rest intervals, and moderate load, this method produces a very anabolic natural growth hormone response.

The idea, as Poliquin has written, is to attack the same muscle fibers over and over with the same movement for extremely high volume, and this will force the muscle fibers to experience major growth.

This happens by doing multiple sets. Your fatigued muscle fibers no longer are recruited; instead, new ones will be called to action, equating to more growth. The idea is that fast-twitch and growth-resistant slow-twitch fibers will both experience growth from this demanding regimen.

Powerlifters have used a similar approach with much lower reps with the same idea, and have become neurologically efficient in the competition lifts.

Many strength coaches now advocate supersetting German Volume Training with an antagonist muscle movement, so for the bench press this could be a dumbbell row, or for the overhead press this could be a chin-up.

Australian Strength Coach Dan Barker recommends a 3-minute recovery between each superset complex. For well-conditioned athletes, an abdominal exercise could be added into the complex, so a complex could be shoulder press–chin-up–leg raises (rest 3 minutes, repeat 9 more times).

When performing squats or deadlifts, because of the core involvement and massive loads they require, it would not be wise to add an abdominal exercise. Because of the neuromuscular complexity, I do not recommend using Olympic lifts or their variations for German Volume Training.

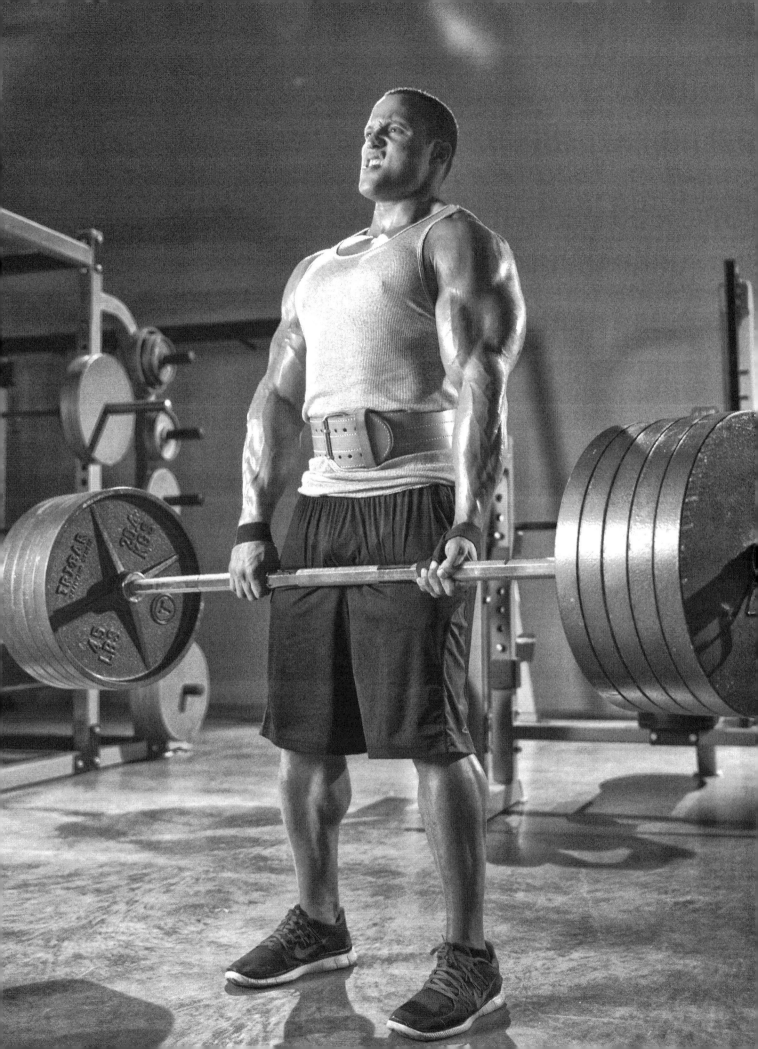

Practical Examples of German Volume Training

Complex 1

1a. Bench Press: 10 sets 10 reps (rest 20 seconds before 1b start @ 60% one-rep max)

1b. Inverted Row: 10 sets 10 reps (rest 20 seconds before 1c; if bodyweight becomes too difficult, go band assisted)

1c. Leg Raises (rest 3 minutes before repeating the complex)

Complex 2

1a. Overhead press (OHP): 10 sets 10 reps (rest 20 seconds before 1b start 60% one-rep max)

1b. Chin-ups: 10 sets 10 reps (rest 20 seconds before 1c; if bodyweight becomes too difficult, go band assisted)

1c. Leg Raises (rest 3 minutes before repeating the complex)

Complex 3

1a. Squats: 10 sets 10 reps (rest 20 seconds before 1b start 60% one-rep max)

1b. Glute Ham Raises: 10 sets 10 reps (rest 3 minutes before repeating complex; if bodyweight becomes too difficult, go band assisted)

Besides muscle hypertrophy, German Volume Training can benefit the cardiovascular system. Daniel Barker and Robert Newton showed this to professional Rugby players performing a German Volume Training bench press routine; by their last set, their heart rates climbed to 160 beats per minute and never dropped below 120 during the recovery phase.

It would be interesting to see how high athletes' heart rates would climb performing a German Volume Training workout with a squat or deadlift emphasis. Because of the cardiovascular demands, athletes with poor conditioning will not be able to effectively benefit from a German Volume Training routine.

20-REP BREATHING SQUATS

The 20-rep breathing squat routine has been used by athletes for over three-quarters of a century. J. C. Hise gained nearly 100 pounds in two years using this routine; Hise was heavily influenced by iron pioneer Mark Berry.

Peary Rader, founder of *Ironman Magazine* and a self-described hard gainer, credits this routine with adding 100 pounds to his frame. Rader was the first to publish the 20-rep breathing-style squat routine. Breathing squats are done for 20 repetitions with a weight you would typically do for 10 repetitions. It is one all-out set! Each time you think you will fail, take 3–4 deep breaths and continue until you reach 20 reps. These sets should be a very painful and unpleasant experience. If you find that they are not, add some weight to the bar.

Rader advocated the Valsalva Maneuver (holding your breath) while performing the squat movement and between reps taking deep breaths of air. Start off with a weight that you can complete, and add weight each session; the best gains will be made when the set of 20 reps is an all-out effort.

Initially, the breathing may make the weight seem more difficult to lift; but over time, as you familiarize yourself with this technique, you will actually be able to lift more weight for more reps this way.

This routine is not one for the faint of heart. A massive degree of mental toughness is required to squat an all-out set of 20 reps to full depth. Your mind will want your body to stop at 12 reps; this is where you really challenge your intestinal fortitude. Don't focus on how many reps you have left, focus on the next rep breath and block out the voice in your head urging you to quit.

To reap the intended benefits of this protocol, the squats must be performed with a full range of motion going below parallel on every squat.

Let's say you use 225 for 20 reps all-out and it was a gut buster. Next workout, try the same weight with half squats; it will not be a challenge.

If your full-range-of-motion squat is 20 inches and you use 200 pounds, look at the amount of mechanical work you do: 200 x 20 = 4,000. Now, if you do a half squat, look at how that equation has changed: 200 x 10 = 2,000. Not to mention the work your glutes and hamstrings are robbed of because of the insufficient range of motion and, of course, you spend less time under tension.

Here is the original 20-rep routine printed in *Ironman Magazine* in 1968:

- Behind-the-Neck Press: 3 x 12
- Squat: 1 x 20
- Pull-Overs: 1 x 20
- Bench Press: 3 x 12
- Bent-Over Rows: 3 x 15
- Stiff-Legged Deadlift: 1 x 15
- Shrug: 1 x 15
- Pull-Overs: 1 x 20

This routine would be performed two to three times a week, which would be a bit much for many trainees, especially without cycling in heavy, medium, and light days/exercises. Bodybuilders have used this routine on their leg days, doing an all-out set of 20 reps of breathing squats with more traditional lower-body accessory work.

Such a routine would look like this:

- Squat: 1 x 20
- Lunges: 3 x 12
- Leg Curls: 3 x 6
- Leg Ext: 3 x 15
- Calf Raises: 4 x 20
- Abdominal Work

There have been no peer-reviewed studies on the 20-rep breathing squat routine, only the amazing anecdotal reports of lifters who have claimed to gain massive amounts of muscle with this routine.

This routine for bulking is advocated with a very high-calorie diet and a gallon of whole milk a day. When you work out only a couple of hours a week and drink seven gallons of whole milk weekly, you will gain weight.

Regardless of routine, this is not to downplay the effectiveness of this routine; it is just important to consider all of the variables at play.

FORCED REPS

We talk a lot about the risk-to-benefit ratio. Forced reps offer a huge benefit when properly implemented. However, you run the risk of overtraining when using this system of training too frequently because of the ultra-high intensity and the trauma-to-the-muscle experience. Forced reps propel you past your pain threshold. Some believe this lowers the excitation threshold of hard-to-stimulate motor units in ways that would never be possible otherwise.

William J. Kraemer, Ph.D, one of the world's foremost resistance training experts, had this to say about forced reps in the August 2002 edition of *Muscle & Fitness:*

> During a set, as a muscle is trained, it produces force. Motor units (muscle fibers activated by nerve impulses) are recruited, starting with the smaller ones. With each succeeding repetition, progressively larger fibers—which take more stimulation to activate—come into play. By the time you reach positive failure, theoretically all of the fibers of a muscle have been recruited.

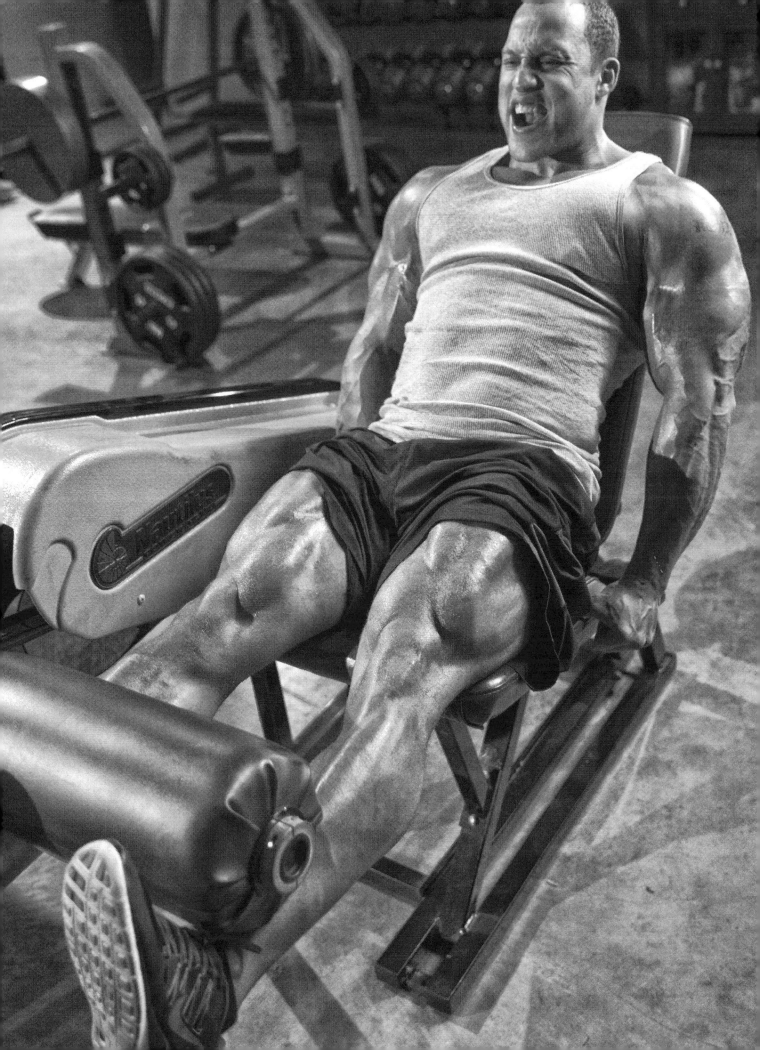

Kraemer went on to say:

> In the past, it was thought that the use of forced reps would provide continued use of the already-activated motor units. This is called "continued activation." But what we've found is that certain large muscle fibers cannot be re-activated without rest, and forced reps don't continue to activate these fibers. Instead, forced reps challenge smaller motor units, which have "recycled" during the set.

It is also believed that forced reps can condition a less inhibitory response by the Golgi Tendon Organ during high-intensity training. When you can no longer complete a rep by yourself, you have reached the point of failure; going beyond this point with assistance for additional reps, generally 1–4, is forced reps.

This is a great way to help bring up lagging body parts, but this method must be used with caution.

I have found it effective to perform this no more than once per week on the last set of a given exercise. Remember, this a great way to build muscle, not necessarily strength. Although strength is built from increases in cross-sectional muscle mass, it is developed by ingraining more efficient motor patterns. Going to failure potentially inhibits motor patterns.

What does science say?

One 2003 study published in the *International Journal of Sports Medicine* consisted of 16 weight-trained men who completed a leg workout of four sets of leg presses, two sets of squats, and two sets of leg extensions.

On the first trial, the subjects performed the set of each exercise with their 12-rep max, taking each set to momentary muscle failure. On the next trial, they went slightly heavier and had spotters assist them with forced reps until 12 reps were completed.

The results were amazing.

When the subjects trained with forced reps, their growth hormone levels were three times as high as when they trained to momentary muscular failure. Growth hormone is very anabolic and is a potent, fat-burning hormone, so this demonstrates the effectiveness of this method for promoting fat loss and gaining muscle.

Another study showed that collegiate football players who performed three sets of 6–10 repetitions per set, taking each set to momentary muscular failure, lost less body fat over a 10-week period than collegiate football players on the same routine with the last set including forced reps.

Here is an example of a forced reps chest routine:

Bench Press: 12, 8, 8, 8 (2–3 forced reps)
Incline Press: 8, 8, 8
Chain Flyes: 15, 12, 10, 10 (2–3 forced reps)
Cable Cross-Overs: 12, 12, 12
Machine Press: One set to failure

This method is effective, but it causes a significant amount of peripheral and central fatigue. Proceed with caution!

NEGATIVES (ECCENTRIC TRAINING)

Some bodybuilders, in effort to increase intensity, use supramaximal weights and have their partners stand by as they lower the weight.

If your bench press max is 250 pounds and you put 275 pounds on the bar and slowly lower the weight, you have performed a negative in the traditional sense. After the weight is lowered, your partner will assist you by helping you lift the weight back to arms extension or the starting point; the weight is lowered once again and the muscles are engaged in an all-out fight against all-mighty gravity. Some athletes can handle an excess of 160% of their one-repetition maxes on negatives.

Here is how that same lifter could implement negatives into his training:

Set 1: 200 x 10
Set 2: 215 x 6
Set 3: 240 x 2
Set 4: 275 x 3 negatives (4-second negatives)
Set 5 160 x 15

Some athletes anecdotally report doing heavy negatives in the bench prior to doing traditional barbell bench press, which allows them to lift more weight and perform more reps.

One could argue a PAP-like effect is possible, but most studies on the effects of PAP show its effects on reversible muscle actions eccentric-amortization-concentric to the same type of movements, not necessarily a maximum negative to a positive.

If you did just handle 330 pounds on the bench press with a negative and your max is 300 pounds, it would not be unbelievable that performing reps with 260 pounds would feel lighter than usual.

Other examples of negative exercises are eccentric emphasis exercises like Smith Machine bench press, where the athlete hypothetically bench presses 225 pounds for six reps; however, an additional 25-pound plate is placed on the bar, making the total weight 275 pounds.

Once the bar is lowered, two side spotters will quickly pull off the 25-pound plate and the athlete will proceed to push up the 225 pounds, so he handled 275 pounds on the negative portion of the lift and 225 pounds on the positive portion, the limiting factor.

That is why this is called *negative emphasis training*. With this type of training, it is important to ensure you have competent spotters who can quickly pull the weight off the bar. *Never attempt this with a barbell or any free-weight apparatus.*

Sticking with the bench press, another example of negative emphasis training is using a slow tempo to lower the bar, then pushing the bar to lockout forcefully. The advantage here is we can handle more on negatives, we will not tire out as easily because of higher-force production capabilities on negatives, and we still get the benefit of an explosive positive rep. We also lengthen the time under tension—an important variable in the road to anabolism.

Another example of a negative movement for the biceps is the one-armed eccentric barbell curl. It is performed by sitting at a preacher-curl bench and grasping the center knurling of an Olympic barbell with your left hand; the back of your upper arm rests on the preacher bench in front of you with your arm supinated (palm up). The barbell should be in the finished position of a biceps curl with your palm in front of your shoulder.

Next, lower the barbell for a count of 8 seconds and pause for a second at the bottom. Have a spotter assist you to the top, or you can use your right hand to assist you in curling the weight up. Repeat for reps, and then switch sides.

An example of how to use the one-armed eccentric barbell curl would be:

3–6 sets of 3–6 reps

Repetitions are kept low because just five reps will produce 40 seconds under painful eccentric tension!

The world of negatives is endless.

You can also push a weight to momentary muscle failure (positive failure) and have a spotter assist you on the positive portion of the rep; but because we are stronger on negatives, we can continue to do 3–4 more additional negative reps unassisted and only receive assistance on the positive portion of the lift.

An example of this type of training for the Seated Barbell Military Press would be for an athlete capable of doing 155 pounds for eight repetitions.

Set 1: 155 x 8
Set 2: 155 x 8
Set 3: 155 x 8 (after failure do three more negatives with spotter assistance on the positive portion of the rep)

A study in the August 2009 *British Sports Medicine Journal* demonstrated high-intensity eccentric training was more effective in promoting increases in muscle hypertrophy than high-intensity concentric training.

Remember, we are comparing a negative to a positive, not an entire rep, a reversible muscle action. Furthermore, eccentric training has shown an increased muscle cross-sectional area measured with magnetic resonance imaging or computerized tomography.

While heavy eccentric training can increase muscle mass, strength adaptations are highly specific; in other words, heavy eccentric training gets you stronger in eccentric movements, not in the concentric or positive portion of the lift.

This was confirmed in that same 2009 study published in the *British Sports Medicine Journal*.

That is why it is an effective strategy for athletes wishing to maximize strength-to-bodyweight ratio. In other words, to not gain too much mass and to avoid the delayed onset of muscle soreness (DOMS) to include concentric-only training.

You can handle more weight on an eccentric contraction than a concentric contraction, as we discussed earlier. Interestingly enough, far fewer motor units are activated in an eccentric contraction than in a concentric contraction. This is a recipe for muscle soreness! During negative reps, the force distributed is spread across a much smaller area of cross-sectional muscle fiber area than during a positive rep with more weight being handled.

PARTIAL REPS

Full range of motion for full development is generally a good rule of thumb, but like the old proverb says, there is a time and a place for everything.

Partial reps are a movement performed in a specific range of motion. For the bench press, an example would be a board press; for the deadlift, a rack pull; and for a military press seated, a military press to the top of the head, or presses from pins in a power rack.

Partial reps allow for an overload. In other words, you can use more weight in a partial range of motion than a full range of motion, which will help your central nervous system adapt to heavier weights, along with providing a huge psychological boost as you climb the intensity ladder of heavy weights. After all, how intimidating is 300-pound bench press if you have done a 405-pound bench press off of four boards?

Partials can additionally work specific range of motion, i.e., attacking sticking points.

Let's use the bench press as an example.

If you have a sticking point at the four-board height, your training weights could potentially be held back. By overloading that sticking point and eliminating it, you can now handle heavier weights on a full-range-of-motion bench press, which means fully developed pecs. Additionally, by handling supramaximal weights, you will also strengthen connective tissue.

Remember, while partials reps are great for handling heavier weights, you should also work them at your weakest points. Many times this might mean using less weight than you could perform through a full range of motion.

That's because you're in your individual worst leverage point, but this will ultimately help you blow past your sticking point and eventually handle more weight throughout the full range of motion.

Partial rep training guidelines:

- Partials are very demanding and, if overdone, can induce central and peripheral fatigue because you are lifting beyond your one-rep max. Do not do partials more than three weeks in a row without a deload (period of lower intensity).

- Keep full-range-of-motion movements in your program; do not use exclusively partials or include partials every single session. Ultimately, our base training is a full range of motion, and we do not want to adversely affect neurological adaptations to full-range-of-motion movements. In other words, if you do too many partials, your full-range-of-motion movements will feel extremely awkward.

- Use periodization training with partial movements. Do not perform partials more than 3 weeks in a row without a deload. After the deload, one more 3-week mesocycle can be completed, and then you can take time off from partials.

- Overload and work weak points.

- Make sure you are mentally and physically prepared for partial reps. You have to make sure you are tight; you are lifting more than your max!

Here's an example of a back routine including partial movements:

Rack Pull 18 inches (working a sticking point): 3 sets of 3 reps
Rack Pull Overload 8-inch range of motion (great for upper back development): 3 sets of 5 reps
Deadlift: 3 sets of 6 reps
Rest-Pause Chin-ups with Weight: 1 set (3 rest pauses)
Wide Grip Lat Pull-downs: 3 sets 12 reps
Meadows Rows—3 sets of 8 reps

If you train only with partials, you will experience only partial development. Correct implementation of partials can be an integral part of building a championship physique.

DC TRAINING

Doggcrap Training (DC Training) is the training philosophy of southern California bodybuilder Dante Trudel. Trudel invented this training philosophy as an alternative to more traditional high volume approaches.

According to Trudel, he was unable to gain muscle mass taking a more traditional approach, and because of this he developed DC Training, which Trudel believes helped take his muscle mass to the next level.

Others have echoed this claim, while some are loud to pontificate the ineffectiveness of what they tout as "Trudel's haphazard training philosophy." There seems to be a love/hate relationship in muscle building with DC Style Training.

The concept behind DC Training is to *train heavy*. The idea is your limit strength is your base. Stronger muscles generally equal bigger muscles. Although the correlation is not always that direct, getting stronger is a surefire way to increase neuromuscular efficiency and set the stage to increase muscle mass.

For bodybuilders, getting stronger by way of increasing neural drive will eventually lead to increased muscle mass. You'll be able to work at greater percentages of your newfound one-rep maximums.

Although countless folks who have trouble filling out a size medium compression shirt tout the mantra of not needing to lift heavy to get big, scores of scientific studies and countless stories originating from the trenches say otherwise.

Observations in the battle-hardened bodybuilding trenches of the most muscular men in the world at Metroflex Gym, like Johnnie Jackson, Branch Warren, and Ronnie Coleman, and the behemoth poundages they use, would literally squash the notion of not needing to lift heavy to get big. Lifting heavy is the foundation of DC Training and nearly every successful bodybuilding program.

The rest-pause method, discussed earlier in detail, is performed by using a heavy weight with all-out intensity and completing as many reps as possible. After failure is reached, take deep breaths while you rest 20–30 seconds, and then repeat the process. Do this one more time for a total of three sets. This rest-pause method is used not just for the primary lift but even for accessory movements.

DC Training is different from many traditional bodybuilding programs because it uses a much lower volume. The reason more people succeed with this training program over Mike Mentzer's Heavy Duty system is the emphasis of heavy training with compound movements.

Also, while the volume recommendations may not be in line with scientific studies that show the superiority of high volume programs for muscle hypertrophy, because of increased frequency, weekly total volume may be closer in line with traditional recommendations.

A DC split would look something like this:

Monday
Bench Press (Chest), Upright Rows (Shoulders), Triceps Extensions (Triceps), Wide Grip Chin-ups, Bent-Over Rows

Wednesday
EZ Curl Biceps Curls (Biceps), Wrist Roller (Forearms), Calf Raises (Calves), Hack Squats (Quads)

Friday
Repeat Monday Workouts

Monday
Repeat Wednesday Workouts

Wednesday
Start cycle over; alternate exercises every 1–3 weeks

PEAK CONTRACTION TRAINING

Anybody who has been around bodybuilders for any length of time has heard them refer to doing shaping exercises or even dedicating a workout or training cycle to focus on "shaping." The reality is you are not truly shaping, you are making your best attempt at isolating a muscle by minimizing the contribution of synergist muscles engaging the overload principle of isolation.

In other words, peak contraction training would call for a cable flye over a dumbbell flye because of the continuous tension offered, and this would be done at a slow speed, purposely feeling out the tension placed on the pectorals and holding the cables together at the top, or "peak" of the movement, where tension is greatest, for 1–2 seconds, maximally contracting the chest.

The same movement would be done over any sort of pressing movement, whether at maximum speed or even at a slower speed, purposefully trying to feel the movement; the idea here is to stress the pecs, feel the movement, and have as little help as possible from assisting movements.

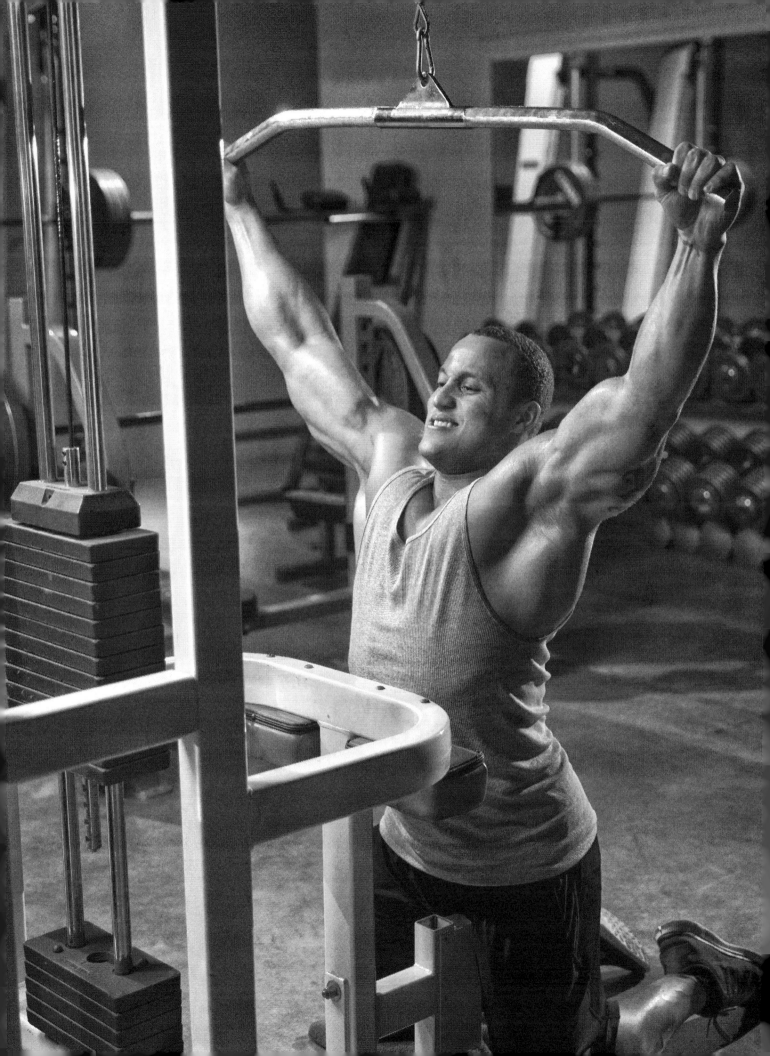

Because this not a natural movement pattern like a pushing/pressing movement, training this way frequently enough and with adequate volume can, to the naked eye, appear to cause a morph in muscle shape; the reality is that you have unnaturally isolated a muscle, and because of the isolation it grows out of proportion to the synergist muscles that are no longer assisting as they would in a pressing movement. This can help you or hurt you, depending on your proportions; to an untrained eye you have "shaped" your chest.

Generally, when bodybuilders talk about the mind-to-muscle connection or "feeling" a movement, they are referring to peak contraction training.

Others believe the mind-to-muscle connection is a product of training as explosively as possible and using as heavy weights as possible because bodybuilders will improve neural drive to their muscles.

Who's right? Actually, both.

To maximize the mind-muscle connection, you must not shy away from moving the heavy pig iron fast. You'll also have to feel some weights with peak contraction training.

Peak contraction in bodybuilding training refers to a maximum amount of resistance placed on the muscle in a contracted position.

An example for the chest would be a cable flye over a dumbbell flye. The reason is the dumbbell provides great resistance in the abducted (stretch part of the flye) movement; but as you perform the adduction phase, (bring your arms together) where the chest is fully contracted as the dumbbells are about to touch, the movement eases up because of the natural strength curve.

Studies have been performed on barbell movements like the squat, bench press, and deadlift that show barbells significantly reduce over the final portion of the lift, and this is known as the negative acceleration phase.

This is the same concept applied here to the dumbbell flye. One way to circumvent this potential roadblock to hypertrophy heaven is using cables or a pec deck because of the constant tension they provide on the muscle.

The problem with using only machines is that they are designed for a specific body type, which many times will not be yours. Cables provide much more freedom of movement, so for this purpose they would be a better choice.

One technique I have currently been using with IFBB Pros Johnnie Jackson and Branch Warren, as well as other bodybuilding clients, with great results, is the addition of accommodated resistance techniques to traditional bodybuilding movements, such as chain flyes; these take a lot of stress off the pecs and shoulders in their most vulnerable position, yet allow for a true peak contraction of the pecs with the benefits free weights provide.

Yes, this is greedy, getting so much accomplished with one movement, but that is the name of the game. Another variation of the dumbbell flye for peak contraction is to put a rubber EliteFTS resistance band around your back and hold it in your hands with the dumbbell. Again this is a great way to provide peak contraction, lessen stress in the body's most vulnerable position, and complement the strength curve of the lift.

Bands and chains can be used in pressing, squat, rowing, extending, curling, you name it; and if you are innovative not only will they help you get stronger, which powerlifters have known for decades, but they will enhance your physique. For more on bands and chains, see Chapter 6, which is devoted to their use in bodybuilding.

Any peak contraction movement should be held in the contraction position for 1–3 seconds but keep continuous tension on the muscle throughout the entirety of the movement.

For example, for a leg extension movement, it's holding the top of the movement. This is generally what well-meaning bodybuilding gurus are referring to when they pontificate about shaping exercises. Peak contraction techniques are great for single-joint exercises; after all, the sole purpose is growth of the muscle you are focused on!

Some examples of exercises that are great for peak contraction are:

> Quads: Leg Extensions
> Hamstrings: Leg Curls
> Chest: Chain Flyes
> Triceps: Single Armed Band Push-downs
> Biceps: Cable Double Biceps Curls Standing
> Delts: Lateral Cable Raises
> Abs: Crunches
> Lats: Straight Arm Pull-downs
> Mid Back: Band Resisted Chest Supported T-bar Rows

WEIDER SYSTEM/PRINCIPLES

The Weider Principles have guided bodybuilders for over a half a century. A common criticism of the Weider System is that it is not a true system of training but in fact is more a collection of crypto-scientific muscle-building methods and guidelines based on tradition.

While some of the criticism might hold some weight, the bottom line is that most effective training methods are born in the trenches and after anecdotal reports surface of their effectiveness, then the ivory tower orders the boys in the lab to perform a study on untrained graduate students to confirm their effectiveness.

Look at bands and chains used in training by powerlifters for decades. Science is just now "telling" us they work and celebrity trainers are now using them. But those in the trenches could have told us this decades ago. Many want to classify Weider's Principles as bro science, antiquated, or even as one man's attempt to monopolize the industry; there is no doubt these principles have helped thousands, and Weider was truly ahead of his time.

Weider's ideas are a collection of training philosophies and programs he gathered from iron athletes of the day, the top coaches and, of course, independent writers. Joe had access to all of these people, and fortunately he shared this information with everyone else.

Joe analyzed the methods he accessed to present them in a way they were applicable to the lay public and, of course, the competitor. He then went on to name the principle/methods as the Weider Principles. This has had a major impact on how bodybuilders have trained and do train. That was the concept of splitting your workouts to train specific body parts. The split system, double split system, and triple split system have been used since the 1950s; the split system is one of many contributions Weider made to bodybuilding science.

There are three broad categories of Weider Principles:

1. Principles to help you plan your training cycle
2. Principles to help you arrange your exercises in each workout
3. Principles to help you perform each exercise

Anyone serious about training knows these three categories are applicable today and are the basis of good program design.

HEAVY DUTY TRAINING

1978 Mr. Universe, the late Mike Mentzer, had some radical ideas when it came to building the body. Whether you loved him or hated him, there is no denying his ideas have influenced gym rats worldwide.

Mentzer's training system was a form of High Intensity Training he named "Heavy Duty Training." A similar method had been the brainchild of Nautilus Founder Arthur Jones. Mentzer did a much better job of marketing his training system along with building a physique many considered to be the best of all time in his heyday; after all, at the 1978 Mr. Universe he received a perfect 300 score, the first person ever to do so.

In a nutshell, Mentzer's system was based on believing virtually every bodybuilder was severely overtrained. Mentzer called for infrequent, brief and very intense workouts. Every set was taken to absolute failure and the goal was to always use more weight than the previous workout. Many times, just one set per bodypart was taken to total failure. Heavy

Duty routines are generally performed for the whole body 2–3 times a week, and some go as infrequently as a single session every 9–10 days.

As the 1990s rolled around, Mentzer advocated an even more extreme reduction in volume. He encouraged using fewer sets and more days of rest, working out once every 4–7 days and with each workout consisting of only five working sets. Mentzer believed hypertrophy was not a product of volume, but rather intensity.

Mike Mentzer was a training fundamentalist; he believed his way was the Holy Grail that led to the promised land of perfect size and symmetry, and all other methods led to eternal training damnation!

What does science say? Not much.

There have been no peer-reviewed studies on traditional higher volume approaches versus heavy duty training. Some of the advantages of heavy duty training are that it saves time and it allows fully recovery and much lower probability of overtraining.

One of the disadvantages is lack of exercise variety. With only one all-out set, it is impossible to attack the muscle from multiple angles. After all, should you choose a compound exercise or a peak contraction effort exercise? You must think long and hard if you only get one set of one exercise. It is much more difficult to achieve a pump, and the internal satisfaction of completing a workout is much less if all you do is perform five total sets.

A vast majority of champions, from natural, local level to juiced-up professionals, have built their physiques with a much more high volume approach than the heavy duty system. A plethora of studies show the advantage of high volume training for adding muscle. Unfortunately, none of them have ever been directly compared to the heavy duty training system.

Anecdotally, this system would not appear to be superior by any means. You might be thinking, well I have a friend who put on eight pounds of muscle in a month using this workout system, but odds are he changed his diet or added in some quality muscle-building supplements and maybe even some not-so-legal muscle-building supplements.

Another explanation may be your friend was severely overtrained, and this short stint off heavy duty training essentially served as a deload (a reduction in volume); because of this, super compensation took place and he grew. Odds are, this rate of muscle hypertrophy dissipated rather quickly.

Could heavy duty training be cycled in a bodybuilder's arsenal from time to time? Certainly. Should the bodybuilder abandon all other forms of training and become a devout heavy duty disciple? Absolutely not!

PERIPHERAL HEART ACTION TRAINING

This system of bodybuilding circuit training was popularized to the masses by Bob Gajda, a Mr. Universe and Mr. America winner in the 1960s, but it was actually the brainchild of Chuck Coker.

The idea with peripheral heart action (PHA) training is to keep circulating blood through the body throughout the entire workout, done by attacking the smaller muscles around the heart first, then moving outward. This system is vigorous and requires continued intense exercise for a prolonged period with no rest. For these reasons, the poorly conditioned bodybuilder and the faint of heart will not do well with this training system.

The idea is to use primarily compound movements for efficiency. The system is made up of four different sequences of exercises, and each sequence is designed to encompass every major body segment. The goal is to "shunt" blood up and down the body. This is extremely taxing on the cardiovascular system, for which the obvious benefits are a reduction in body fat and, of course, improved metabolic rate.

Because each sequential body part covered in each sequence is getting adequate rest between each circuit, strength will be conserved, allowing close to maximal strength to be exhibited on the sequential bout.

Even though your heart will likely beat at over 150 beats per minute throughout the entire workout, this does not give a license to reduce the weights used—unless of course, you don't possess the intestinal fortitude of a successful bodybuilder.

Here is an example of PHA Training designed by Fred Hatfield, Ph.D., aka "Dr. Squat," legendary trainer, former world record holding powerlifter, and ISSA Co-Founder.

Sequence 1
Partial Press
Crunches
Squats
Triceps Extensions

Sequence 2
Pull-downs
Back Raises
Leg Curls
Biceps Curls

Sequence 3
Bench Press
Side Bends Left

Leg Extensions
Dips

Sequence 4
Bent Rows
Side Bends Right
Toe Raise
Shrugs

Dr. Hatfield provided these guidelines:

- Perform the exercises in sequence 1 for the required number of reps sequentially, and do not stop!

- Repeat the sequence two to three more times, then move on to sequence 2, performing it the same way you performed sequence 1.

- Do the same thing for sequences 3 and 4; do not rest during a sequence and do not rest between sequences unless absolutely necessary. After all, long breaks defeat the purpose.

- Maintain your heart rate at 80% of your heart rate max; wear a monitor so you can adjust the pace accordingly.

- If you are in shape, you will not have to trade heavy weight for a slower pace or longer rest.

CIRCUIT TRAINING

Circuit training is similar to PHA training, only it's sort of an easier, poor man's version. The objective in PHA training is to keep the heart rate at 80% of your maximum. With circuit training, your goal is to complete the prescribed exercises within a time limit.

Circuit training is supposed to increase your metabolic rate and raise your heart rate, so the emphasis should be on larger muscle groups. You do not want to give up the strength aspect, so it is recommended to perform circuits with an emphasis on opposing muscle groups, preferably with emphasis on compound movements.

An example would be that the Romanian deadlift/close grip bench press/chin-up/front squat circuit is superior to a leg curl/triceps pushdown/biceps curl/leg extension superset.

The objective is to move through the circuit fast and non-stop; you want to beat your target time!

TIME UNDER TENSION (TUT) TRAINING

In layman's terms, Time Under Tension (TUT) means how long it takes to complete a set. Traditionally, hypertrophy sets have been advocated simply by performing 6–15 repetitions in a given set. While this is great for simplicity, it doesn't tell the whole story of the adaptations that are truly taking place.

Just think, if you bench press 50% of your max for 10 repetitions in 8 seconds, it is not the same as using 80% of your one-rep max for 8 repetitions and the set's taking 40 seconds; just by looking at the variables presented, a different speed of contraction took place, more weight was used and, of course, the muscle was under tension much longer.

Muscular adaptations are much more complicated than a simple rep scheme. One measurable variable we have that can help induce a hypertrophic response is Time Under Tension (TUT).

A typical set of 10 repetitions with a challenging weight will take approximately 20 seconds. What if that set took twice as long? Well, longer strain equals more muscle breakdown, which in turn will lead to more muscle growth when used correctly. How long your muscle is under tension is extremely important to how much it will grow!

Studies generally show the most effective time under tension for maximal hypertrophy is 30–50 seconds per set. The total length of time is important; however, avoid spending maximal time in the portion of the lift that is the easiest.

If you are leg pressing, don't spend 5 seconds at lockout between reps, because this compromises the amount of tension on your muscles; if you feel like you are resting, you are! In turn, you are compromising your results. Because you can handle much heavier lifts on the eccentric (negative) portion of a lift, instead of sitting at lockout cheating the clock and yourself, draw out the eccentric—make it take 3–5 seconds.

With time under tension, it is important to use the heaviest weights possible while maintaining good form, but you are better off doing a partial movement with maximum intensity once you have reached failure than to just hold a weight in a locked-out position and resting to conserve energy.

Many advocates of time under tension training advocate a prescribed tempo such a 4-second negative, 1-second isometric hold at the bottom, 2 seconds on the positive, and a 1-second hold at the top of the movement. They believe perfect form must be maintained the whole time and, if it deviates, one must stop and reduce the amount of weight being used. The key, after all, is to use full range of motion for full development, right? In most cases, absolutely; and that's the way these sets need to start off.

I believe a more effective approach is to go for maximum reps in a prescribed amount of time using a moderate pace, doing as many as possible within that time frame and, if momentary

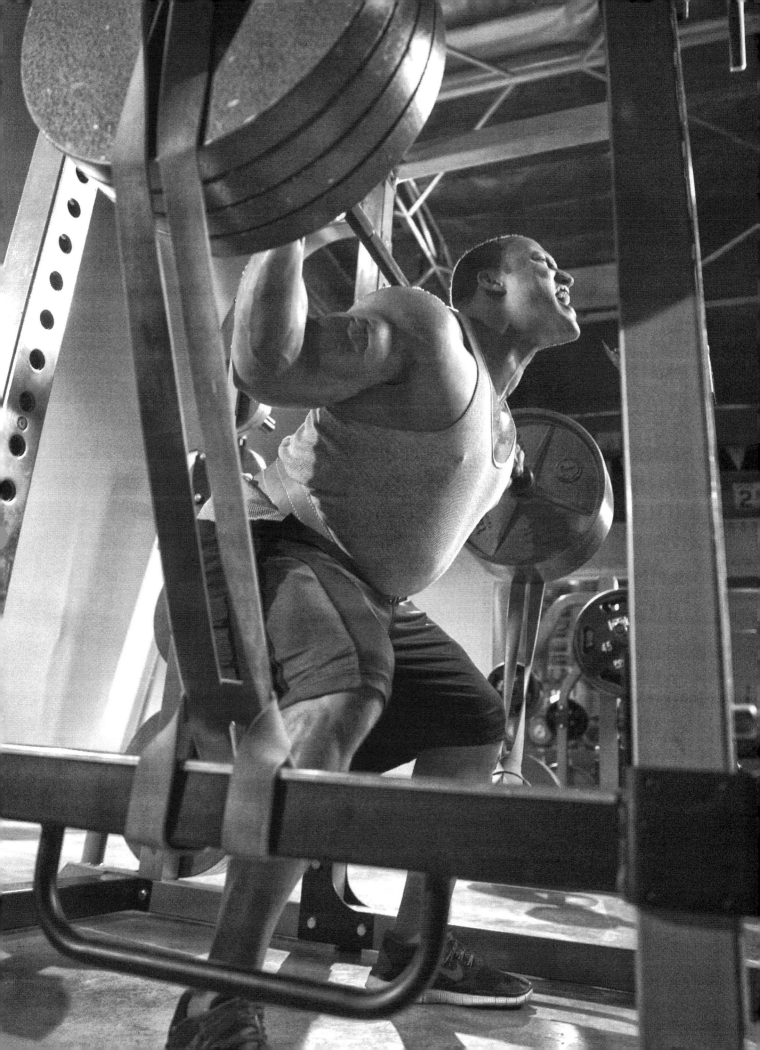

muscular failure is reached, cheat—do an isometric hold, partial movement, whatever—just keep that maximum tension going the whole time, and do not rest by dropping weights or rest-pausing. This training is intense, and I recommend starting each set with a weight you can complete for 10–12 reps, then taking a rest interval that is three times as long as the previous set; for example, 30 seconds under tension would call for a 90-second rest interval. Each set, because generally failure will be reached, calls for a one-third reduction from the previous set, so each exercise should be performed for no more than 3 sets.

Here is a 3-week wave of time under tension training; a deload, or period of reduced intensity, is recommended after 3 weeks of this intense training.

Week 1 (30 seconds time under tension, 90-second rest interval):

Day 1 (Chest & Triceps)
Incline Dumbbell Bench Press: Set 1–90s, Set 2–60s, Set 3–40s
Cable Flyes: Set 1–60, Set 2 40, Set 3–30 (rounded)
Close Grip 3 Board Press: Set 1–210, Set 2–140, Set 3–100
Triceps Push-downs: Set 1–75, Set 2–50, Set 3–35

Day 2 (Back & Biceps)
Cambered Barbell Rows: 240, 160, 110
Wide-Grip Lat Pull-downs: 180, 120, 80
Zottman Curls: 30s, 20s, 15s
Scott Curls: 60, 40, 25

Day 3 (Legs & Shoulders)
Hack Squats: 300, 200, 140
Stiff Leg Deadlifts: 240, 160, 100
Dumbbell Military Presses: 60s, 40s, 25s
Lateral Raises: 30s, 20s, 15s

Here is the way this program would progress over the next two weeks. During **Week 2**, the same weights would be used, but the time under tension would increase to 40 seconds. This would also add another 30 seconds to the rest interval, so that it's now 120 seconds.

For **Week 3**, the same weights would be used, but the time under tension would increase to 50 seconds; and because of this additional 10 seconds under tension, the rest interval would increase to 2.5 minutes.

This is a great way to add mass! This is intense, and you must reduce intensity after this tough mesocycle.

TEMPO TRAINING

We just learned about the importance of time under tension and the potential hypertrophic response this training variable can induce. Tempo training has been popularized by the legendary Charles Poliquin.

In essence, your goal is not only to perform a specific set in a predetermined amount, but also to perform the reps at a prescribed cadence. Different speeds of contraction cause different adaptations to resistance training. A shot putter needs to train fast contractions; you, the bodybuilder, need to train a wide array of speeds.

Four numbers make a tempo; let's look at a 4-1-2-1, a common prescription for hypertrophy.

The first number 4 is the negative (eccentric phase). Let's say you are bench pressing; this means take 4 seconds to lower the weight to your chest.

The second number is a 1, meaning a 1-second pause at the bottom of the lift between the negative and positive portion, rather than an isometric hold of the weight on your chest for 1 second.

The third number is the amount of time it will take to perform the positive or concentric portion of the lift, in this case, 2 seconds.

The last number, 1, is the isometric hold of 1 second at the top of the movement before beginning the negative portion of the lift. One complete repetition will take 8 seconds, so six repetitions will produce a total of 48 seconds under tension. This makes prescribing repetitions much easier if you are after a certain amount of time under tension.

Some swear to the tempo prescription as the Holy Grail to muscle building and strength gain supremacy, while others view it as an unnecessary variable that at best detracts from maximum intensity.

So who's right? Both.

There is a time and a place for the tension variable in training. Could it be valuable for a peak contraction set of cable flyes?

Yes!

What about for a max triple in the deadlift? No, it will just detract from intensity. As bodybuilders, we have to take a holistic training approach; tempo is one more variable that can have a place in your training.

POWERBUILDING

This method was popularized by yours truly in the groundbreaking book *Metroflex Gym Powerbuilding Basics,* which I co-authored with Brian Dobson. In it, we wrote: "In the past, the founding fathers of bodybuilding were required to perform feats of strength in addition to their posing routines. This meant men with great physiques also possessed great strength and power, and those who possessed great strength and power did not look like total 'slobs.'"

Even if bodybuilding is your goal, your limit strength—or how much force you can exert in one all-out effort—is the base of both athletics and physique building.

For strength athletes, it is important to include the small exercises that assist in the core lifts. Remember that Branch Warren, Johnnie Jackson, and Ronnie Coleman all started out as powerlifters. That foundation of limit strength set the stage for their superhuman physiques.

Powerbuilding is a hybrid of powerlifting and bodybuilding. Successful powerlifters are part bodybuilder, and successful bodybuilders build their base with powerlifting.

Studies confirm that exercise sequence is extremely important for the desired adaptations of training to take place. In other words, the most important exercise needs to be the first exercise in your routine.

The difference between powerbuilding and post-exhaustion training is that powerbuilding emphasizes the big three, the competitive powerlifts: squat, bench press and deadlift, the cornerstone of your training.

Essentially, the workout starts off with a heavy core lift and the assistance work, and more traditional bodybuilding techniques follow suit; so, a back day begins with the deadlift, a chest day with the bench press, and a leg day with the king—squats!

Powerbuilding is traditionally much higher volume than many powerlifters use in preparation for meets. Many use this form of training in the off season, and some even do it leading up to a powerlifting contest.

Three of the most famous powerlifters who were avid powerbuilders are the legendary Ed Coan, Dave Pasanella, and, of course, the immortal Bill Kazmaier.

Some bodybuilders train this way right up to contest time, whereas others do it in the off season. After all, how can we forget Ronnie Coleman's deadlifting 800 pounds, three weeks out from the Olympia?

Johnnie Jackson, under my guidance, competed and won the Raw Unity Deadlift Meet with an 832-pound deadlift, without any assistive gear! Johnnie also pulled 800+ at 41 years old, which is another tremendous accomplishment.

If a bodybuilder is big and freaky but never trains with heavy core lifts, at some point— whether it be post-exhaustion, reverse pyramid or powerbuilding—odds are he is primarily a product of great drugs and/or great genetics. Dr. Fred Hatfield once said, "When all else fails, don't get cute, pile on the pig iron." That sums up powerbuilding.

Here is a sample powerbuilding routine:

Day 1–Back
Deadlift: 3, 6, 6, 6, 6
Cambered Bar Bent Over Rows: 10, 8, 6
Straight Arm Pull-down/Wide Grip Chin-up superset: 3 sets
Hyper Deadlifts: 8, 8, 8
Seated Rows, Slow, Continuous Tension Training: 2 minutes
Abs/Calves

Day 2–Chest
Bench Press: 4, 6, 8, 10
Neutral Grip Incline Press: 12, 12, 12
Weighted Dips: 8, 8, max reps 1 minute (bodyweight)
Chain Flyes: max reps x 3 sets
Pec Deck: 1 set (3 rest pauses)

Day 3–Off

Day 4–Arms
Decline Close Grip Bench Against Chains: 6, 6, 6
Floor Barbell Paused Triceps Extension: 12, 10, 8
Triceps Kickback/Diamond Push-ups superset: 3 sets
Chin-ups/Biceps Curl: 5-second eccentric superset x 3
Zottman Curls: 12, 12, 12, 12
Cable Preacher Curls: 12, 12, 12

Day 5–Legs
Squats: 6, 6, 6, 10
Dead Stop Leg Press: 15, 15, 15
Leg Curls: 6, 6, 6, 12
Glute/Ham Raises: 8, 8, 8
Leg Extension: 15, 15, 15
Dumbbell Lunges: 12, 12, 12
Abs/Calves

Day 6–Shoulders
Overhead Press: 5, 5, 5, 12
Lateral Raises Seated: 15, 15, 15, Rest Pause
Face Pulls: 12, 12, 12
Reverse Flye: 12, 12, 12
Abs

Day 7–Off

COMPENSATORY ACCELERATION TRAINING (CAT)

Compensatory Acceleration Training (CAT), popularized by Dr. Fred Hatfield, simply means lifting sub-maximal weights with maximal force.

CAT training provides the bodybuilder with great neural adaptations, a true mind-muscle connection; because CAT training is performed in basic core lifts, the learning curve is virtually non-existent, especially compared with Olympic lifts designed to improve speed strength.

If we look at the force velocity curve, the speed of muscle contraction is proportional to the intensity of the load. Large forces cannot be produced at extremely high speeds.

Conversely, maximum acceleration cannot be achieved with near-maximum weights; however, neuromuscular efficiency can be enhanced without the stress imposed on the central nervous system by lifting maximal weights, allowing similar neural adaptations to take place.

In the long run, you will get stronger implementing CAT in your program. Higher limit strength means heavier sets of 10–12 reps on core movements and heavier weights used on single-joint movements. Bodybuilders have to train slow and fast, unlike many other athletes.

Even if you are new to bodybuilding, this term is pretty self-explanatory. Think of the studies we examined earlier; the conclusion was to work whatever is most important in your workout first. Generally, in this context, it is working your weakness first; after all, once all weakness is eliminated, you will proudly sport an armor-clad, prize-winning physique.

Your weakness needs to be priority one. That is, of course, within reason. If you are training your arms and your biceps are weaker than your triceps, it will not serve a good purpose to pump up your biceps so much you cannot get a good range of motion on triceps extension exercises.

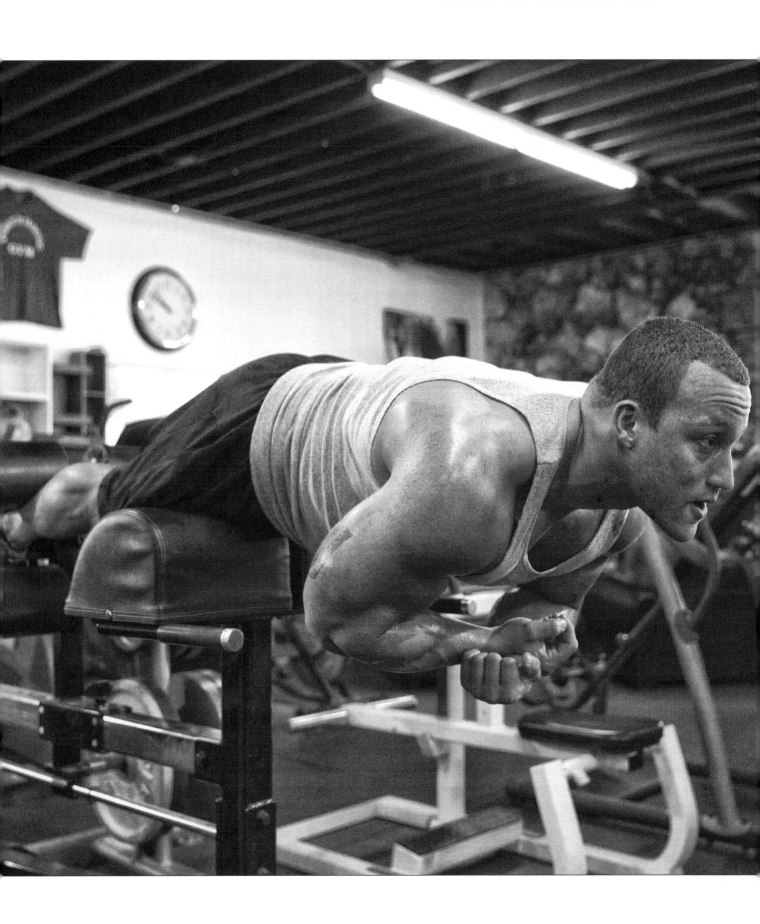

If less-than-adequate-sized triceps are your arch nemesis, you are going to start off with an exercise like heavy close grip 3 board presses with bands or chains. A compound movement builds the most size; this would not be done after 100 reps of cable push-downs.

Know your priorities and organize your training around them and what you hope to accomplish.

CHEATING EXERCISES

Brian Dobson, world famous Metroflex Gym Owner and trainer, said this in the book he co-authored, *Metroflex Gym Powerbuilding Basics:*

> Whenever I train a person who is not into bodybuilding or powerbuilding, they act as if it is wrong to heave up heavy iron on the cheat curl, usually citing how their last trainer at Pansy Inc. Fitness said to stay perfectly straight and not to lean back. These trainees usually have arms that are less than 14" and the trainers' arms are usually less than 15"! Trust me on this: Heavy cheat curls build big, strong arms.

This makes sense. After all, if you need financial advice, are you going to look for it at a homeless shelter? Certainly not. If you are hell-bent on getting big and muscular, you are going to look at what such greats such as Arnold, Ronnie Coleman, Bill Kazmaier, Johnnie Jackson, Branch Warren, and Ted Arcidi have done.

The bottom line is this: Big, muscular, strong people have demonstrated the effectiveness of the cheat curl repeatedly. While I am citing the curl as an example, cheating is an advanced bodybuilding principle that, when used correctly, can open up the gates to an anabolic paradise.

What does cheating mean exactly?

Generally, it means swinging a weight past a sticking point; on a front raise it might be a slight hip bump out of the bottom; on a bent-over row it might be a slight vertical pull on the way up; it may be a "kip" to finish off your last rep on chin-up.

The philosophy is similar to a drop set: On a drop set, you reduce resistance to continue the set; on a cheating movement, you get outside swing help to complete the movement. Cheating does not require the assistance of a partner.

When performing a cheating movement, using the curl again as an example, while you do use some swing to complete the movement, you finish the movement with the target muscle, the biceps, which have effectively been overloaded. Swinging the weight all the way up is counterproductive and serves no real purpose in bodybuilding training.

Although some bodybuilders have used this technique, they always started the workout with lighter, stricter reps.

It is also very important to perform the negative portion of the lift under control, because not only do you have the capabilities to handle up to 160% of what you can on a positive, but you would rob yourself of the hypertrophy that can be gained on a controlled eccentric; a controlled eccentric takes a couple of seconds to lower the weight. An uncontrolled drop not only will kiss maximal hypertrophy goodbye but will open the door to a life of arthritis and getting to know your local orthopedic surgeon on a very personal level.

Cheating is an advanced high-intensity technique; it should not be used every workout! Use it infrequently on body parts you are trying to bring up; you know, those stubborn ones that just can't figure out they are supposed to grow.

Here are some cheat exercises that advanced bodybuilders have used effectively:

> Shoulders: Front Raises
> Arms: Cheat Curls
> Back: Bent-Over Rows

With proper implementation, this advanced training principle can help you cheat your way to the top!

PERIODIZATION TRAINING

Periodization training is not the latest 12-week program you saw on an infomercial at 3 a.m. or the glossy *Flex Magazine* foldout you read on the can at the gym. Periodization is a logical, sequential organization of purposeful training toward one's goals.

Periodization refers to how one's training is broken down into discrete time periods called macrocycles, mesocycles, and microcycles. Essentially, we look at long-term as well as short-term planning by systematically cycling methodology, volume, and intensity toward one's goals.

Some might ask, "Why not just train all-out year round, trying to maximize muscular size, symmetry, and limit strength, bring up lagging body parts, minimize body fat, and be in peak aerobic condition?"

While this may be the training objective of the cross-fitter or recreational gym rat, it is not possible to accomplish these objectives simultaneously. Just take a gander at the poor misguided souls who continue to spin their wheels and fail to make progress in any of the above objectives.

For you, the competitive bodybuilder or serious iron athlete who has long-term goals of balancing size and symmetry and minimizing body fat, there is a better way—it's called periodization! Chapter 4 is dedicated to periodization; I highly encourage you to study it.

Training with purpose and managing objectives is what you must understand. For some bodybuilders, working on a limit strength base may be a major off-season priority; for others, it might be to add overall mass; yet others may have a lagging body part that needs extreme focus.

Then there is contest prep and different phases that apply to different bodybuilders' nutritional strategies, cardio training, and posing routines. The bottom line is, you can't do it all at once, if you want to be the best!

Remember the three basic tenets to the Weider Principles:

- Principles to help you plan your training cycle
- Principles to help you arrange your exercises in each workout
- Principles to help you perform each exercise

A FEW LAST WORDS

To maximize muscular development, it is important to have knowledge of various bodybuilding methods. If you decide to use a new method, it is important to know why. If you avoid a certain method, you should have a reason for doing so. Take this knowledge and build with it.

SOURCES

Augustsson, J., R. Thomee, P. Hornstedt, J. Lindblom, J. Karlsson, and G. Grimby. "Effect of Pre-Exhaustion Exercise on Lower-Extremity Muscle Activation During a Leg Press Exercise." *Journal of Strength and Conditioning Research* 17, no. 2 (2003): 411–16.

Barker, Daniel. "German Volume Training: An Alternative Method of High Volume Load for Stimulating Muscle Growth." *NSCA Performance Training Journal* 8, no. 1 (2010): 10–13.

Dias, Ingrid, Roberto SimÃ£o, and Jeffrey Willardson. "Exercise Order in Resistance Training." *Sports Medicine Journal* 42, no. 3 (2012): 251–66.

Gentil, P., E. Oliviera, V. de Araújo Rocha Júnior, J. do Carmo, and M. Bottarro. "Effects of Exercise Order on Upper-Body Muscle Activation and Exercise Performance." *Journal of Strength and Conditioning Research* 21, no. 4 (2007): 1082–86.

Hatfield, Frederick. *Bodybuilding: A Scientific Approach.* Chicago: Contemporary Books, 1984.

Labrada, Lee. "Muscle by Force: How to Use Forced Reps to Stimulate Your Growth." *Muscle & Fitness* (August 2002): 120–24.

Marshall, P. W., D. A. Robbins, A. W. Wrightson, and J. C. Siegler. "Acute Neuromuscular and Fatigue Responses to the Rest-Pause Method." *Journal of Science & Medicine in Sport* 15, no. 2 (2012): 153–58.

Mosey, Tim. "The Effects of German Volume Training on Lean Muscle Mass and Strength and Power Characteristics in Elite Wild-Water Canoeists." *Journal of Australian Strength & Conditioning* 18, no. 2 (2010): 179.

Poliquin, Charles. "German Volume Training!" *Bodybuilding.com* (27 November 2002). http://www.bodybuilding.com/fun/luis13.htm.

Stoppani, Jim. "Forced Reps." *Muscle & Fitness* (September 2009): 46.

Wolff, Robert. *Bodybuilding 201: Everything You Need to Know to Take your Body to the Next Level.* Chicago: Contemporary Books, 2004.

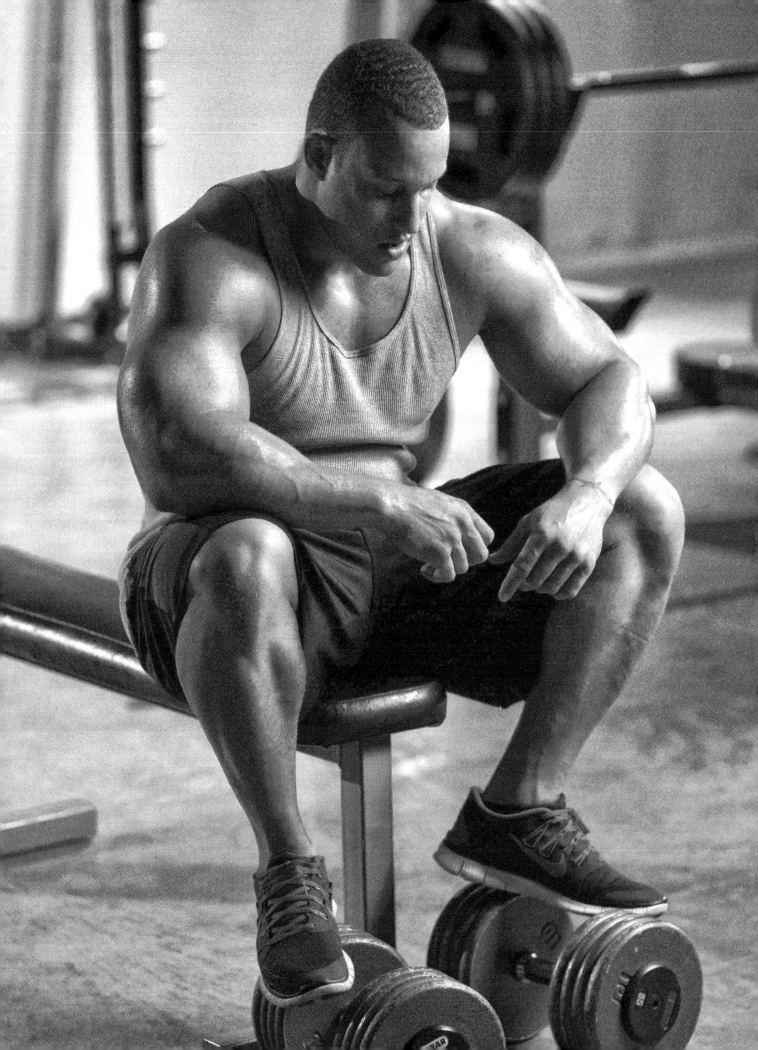

CHAPTER 2.

Hypertrophy and Adaptations to Strength Training

Bodybuilders are known for having one thing on their mind: How do I get big?

Let's take a look at what happens to your body behind the scenes.

IT'S ALL ABOUT THE MUSCLE

The human body has three types of muscle: Smooth muscle, which is governed by the autonomic nervous system, includes the muscles that line the digestive tract and protect the blood vessels. Cardiac muscle, which includes the heart, like smooth muscle is modulated by the autonomic nervous system. The functioning of smooth and cardiac muscle is largely involuntary. Skeletal muscle, the type anyone reading this book is concerned with building, blends into tendinous insertions that attach to bones, pulling on them, which generates desired movement.

When the body has to move, it responds by activating a slew of muscles. The forces generated by the body internally must overcome the forces imposed on the body externally.

During strength training, the body must overcome gravitational and inertial forces, which are magnified when a barbell is in people's hands, on their back, or overhead. Cumulatively, strength training will make skeletal muscles stronger, make cardiac muscle more efficient, and enhance the functioning of smooth muscle.

MUSCLE STRUCTURE AND FUNCTION

Mircrostructure

Muscles are composed largely of proteins, which are hierarchically organized from large groups to small fibers. A muscle is a group of motor units physically separated by a membrane from other groups of motor units. A muscle is connected to bones through tendons.

A motor unit consists of a single neuron and all of the muscle fibers innervated by it. The ratio of nerves to fibers determines the fine motor control available to that muscle. For example, the hand has fewer fibers per motor unit than do the muscles of the calf.

The muscle fiber is composed of myofibrils, which are small bundles of myofilaments. Myofilaments are the elements of the muscle that actually shorten upon contraction. Myofilaments are mainly made up of two types of protein: myosin (short, thick filaments) and actin (long, thin filaments). Two other important proteins comprising myofibrils are troponin and tropomyosin.

Reciprocal Innervation

When a prime mover muscle (or group of muscles) contracts, the opposing muscle (or group) relaxes. When locking out a bench press, the triceps are the prime mover; the biceps relax as you push the weight to completion. This phenomenon is called reciprocal innervation. Without this reciprocity, muscle actions would be very jerky and weak at best, or at worst result in no movement at all. The contracting muscle is referred to as the agonist, while the relaxed is the antagonist.

Sliding Filament Theory

The strength of contraction in a muscle depends, in large part, upon the number of muscle fibers involved; the more muscle fibers, the stronger the contraction.

The sliding filament theory states that a myofibril contracts by the actin and myosin filaments sliding over each other. Chemical bonds and receptor sites on the myofilaments attract each other, allowing the contraction to be held until fatigue interferes.

Muscle Fiber Pennation Arrangement

The alignment of the muscle fibers has a distinct effect on the ability to generate force. Fusiform arrangement occurs when the fibers are parallel to the tendons and therefore can contract at great speeds without a loss in total force output.

A unipennate muscle will have fiber alignment going from one side to the other in regards to the tendon, while a bipennate muscle will have alignment of fibers on both sides of the muscle.

Muscles with a unipennate, bipennate, or multipennate arrangement are capable of producing higher amounts of force than a fusiform arrangement can, but at the expense of contractile velocity. It is believed that fiber arrangement is determined by genetics but it may be altered somewhat with training.

Muscle Fiber Types

Three distinct types of muscle fiber are found in skeletal muscle: Type I, Type IIa, and Type IIx. The percentage of each varies from person to person and from one muscle to another in the same person.

Type I muscle fibers (slow-twitch or red fiber) are highly resistant to fatigue and injury, but their force output is very low. Activities performed in the aerobic pathway call upon these muscle fibers.

Type IIa muscle fibers (fast-twitch or intermediate fibers) are larger in size and much stronger than Type I fibers. They have a high capacity for glycolytic activity—they can produce high-force output for long periods.

Type IIx muscle fibers (fast-twitch muscle fibers) are often referred to as "couch potato fibers" because of their prevalence in sedentary individuals.

Research has shown that 16% of a sedentary person's total muscle mass is of this fiber type. It's been hypothesized that Mother Nature gave deconditioned folks these explosive fibers so they could cope with emergency situations.

Type IIx fibers are extremely strong, but they have almost no resistance to fatigue or injury. In fact, they are so strong and susceptible to injury that when they are used, they often are damaged beyond repair. Unless the body can repair the muscle cell, it is broken down and sloughed off into the amino acid pool. In most cases, sedentary people immediately lose their Type IIx fibers when beginning a training program. However, neural efficiency is increased via strength training, resulting in the production of higher forces for longer periods.

A fourth type of fiber (Type IIc) is the result of Type IIx fibers' "fusing" with surrounding satellite cells.

As noted earlier, Type IIx fibers are destroyed when they are used because of their fast-twitch capacity and poor recovery ability. When muscle fibers are damaged from training stress, a highly catabolic hormone called cortisol is released to facilitate the cleanup operation.

However, if cortisol is blocked, the Type IIx fibers will fuse with surrounding satellite cells (non-contractile muscle cells which help support or bulwark the tenuous IIx fibers). The result of fusion is a Type IIc fiber. Insulin-like growth factor-1 (IGF-1) stimulates the fusion process, which has huge implications for bodybuilders.

Fast-twitch fibers are serviced with thicker nerves, giving them a greater contractile impulse (measured in number of twitches per second). Slow-twitch fibers have smaller nerves (thus twitch fewer times per second) but have a high degree of oxygen-using capacity stemming from the greater number of mitochondria (the cells' "powerhouses" where adenosine-5'-triphosphate, or ATP, is synthesized), and a higher concentration of myoglobin and other oxygen-metabolizing enzymes.

CONNECTIVE TISSUE

The primary function of connective tissue is to connect muscle to bones and to connect joints together. Consisting of fiber called collagen, mature connective tissues have fewer cells than other tissues and therefore need (and receive) less blood, oxygen, and other nutrients than other tissues.

The positive effects of exercise on connective tissue have been well documented. Physical training has been shown to cause an increase in tensile strength, size, and resistance to injury, as well as the ability to repair damaged ligaments and tendons to regular tensile strength.

Tendons

Tendons are extensions of the muscle fibers that connect muscle to bone. They are slightly more pliable than ligaments but cannot shorten as muscles do. Various proprioceptors, the sensory organs found in muscles and tendons, provide information about body movement and position, and they protect muscle and connective tissue.

The Golgi Tendon Organ is embedded in tendon tissue and can be thought of as a safety valve. Increasing levels of muscular contraction result in feedback to the nervous system from the Golgi Tendon Organ.

When tension becomes too great—greater than your brain can handle—this signal inhibits the contraction stimulus, thereby reducing the likelihood of injury. This protective response is called the feedback loop.

While this may sound debilitating to the intense weight trainer, there is some good news: Training with high-speed contractions and with bands and chains can train you to somewhat inhibit the response of the Golgi Tendon Organ.

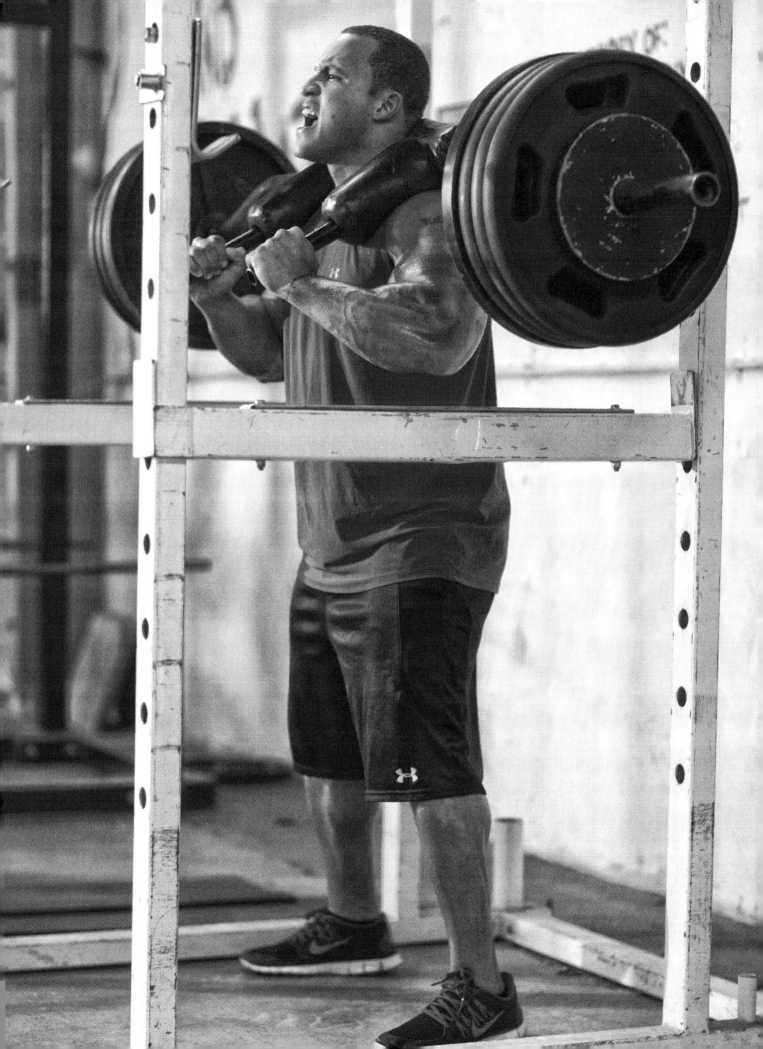

Ligaments

Ligaments connect bones to bones at a joint and, along with collagen, contain a somewhat elastic fiber called elastin. While ligaments must have some elasticity to allow for joint movement, this elasticity is limited.

Cartilage

Cartilage is a firm, elastic, flexible, white material. It is found at the ends of ribs, between vertebral discs, at joint surfaces, and in the nose and ears. As a smooth surface between adjacent bones, cartilage provides both shock absorption and structure. It also lubricates the working parts of a joint.

Unlike tendons and ligaments, cartilage has no blood supply of its own. The only way for cartilage to receive oxygen and nutrients is through synovial fluid. Because of this lack of nutrients, damaged cartilage heals very slowly.

NERVOUS SYSTEM: THE MIND AND BODY LINK

Your nervous system is made up of two major parts. The central nervous system (CNS) consists of your brain and your spinal column. You should think of them as being an integrated unit, not separate.

The CNS receives messages and, after interpreting them, sends instructions back to the body. The peripheral nervous system (PNS) does two things: (a) It relays messages from the CNS to the body (the efferent system), and (b) it relays messages to the CNS (the afferent system) from the body. (For a deeper understanding of how Central and Peripheral fatigue affect your performance, study Chapter 11, Recovery.) The CNS does the following:

1. It senses changes inside and outside your body.
2. It interprets those changes.
3. It responds to the interpretations by initiating action in the form of muscular contractions or glandular secretions.

Obviously, all the strength-training vernacular you've been exposed to over the years regarding the crucial link between your mind and your body all boils down to the fact that your central nervous system is linked with your peripheral nervous system.

THEORY OF NEUROMUSCULAR ACTIVITY

With the basic understanding of the neuromuscular system's structure and function, the next step is understanding exactly how it works.

One of the most important theories of neuromuscular activity, the Sliding Filament Theory, was discussed earlier. Now let's take a look at the other theories of neuromuscular activity.

The "All or None" Theory

When a nerve carries an impulse of sufficient magnitude down to the muscle cells that comprise the motor unit, the myofibrils do the only thing they know how to do—contract, or shorten.

Each myofibril could be described as a fundamentalist in its functioning. It knows nothing less than total contraction, as it responds with an all-or-none reaction. A key point here is that a motor unit is either completely relaxed or fully contracted.

Because muscle fiber (including its myofibrils) and the entire motor unit of which it is a part respond to a nerve stimulus with the all-or-none reaction, this means not all the motor units comprising a muscle are activated during any given movement.

Think of the Weider "muscle confusion principle"; this is why it is of paramount importance to hit muscles at different angles, speeds, and ranges of motion. Not only that, but doing the same movements habitually means becoming more and more proficient at that movement, which is great for the strength athlete but handicaps the potential of maximal muscle growth.

This means you are able to exercise a gradation of response by increasing or decreasing the amount of chemo-electrical impulse to the muscle. In other words, you are coordinated enough to produce sufficient force to lift a fork to your face or curl a heavy dumbbell. Being unable to control force production by lifting a fork to your face would invoke a bloody disaster.

Both are similar movements, but curling a fork involves only those motor units with a very low excitation threshold, while curling the dumbbell requires many more motor units. The principle that allows this to happen is known as the Size Principle.

The Size Principle of Fiber Recruitment

Force output of muscle is related to the stimulus it receives. Different muscle fibers have different liability to recruitment, with Type I fibers having the highest liability, Type IIa and IIc having a moderate liability, and Type IIx having a low level of liability.

The Size Principle of Fiber Recruitment (also called the Henneman Principle) states that those fibers with a high level of reliability (slow twitch fibers with the fewest motor units) will be recruited first, and those with lower levels of reliability (fast-twitch fibers with the greatest number of motor units) will be recruited last. This is why you are able to eat using Type I fibers, which allows you to safely put your fork into your mouth.

To recap, Type I (slow twitch) muscle fibers are smaller and more endurance based than Type II (fast-twitch) muscle fibers. Type II muscle fibers begin to be recruited when you use more than 25% of your maximum strength. Although a one-repetition max in the squat may be performed slowly, you will still be using all of your fast-twitch muscle fibers along with your slow twitch ones to move the heavy barbell on your back.

The Stretch Reflex

As a muscle is stretched, muscle spindles become activated and the brain receives a message that tells the muscle to contract. A rapidly stretched muscle stores elastic-like energy; this stretch reflex sparks a quick contraction.

Take a look at a vertical jump from a held squat position compared to one where the athlete rapidly drops his butt and reverses the action as fast as possible. Numerous studies confirm athletes can jump higher using a counter movement than from a squat position. The stretch reflex is similar to how a rubber band works.

For the bodybuilder, an example of the stretch reflex in action is aiding a lift like the bench press. A full range of motion is much easier than a dead bench press starting at chest level, due to the contributions from the stretch reflex.

A more scientific look at the stretch reflex shows it is a built-in protective function of the neuromuscular system in the muscle spindle, a proprioceptor found in the bellies of muscle.

In contrast to the Golgi Tendon Organ, which is in series with the force plane of the muscle, the muscle spindle is in parallel with the force plane. The action is similar to that of the Golgi Tendon Organ, in that it protects against overload and injury in what is known as the "stretch reflex" action (medical example: the knee-jerk response used by physicians to test your muscle's response adequacy).

Neural Adaptations

It is universally accepted that intense resistance training causes morphological changes to the physique by increased muscle mass. The question remains, can the nervous system be modified to your advantage?

The answer is Yes! Not only can you modify certain aspects of your nervous system function, but the rewards in terms of training are significant.

The greatest advantages for the bodybuilder are improved strength output, better mental concentration, greater training intensity, pain management, and glandular secretions. All of these areas are modifiable to at least a measurable degree and will aid you in your muscle-building quest.

Hypertrophy

Mechanical tension, muscle damage, and metabolic stress are the three factors that induce muscle hypertrophy from exercise, according to Brad Schoenfeld in *The Journal of Strength and Conditioning Research*. Mechanical tension is a product of intense resistance training and muscle stretch.

Muscle damage induces the delayed onset of muscle soreness that sets in approximately 24 hours after a workout and can peak out 2–3 days after weight training. Metabolic stress results from the byproducts of anaerobic metabolism; this, in turn, promotes hormonal factors that induce hypertrophy.

"Everybody wants to be a bodybuilder but nobody want to lift heavy ass weight. But I do," said Mr. Olympia Ronnie Coleman.

The human body desires to be in a state of stability known as homeostasis; when the state of stability is disrupted, adaptations take place.

This is how your muscles grow!

Stress from resistance training is placed on muscles they are not accustomed to; the response is increased growth "hypertrophy."

Time and time again, research has confirmed that heavy resistance training is the most beneficial method of achieving hypertrophy. The reason seems to be that the Type II fibers are most affected by heavy resistance training (as noted in the Size Principle) and ultimately have the greatest potential for growth.

That is why I recommend starting off with powerlifting to build a base, just like Ronnie Coleman and "The Austrian Oak."

Muscle hypertrophy, to those outside of the iron game, sounds like useless, scientific jargon, but to the bodybuilder it's gospel.

What exactly is muscular hypertrophy?

It is the increase of the muscle's cross-sectional area, involving the concurrent increase in myofibrilar content (contractile element).

Myofibrilar hypertrophy results from lifting maximal weights for lower reps, like powerlifters train. Bodybuilders who train heavy have a very dense look.

If maximal muscularity is desired, there is no way around heavy core lifts.

Sarcoplasmic hypertrophy is the accumulation of noncontractile matter, such as water, glycogen, and myoglobin—which are stored in the sarcoplasm of the muscle cell—and the densification of mitochondrial content.

Sarcoplasmic hypertrophy, the result of high volume training, typically associated with bodybuilders, is essential to maximizing your complete physique development. Typically, this type of training and the imposed adaptations do little to enhance limit strength. On the upside, strength endurance will improve because of mitochondrial hypertrophy.

Another benefit of training for sarcoplasmic hypertrophy is the growth and strengthening of connective tissues. The bodybuilder with the complete package will have a synergistic blend of both hypertrophic elements.

Initially, adaptations to resistance training will be neurological. In other words, by performing a movement, you become more coordinated at the movement technically; and by recruiting the right muscles to lift the weight, you become more efficient at the movement. As neurological adaptations start to slow, the muscle will start to grow.

We get stronger by enhanced neural patterns; as you continually overload your muscle, the cross-sectional muscle fiber area increases and your muscles get bigger.

Hyperplasia

Hypertrophy is the accepted mechanism of increased mass. Basically, you are born with a certain number of muscle fibers; these can increase in size but not in number.

But what if the number of muscle fibers could increase?

During the late '60s and early '70s, European scientists discovered that the muscle cells of some animals adapted to severe overload by splitting in two. This response, called hyperplasia, was subsequently followed by an increase in muscle size. Muscle fibers divided and then multiplied, so the potential implications to the bodybuilder are huge.

Whoa… hold your horses.

Hyperplasia in humans remains controversial.

Studies on animals showed mixed results.

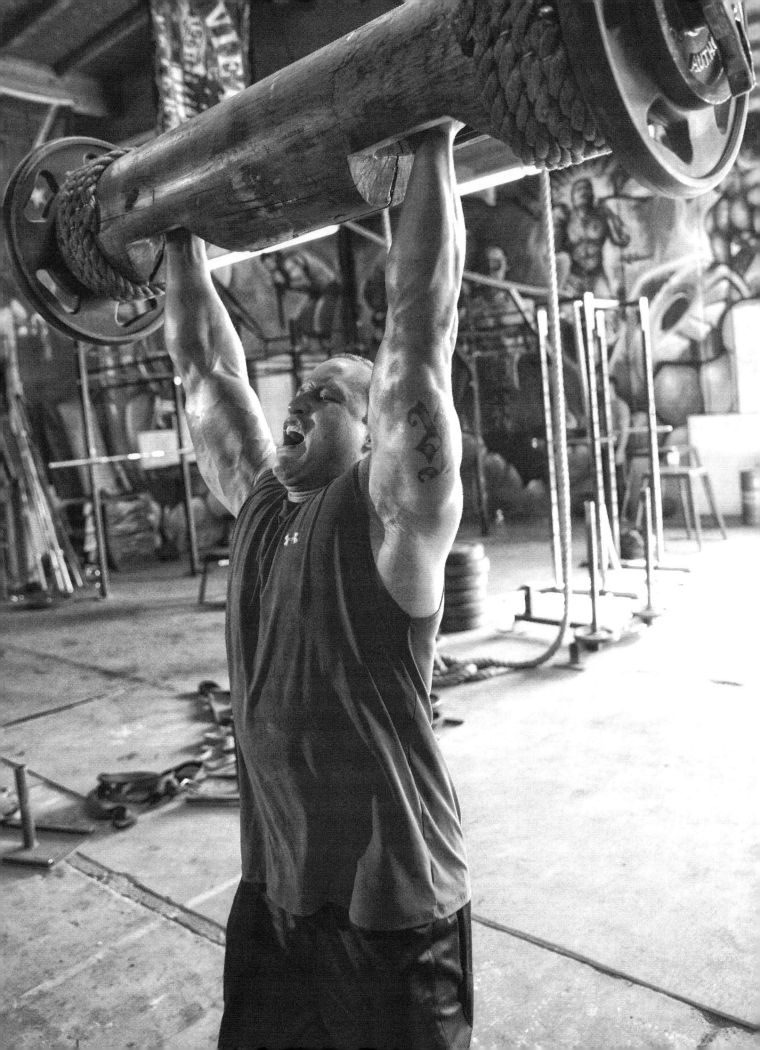

Cats were trained to move a heavy weight with their paw to receive food; hyperplasia took place as a result. Other studies on animals counter these findings: Studies on chickens, rats, and mice found that muscle fibers increased in size but not in number; hyperplasia did not take place.

However, another study performed on birds showed an increase in the number of muscle fibers in their wings as a response of being chronically stretched by attaching a weight on the wings. The cats were subjected to heavy resistance with lower repetitions; the other animals were involved in more endurance-based activities. This might explain some of the discrepancies in results.

According to world-renowned researcher Vladimir Zatsiorsky, in his book *Science and Practice of Strength Training,* both hyperplasia and hypertrophy contribute to muscle size increase. However, the contribution of fiber hyperplasia is rather small (less than 5%).

This may not sound like much, but in the pro ranks this could potentially mean an additional inch on your arms! Research on hyperplasia in people lacks in abundance, but some exists.

A 1978 study reported that muscle fiber size remained constant in swimmers, but the muscle increased in size.

Researchers Nygaard and Nielsen argued increased muscle size was a result of hyperplasia. A 1986 examination of European bodybuilders showed an abnormally high muscle fiber density on the two subjects who had trained intensely with weights for 14 years or longer, while those who had trained for 4–6 years had more normal fiber density. The abnormal fiber density, researchers theorized, may have been a hyperplasic response to long-term extreme weight training.

Assuming hyperplasia *can* take place, it would happen through a few different mechanisms, from what researchers show.

This would mean performing movement with an extreme stretch. Examples are stiff leg deadlifts for hamstrings, sissy squats for quads, dumbbell flyes for chest, incline dumbbell curls (palms supinated the whole time) for biceps, French press for triceps, cable rows for back, and inclined lateral raises or front raises for shoulders. Of course, the list could go on.

You will also need to lift heavy. This means hitting the core lifts hard and, of course, undergoing long-term training. Swimming involves a repetitive high-speed stroke against a relatively low resistance. Holistic, intense, long-term training appears to be the best way to possibly induce hyperplasia.

Satellite Cells

Satellite cells serve to repair damaged muscle tissue, inducing muscle growth after overload from weight training.

Satellite cells are the skeletal muscles' "stem cells." Overload from intense weight training causes trauma to the muscle. This disturbance to the muscle cell organelles activates satellite cells, which are located on the outside of the muscle cell, to proliferate at the site trauma was induced.

After satellite cells are damaged via intense resistance training, damaged muscle fibers are repaired by satellite cells' fusing together and to the muscle fibers, which leads to muscle growth. The satellite cells have only one nucleus and can replicate by dividing.

During the process of satellite cell multiplication, a small percentage of satellite cells stay as organelles on the muscle fibers. However, most will repair damaged muscle fibers or fuse to muscle fibers, forming new myofibrils. For the bodybuilder, this is exciting because the myofibrils of the muscle cell increase in number and size.

What does this mean?

After satellite cells fuse with muscle fibers, muscle fibers are able to synthesize more proteins and create a greater number of contractile proteins, meaning muscle will grow and get stronger.

Let's take a practical look at how you can take advantage of satellite cell proliferation.

A 2006 study in the *The Journal of Physiology* entitled "Creatine Supplementation Augments the Increase in Satellite Cell and Myonuclei Number in Human Skeletal Muscle Induced by Strength Training" for the first time showed that creatine supplementation in conjunction with strength training amplified the effects of strength-training-induced increases in satellite cell number and myonuclei concentration in human skeletal muscle fibers, enhancing muscled fiber growth in response to strength training.

"The Effects of Eccentric Versus Concentric Resistance Training on Muscle Strength and Mass in Healthy Adults: A Systematic Review with Meta-Analysis" was a study published in 2009 in the *British Journal of Sports Medicine*, showing intense eccentric contractions were superior to concentric patterns for increasing muscle size. This is not a surprise, because intense eccentric movements force muscle fibers and surrounding satellite cells to fuse, resulting in muscle fiber growth.

To maximize muscle growth, intense eccentric movements will have to be a part of your regimen. Remember, these induce a greater delayed onset of muscle soreness (DOMS) and should not be a part of a deload *ever.*

IGF-1 is largely responsible for satellite cell proliferation, and that would explain why some bodybuilders are willing to illegally supplement with it.

A 2003 study in the *American Journal of Physiology, Endocrinology, and Metabolism* entitled "Testosterone-Induced Muscle Hypertrophy Is Associated with an Increase in Satellite Cell Number in Healthy, Young Men" studied satellite cell proliferation on subjects using 125 mgs, 300 mgs, and 600 mgs weekly of synthetic testosterone, along with a baseline group that was not using any synthetic hormone assistance. The groups using 300 and 600 mgs of testosterone weekly had significant increases in the number of satellite cells; the baseline and the 125 mg group did not.

While I do discourage any illegal drug use, I believe in presenting factual information.

A FEW LAST WORDS

Fast-twitch muscle fibers have the highest potential for growth. This means to get bigger muscles, you have to get stronger ones, especially as your muscle-building journey commences.

Your limit strength is your base.

Heavy resistance training augments your being able to efficiently recruit the largest high threshold motor units. The more motor units recruited, the more muscle fibers are stimulated. The highest motor unit stimulation is with heavy weights, so you must train heavy.

This all sounds great, but why do the strongest powerlifters in the world have less muscle than bodybuilders who are much weaker?

Powerlifters generally train only in low-rep ranges, enhancing myofibrilar hypertrophy.

The bodybuilder needs to take a holistic approach, developing all components of the muscle. This is done by taking a holistic approach with high reps, low reps, high speed, low speed, compound movement, eccentrics, stretch movements, peak contraction, and time under tension; it's a balancing act to maximize hypertrophy.

SOURCES

Alway, S. E., P. K. Winchester, M. E. Davis, and W. J. Gonyea. "Regionalized Adaptations and Muscle Fiber Proliferation in Stretch-Induced Enlargement." *Journal of Applied Physiology* 66, no. 2 (1989): 771–81.

Antonio, J, and W. J. Gonyea. "Skeletal Muscle Fiber Hyperplasia." *Medicine and Science in Sports and Exercise* 25, no. 12 (1993): 1333–45.

Bubbico A., and L. Kravitz. "Muscle Hypertrophy." *IDEA Fitness Journal* 8, no. 10 (2011): 23–26.

Gollnick, P. D., B. F. Timson, R. L. Moore, and M. Riedy. "Muscular Enlargement and Number of Fibers in Skeletal Muscles of Rats." *Journal of Applied Physiology* 50, no. 5 (1981): 936–43.

Gonyea, W. J., D. G. Sale, F. B. Gonyea, and A. Mikesky. "Exercise Induced Increases in Muscle Fiber Number." *European Journal of Applied Physiology and Occupational Physiology* 55, no. 2 (1986): 137–41.

Holman, Steve. *Train, Eat, Grow: The Positions-of-Flexion Muscle-Training Manual.* Oxnard: Ironman Magazine, 2001.

Larsson, L., and P. A. Tesch. "Motor Unit Fibre Density in Extremely Hypertrophied Skeletal Muscles in Man: Electrophysiological Signs of Muscle Fibre Hyperplasia." *European Journal of Applied Physiology and Occupational Physiology* 55, no. 2 (1986): 130–36.

Nygaard, Berndt, and Berndt Furberg. "Skeletal Muscle Fiber Capillarization with Extreme Endurance Training in Man," in *Swimming Medicine IV* (vol. 6), edited by Bengt O. Eriksson and Berndt Furberg, 282–93. Baltimore, MD: University Park Press, 1978.

Olesen, Steen, Per Aagaard, Fawzi Kadi, Goran Tufekovic, Julien Verney, Jens L. Olesen, Charlotte Suetta, and Michael Kjaer. "Creatine Supplementation Augments the Increase in Satellite Cell and Myonuclei Number in Human Skeletal Muscle Induced by Strength Training." *The Journal of Physiology* 15 (2006): 525–34.

Roig, M., and K. O'Brien. "The Effects of Eccentric Versus Concentric Resistance Training on Muscle Strength and Mass in Healthy Adults: A Systematic Review with Meta-Analysis." *British Journal of Sports Medicine* 43, no. 8 (2009): 556–58.

Schoenfeld, Brad. "The Mechanisms of Muscle Hypertrophy and Their Application to Resistance Training." *Journal of Strength and Conditioning Research* 24, no. 10 (2010): 2857–73.

Tidball, J. G. "Inflammatory Cell Response to Acute Muscle Injury." *Medicine and Science in Sports and Exercise* 27, no. 7 (1995): 1022–32.

Zatsiorsky, Vladimir. *Science and Practice of Strength Training.* Champaign, IL: Human Kinetics, 2006.

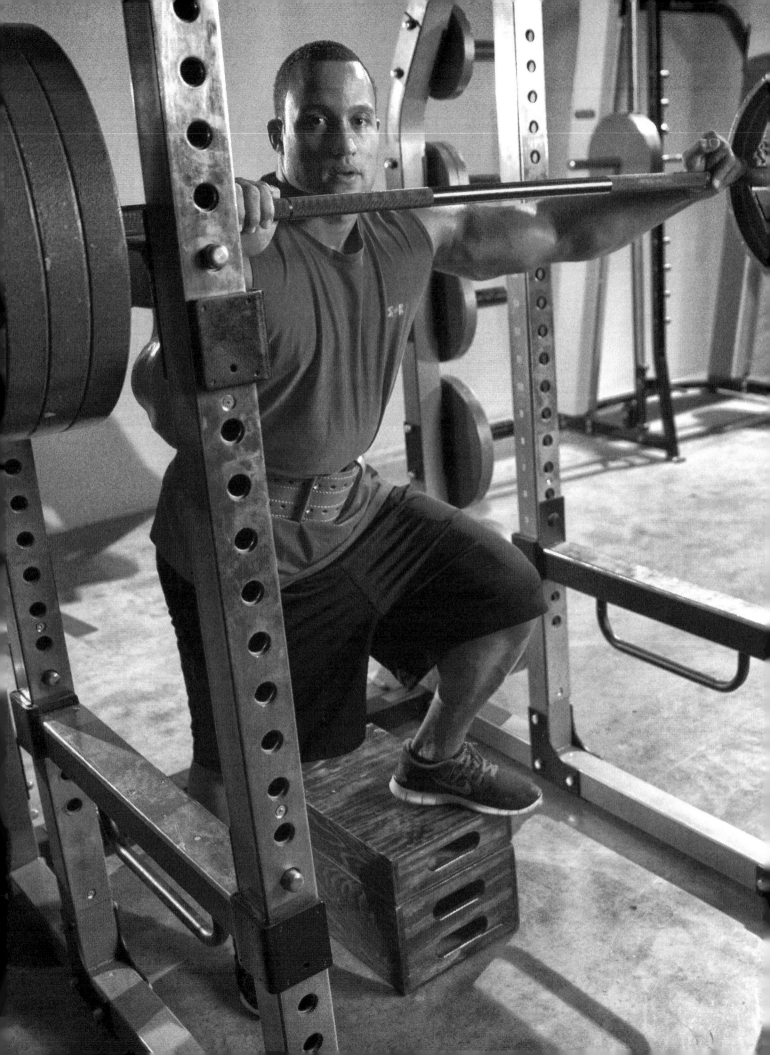

CHAPTER 3.

Back to the Basics

Centuries ago, whenever church leaders felt like the church was headed off course, they would gather in Jerusalem. This pilgrimage back to the Holy Land represented a back-to-the-basics approach.

When a company becomes institutionalized and loses sight of the values spawned in its genesis, often times the solution is go back to the original mission statement.

When bodybuilders train light and only with single-joint isolation movements, taking the path of least resistance, and they find themselves not growing or getting stronger, the situation calls for going back to the basics; we're talking heavy pig iron.

Remember, in the pre-steroid era through the steroid-only era of the 1950s to the early 1980s, before the arrival of synthetic growth hormone and other drugs, most bodybuilders (champion and gym rat alike) with great physiques realized that building strength with basic, compound, multi-joint lifts was the key to size, strength, power, and symmetry.

What has changed? Why do many current bodybuilders not adhere to these time-tested truths?

One reason could be that massive amounts of anabolic agents like growth hormone, IGF-1, Insulin, SARMS, and other strange anabolic agents stacked with absurd amounts of steroids have allowed people to get away with unsound training practices.

Case in point: I have seen some good bodybuilders do a routine for their back that just consisted of:

- Light Lat Pull-downs
- Cable Rows
- Machine Assisted Chin-ups

The combination of great genetics and playing Russian roulette with a massive amount of muscle-building drugs is the only way that aforementioned style of training would build a massive, muscular championship physique.

Just think what would happen if that same bodybuilder used heavy compound movements with the right synergistic blend of single-joint movements and properly periodized the training: A great champion would be in the making! I see it time and time again.

A workout example of such an approach would be:

- Deadlifts
- Various Grip Chin-up Variations
- Peak Contraction Band Resisted T-Bar Rows
- Meadows Rows/One-Armed Dumbbell Rows Superset
- Chest-up Face Away Tempo/Time Under Tension Wide Grip Lat Pull-downs
- Tempo One-Armed Cable Low Rows

Look at the work accomplished here: A heavy compound movement, a peak contraction movement, big movements, small movements, and time under tension are all at the core of the program.

As you can see, this post-exhaustion/powerbuilding style of training does not ignore any of the holistic components of maximizing muscle growth and carving a competition-ready symmetrical physique.

Bodybuilders who ignore the most important part of their training, compound movements, falsely believe their muscular physiques are a product of sound training. Yet the truth is, it's because of great genetics and great drugs.

If you can train like the first bodybuilder I spoke of and happen to be big and muscular, you have great genetics. Now, just think of the amazing metamorphosis that would take place if you trained like the second bodybuilder. Not only would you experience greater internal satisfaction, you would start packing on serious muscle.

GET BIG: TRAIN BIG LIFTS

To get big and strong, you need to keep big compound movements at the core of your program.

For back development, deadlifts beat lat pull-downs; for chest and triceps, weighted dips take precedence over a cable movement; standing presses beat out machine lateral raises; and front squats are superior to leg extensions.

Remember, a great muscle building program will have *both* compound (multi-joint) movements and isolation (single-joint) movements. The key is integrating both to play in concert like a fine orchestra. If we had to choose, we would choose big lifts over small isolation ones… luckily, we do not have to choose!

LIMIT STRENGTH

Limit strength is the ability to produce maximum force voluntarily in a given action. In other words, it's how much force you can produce in one all-out effort, regardless of time. Powerlifting is the best example of a limit-strength test.

There are three kinds of limit strength:

1. *Eccentric strength*—how much weight you can lower without losing control
2. *Static strength*—how much weight you can hold stationary without losing control
3. *Concentric strength*—how much weight you can lift one time with an all-out muscle contraction

Wait, I hear the chorus echoing, "I am a bodybuilder. Limit strength is not important."

To that, folks, I say "Hogwash!"

Limit strength in all athletic endeavors is your foundation and could, in fact, be labeled foundational strength.

Think about it logically.

If you can front squat 450 pounds, you will be able to do more on leg extensions than if your max front squat is 200 pounds.

If you can bench press 400 pounds, you will do more with cable flyes than if your max bench press is 200 pounds.

Think about all the various components of the holistic approach of muscle building—high reps, low reps, and time under tension—or even simply look at the Weider Principles.

Whether it's the principle of isolation or forced reps, you will do more if you are stronger; this in turn is a catalyst for maximizing muscle growth.

Let's go back to the bench press. If your one-repetition max is 400 pounds, 200 pounds is only 50% of your max; you can do a lot more with those 200 pounds than if your max is 250 pounds.

Remember, your limit strength is your base.

It's time to heed the wisdom of Dr. Squat and realize you cannot shoot a cannon out of a canoe; you must shoot it from a sturdy foundation. Start building your base now if you want to build your best physique for the international stage or just because you want it.

Generally, limit strength is best increased for advanced trainees using more than 85% of their one-repetition maximum. Beginners can literally increase their limit strength with less than 50% of their one-repetition max. Limit strength is developed by training heavy compound movements.

Here are some core lifts that can help pave the way for your bodybuilding success.

THE SQUAT

Former Mr. Olympia, Jay Cutler, had this to say about squats in the March 2004 edition of *Flex Magazine:* "Nothing builds quad mass like heavy free weight squats. I recommend all bodybuilders squat."

Many different variations of squat movements are highly beneficial to the bodybuilder. While squatting is a compound movement, meaning multiple joints and muscles are used, it is possible to put a greater emphasis on different parts of the leg development.

This is done by using an assortment of squat variations and foot placements; a narrow stance from squat will be more beneficial for quadriceps development than a wide-stance, West Side Barbell style box squat.

Generally, full range of motion for full development is the name of the game when it comes to squatting. Not only do you rob your glutes and hamstrings of important work by cutting squats high, but you also put undue stress on your patella by artificially stopping at an unnatural point, counter to a full-range-of-motion squat where the muscles of the posterior chain aid you in stopping in the hole. Plus, who can argue with Branch Warren, Tom Platz, and Ronnie Coleman, three men with three of the best pairs of legs of all time, who religiously full squatted.

Bottom line: Partial squats equal partial development.

Full squats provide greater glute activation. And be careful with partials. Once you gain proficiency in partial squats, you may be able to handle hundreds of pounds over your true squat max, but this can cause back problems because of spinal compression with excess weight over your max and, of course, undue stress on your knees.

Your body was created to go through the full range of motion, and we are after full development. Look at Asian and Aboriginal cultures that constantly full squat yet have a low rate of knee injuries.

Here are a few to tips to effectively squatting heavy weights with full range of motion:

- Walk out with one step on each leg; make your walk out as short as possible to safely perform the squat.
- Initiate the movement by breaking at the hips, not the knees.
- Push the knees out as you descend, reverse, and ascend.
- Always keep the knees in line with the toes to avoid unnecessary stress on the knees and connective tissue.
- Hold your breath throughout the entire movement; breathe between reps.
- Come out of the hole by driving your head and upper back into the bar.
- Keep your chest up.
- Keep the back arched and shoulder blades together.

For over a century, the squat has been hailed as the king for gaining size and strength. Various studies have shown that weight training in general increases growth hormone and testosterone levels during and post-exercise. It now appears that this acute response is more important in hypertrophy and tissue remodeling than chronic changes in hormone levels at rest.

To maximize these benefits, training programs that are moderate in intensity with short rest intervals and high volume elicit the greatest acute hormonal elevations.

Compound movements increase testosterone and growth hormone, and squats do the most of any resistance exercise (including the leg press). The body's natural release of testosterone and growth hormone is a catalyst for muscle growth.

What does this mean?

If you have no preexisting injuries and want to maximize the release of anabolic hormones, without using illegal performance-enhancing drugs, *squat!*

If you want your muscles to grow, *squat!*

A study by the University of North Dakota compared muscle recruitment during a leg press and a free-weight barbell squat lift. The study used two groups of subjects. Group 1 was made up of 10 untrained, healthy men, and Group 2 was made up of 16 trained, healthy male athletes. The analysis method used was electromyographic (EMG) activity. EMG activity was recorded from the erector spinae (ES), gluteus maximus (GM), vastus lateralis (VL), and biceps femoris (BF) muscles. The exercises performed were the leg press and the barbell squat.

All subjects in Group 1 lifted 3 repetitions of both exercises using a weight equivalent to their own bodyweight, which ranged from 155 to 165 pounds. In Group 2, each subject performed 3 repetitions of both exercises using a weight equivalent to 80% of their one-repetition max in both lifts, which ranged from 225 to 600 pounds.

The results indicated that in Group 2, the trained group, the squat exercise elicited significantly more EMG activity than did the leg press in the ES, GM, and BF. A significant difference in the VL activity was not observed between the two exercises, but the activity in the VL was still slightly greater. In the untrained group, Group 1, the results were almost a reflection of the trained group. The leg press utterly failed to recruit the ES, GM, or BF to the degree the barbell squat did, and the quadriceps were slightly more stimulated in the squat than in the leg press.

Every single lower body muscle was more active in a squat versus the leg press! So much for the legs getting more direct work in the leg press!

Bodybuilding Squat Variations

Front squats. Front squats are a tremendous exercise for building overall thigh mass and placing a special emphasis on the quadriceps. This exercise requires tremendous core strength because the load is placed on the anterior portion of your shoulders, directly compressing downward on your abdominal muscles. Flexibility of the arms, shoulders, and wrists are required if you hold the bar in a racked position like an Olympic lifter.

For bodybuilders, a crossed arm style is generally preferable.

We are after working the muscle, not direct transference to a push press or athletic movement; but more importantly, there is no reason to put undue strain on the shoulders, elbows, and wrists.

Some important advantages of the front squats is that they force technical proficiency, unlike a back squat. When back squatting, if you lose technique by bending too far forward at the waist or rounding over, you can good-morning the weight up; if this same situation arises on the front squat, you will be forced to dump the weight, reinforcing technical requirements of the lift.

Another advantage of squats is they are more quad dominant, an advantage for paranoid bodybuilders scared of getting their butts too big. Many bodybuilders swear by this movement for development of the vastus medialis, the teardrop muscle of the quadriceps.

Front squats are easier on your back because your torso is more erect, and obviously less weight is being handled. This upright position reduces some of the stress and sheer force on the lower back, making a great alternative for iron brethren who have lower back issues and find back squatting painful. Furthermore, front squats are also a good tool to teach someone to back squat with an erect torso.

Be careful not to do too many reps on the front squat; as strength coach Charles Poliquin advises, "Your rhomboids will tire out isometrically before your quads concentrically. You do not want to get to the point where you are squatting with kyphotic posture. This is when accidents happen."

In other words, don't make the exercise about a futile attempt to maintain proper posture. Instead, make it about building the thighs, as this can become an issue when going beyond 6–8 reps with heavy weight.

What does science say about front squats?

One 2008 study published in the *Journal of Strength and Conditioning* concluded that the front squat was as effective as the back squat in regards to overall muscle mass recruitment during the lift; and, in fact, the front squat produced significantly fewer compressive forces on the back and sheer force on the knees.

The group determined that front squats maybe advantageous for long-term joint health and for individuals suffering from back and knee problems. Remember, during this study subjects used 70% of their bodyweight for front squats and 90% for back squats, so this played a role in measuring sheer and compressive forces.

Another study performed by the University of Texas, Arlington, with loads of 65 pounds comparing front and back squat, showed very similar muscular recruitment patterns for both lifts but significantly more quadriceps; particularly, the rectus femoris was recruited during the front squat.

While it is safe to say most bodybuilders do front squats with much more than 65 pounds, it is interesting to see peer-reviewed science concur with "bro science."

In-the-trenches experience and observations show front squats are a fantastic quadriceps builder, and two of the strongest groups of humans on the planet, Olympic weightlifters and track and field throwers, have relied on this movement for decades to build limit strength.

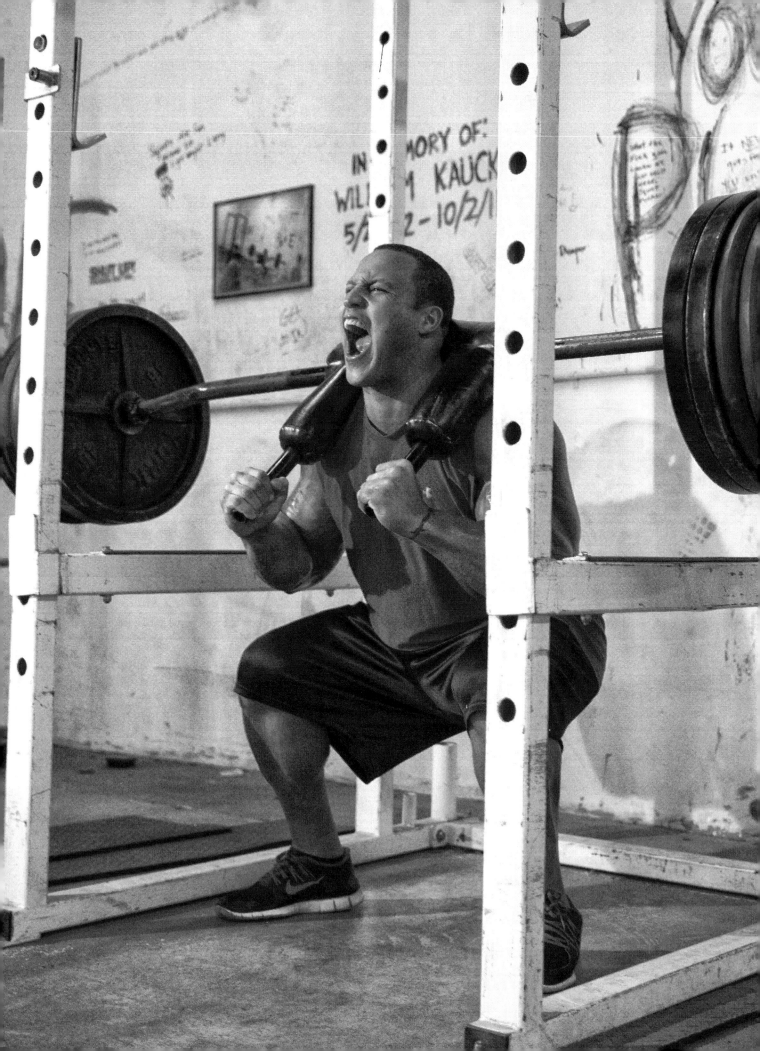

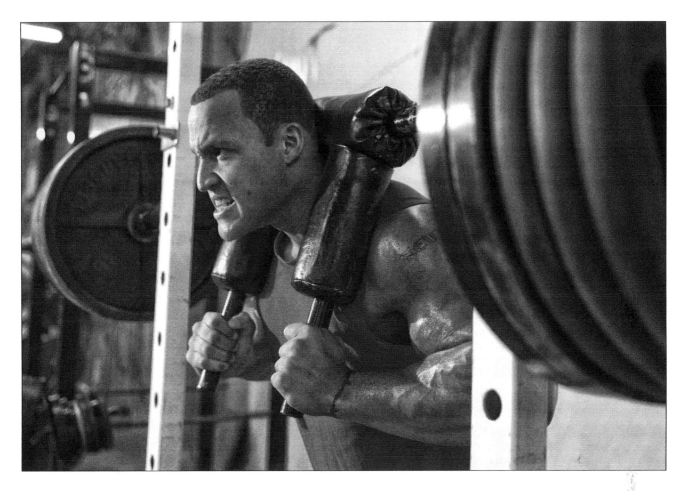

Safety squats. The safety squat bar is an effective training tool that is gaining more and more popularity from top-level pro bodybuilders like Branch Warren and Johnnie Jackson to regular Joes who report less back pain and more thigh development. Properly used, the safety bar, often called the Hatfield bar because of Fred Hatfield's endorsement, is one of the most effective leg training modalities in the bodybuilder's arsenal!

Get ready, because your quadriceps are in for a treat!

When performing safety squats, your hands are not holding the bar. This allows you to grasp the handles on the power rack. Strong athletes will have to use massive poundages to get the most out of squats, and sometimes these enormous loads cause "rounding" of the back, which is way too common and places large amounts of unnecessary stress on intervertebral discs.

The safety bar squat circumvents this by letting the athlete exert pressure against the power rack by grasping the handles and thus maintaining a perfectly straight back throughout the entire squatting motion. Using your hands to spot yourself prevents you from falling forward or backward.

When squatting with a straight bar, you're forced to use a load that you can handle in the weakest position. This results in using an inadequate amount of weight in the strongest position of the squatting motion.

When the "sticking point" is reached, the hands can be used to help you get through it while maintaining optimal form. Furthermore, this will enable you to work with heavier weights in the ranges of movement where you are strongest, and it gives you help when you are weakest. Basically, you get the advantage of continuous tension on the muscle throughout the entire range of motion like a cable offers, but while performing a squat! The fact that you needn't use your hands to hold the bar on your shoulders eliminates wrist, shoulder and elbow discomfort, and that's a good thing.

The pad on the safety bar ads an element of comfort; heavy squatting is not about comfort, but it certainly doesn't take away from the experience.

Because you can use your hands to regulate body position, your posture under the bar can be adapted to suit your leverages so that you can literally "tailor" your squatting style to afford maximum overload.

Go to any powerlifting meet and you'll see that the majority of big squatters with the heavy poundages have a distinct forward lean. This is because regular squatting places the weight behind you, approximately 4 inches behind your body's midline. You are forced to lean or bend forward for balance; to what degree depends on the individual. Using the safety squat bar, the weight is distributed directly in line with your body's midline, so there is no need to lean forward, saving your back.

The disadvantage of the safety bar is that it is tough to quantitatively track data, meaning it is literally impossible to know exactly how much your arms are helping pull you through a sticking point.

A 500-pound safety squat with 50 pounds of pull from the arms is different from one with 120 pounds of pull; keep this in mind when tracking overload and limit-strength gains. Safety bars can also be effective and comfortably used for front squats.

Other specialty bar squats/devices. Many other specialty bars are available that can help eliminate shoulder, elbow, and wrist stress while squatting and, of course, hit the muscles at different angles. Many well-equipped, hardcore gyms will literally have a plethora of bars to choose from.

While variety is the spice of life, some continuity amongst core lifts is required to track progress or lack of progress. Some of the specialty bar/devices are (but are not limited to) the Buffalo Bar, Manta Ray, Yoke Bar, Front Squat Harness, Zercher Squat Harness, Thick Bar, and Cambered Bar. Most of these cambered bars are available at EliteFTS.com.

Dip belt squats. Dip belt squats were popularized by John McCallum in the March and April 1970 issues of *Strength & Health* magazine. This exercise is great for building the thighs, but it mainly offers a great alternative to spinal loading.

While various squat movements may have different levels of downward compressive forces, the dip belt squat does not because the load is placed under the athlete, not resting on the shoulders or even above the head.

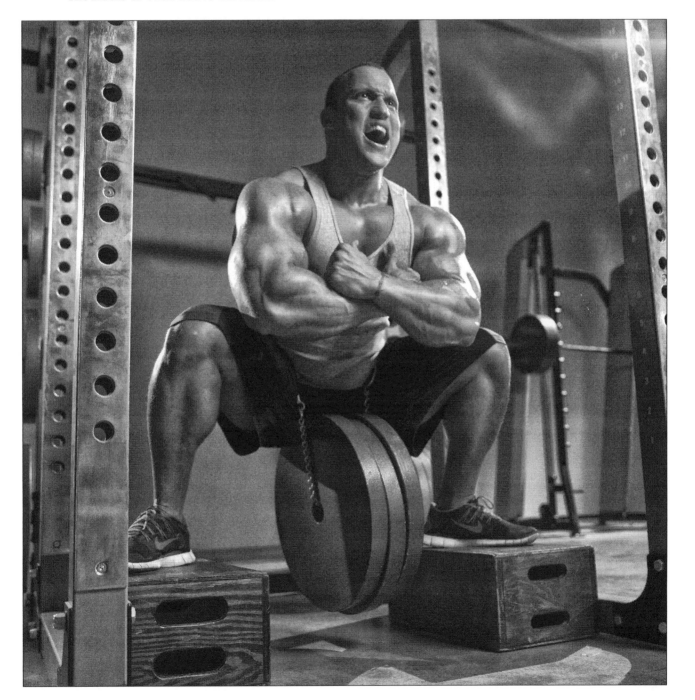

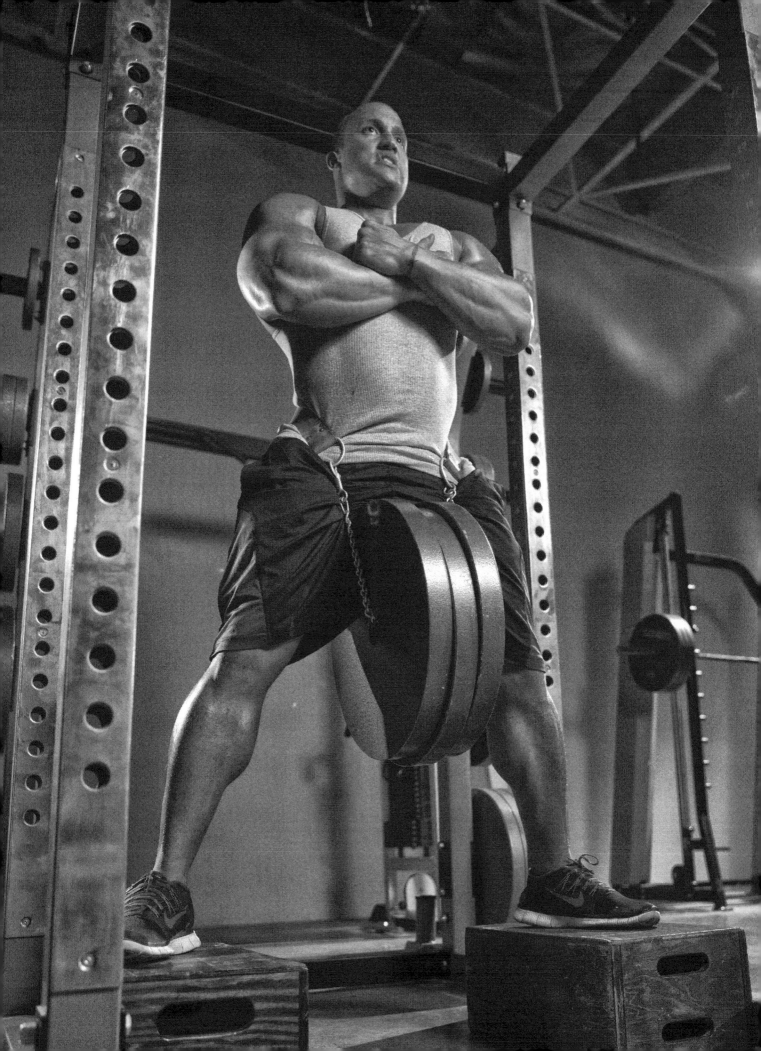

This movement generally should be done for 6–20 reps. This is also a great movement for periods of lower intensity "deloads" because of the lack of spinal compression; and, of course, since the back cannot be used to assist the weight up in a good-morning fashion, less total weight is used but a great overload is still directly applied to the legs.

Performing the belt squat: Preferably place two boxes parallel to one another to accommodate your squat stance; if this is not available, two exercise benches can be placed to perform a v-shaped configuration for you to stand on; however, this is much less safe. Place a solid box between the two boxes you will be standing on; this is where you will place your loading pin with the weight you will use in performing the exercise.

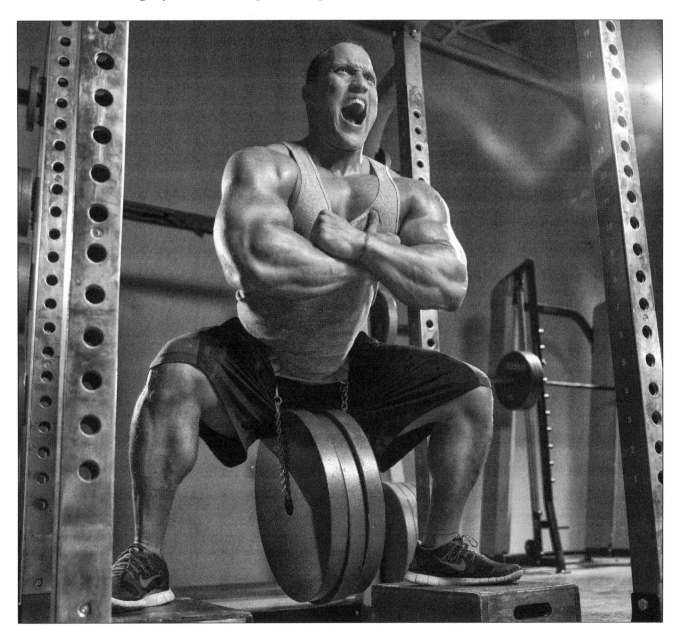

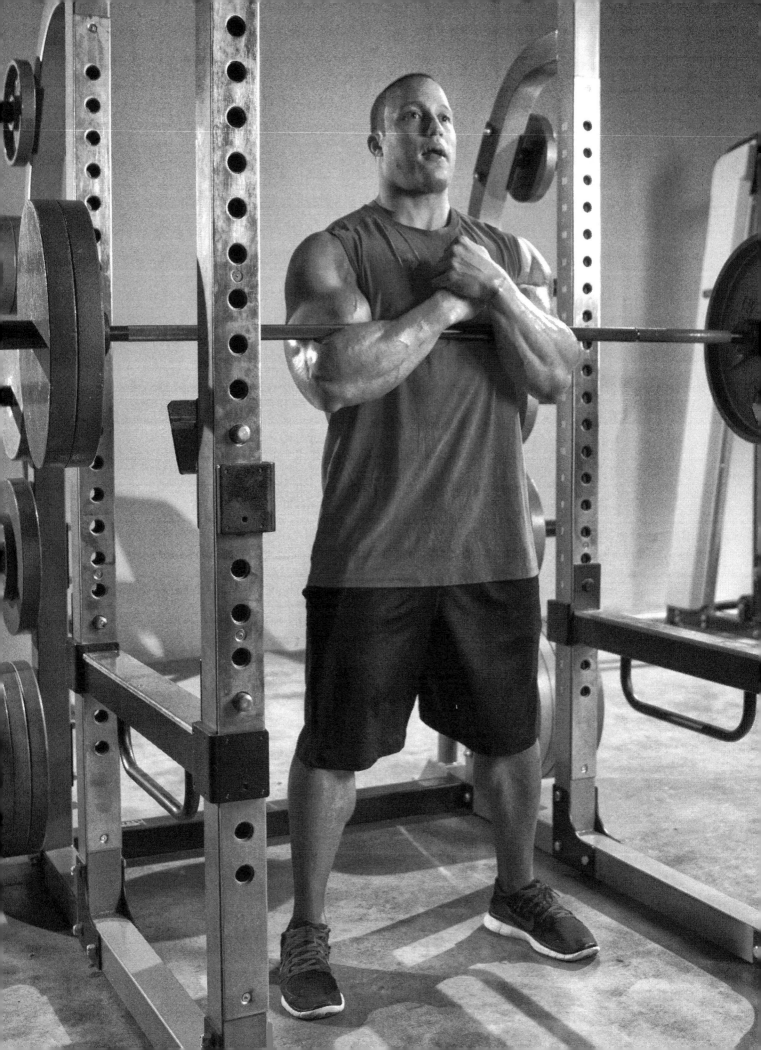

Zercher squats. Zercher squats have showed the most glute work via EMG of any squatting variation, according to Arizona-based strength coach, Bret Contreras.

The Zercher squat was brought to surface by old-time strongman Ed Zercher. This movement is performed simply by placing the bar in the crooks of your elbow. Rack the bar in the squat rack, obviously lower than usual because it is held in the crooks of your elbow.

This exercise is tough and requires a strong core. Because of bar placement, much spinal compression is eliminated. This exercise is unique because of the tremendous glute strength and core strengthening qualities without a large amount of spinal compressive force. You won't see a whole lot of bodybuilders using this exercise, but it can be effectively used to build limit strength and cycled in your training.

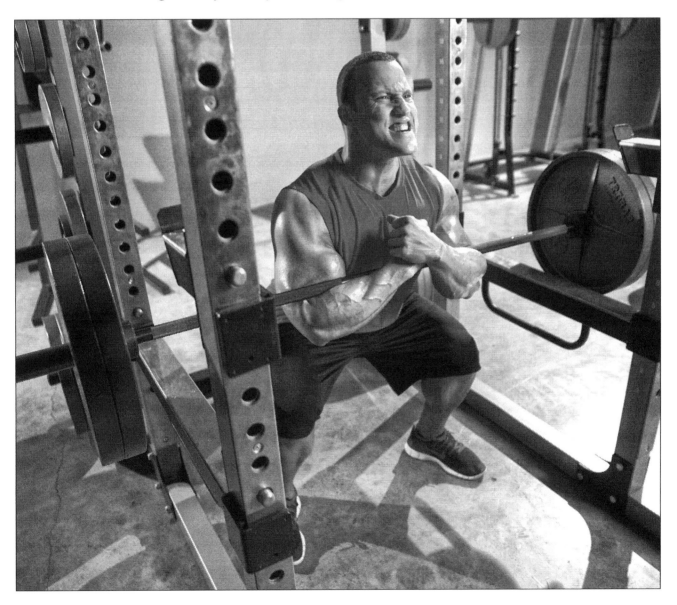

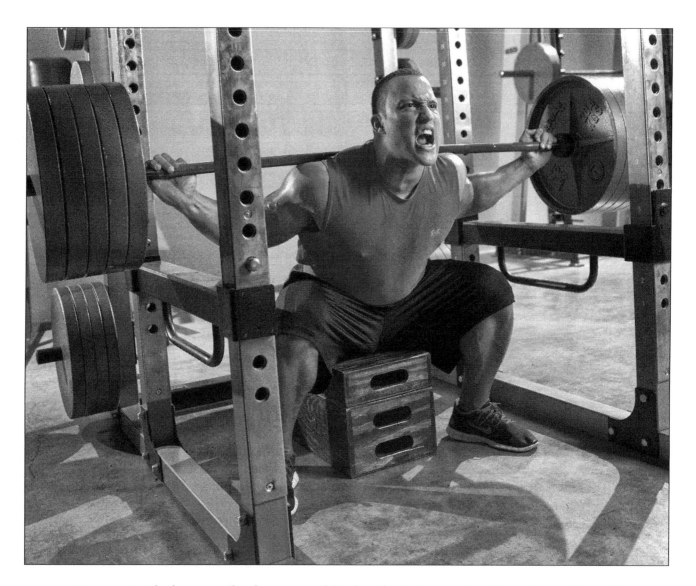

Box squats. The box squat has been around for decades but was not really made popular until the 1990s via the insightful writings of strength coach Louis Simmons (who was heavily influenced by U.S. Olympic Hammer Thrower, the late George Frenn, a world record holder in the squat).

One benefit of box squats is that they require less recuperation time than regular squats. People strive to keep their shins perpendicular to the floor when squatting. Yet box squats allow an athlete to go past this point because it puts the stress on the hips, glutes, lower back, and hamstrings.

These muscles are called the posterior chain. This refers to the backside of an athlete's body. A weak posterior chain is much more common than a weak front side, and box squats are one of the most effective modalities for developing a strong posterior chain.

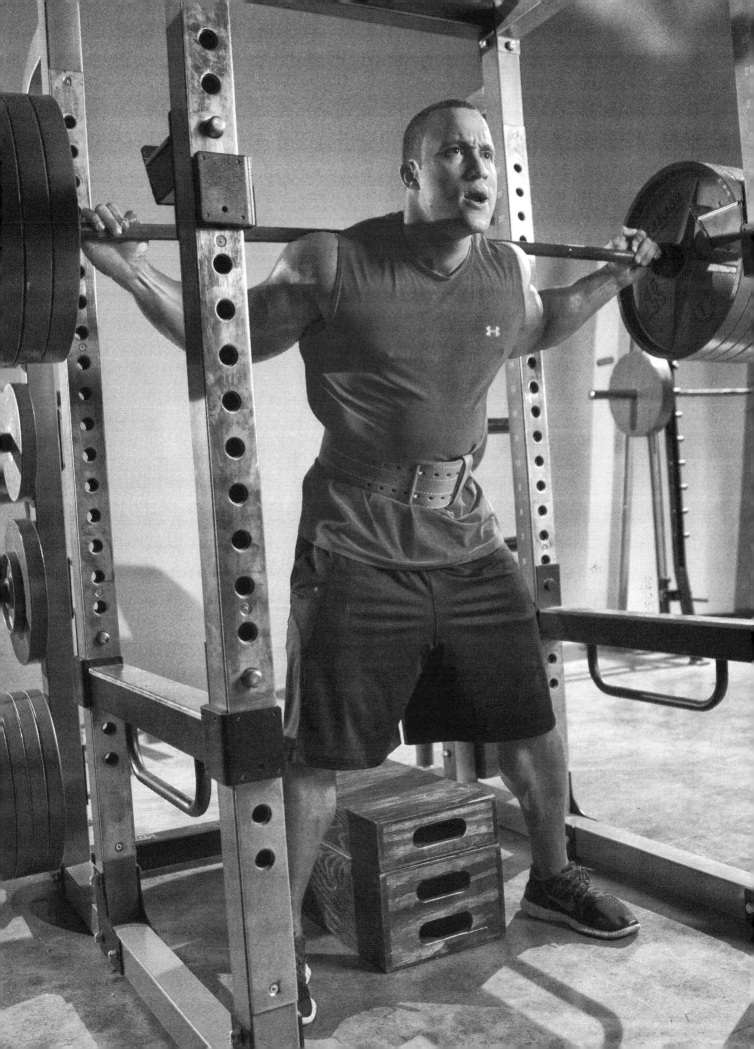

While the bodybuilder may not try to effectively load the posterior chain muscles to aid powerlifting or sport performance, certainly many bodybuilders have weakness in this area from an aesthetic standpoint or from a muscle-weakness standpoint that directly inhibits a movement like the deadlift, which indirectly limits back development.

Generally, we say full range of motion for full development when box squatting depth is not an issue because either your butt was on the box or it wasn't. This eliminates unnecessary guesswork.

Box squats are performed in a similar fashion as regular squats. Some key points to remember:

- Fill your abdomen with air as you push your stomach out (or you could say "abdominals out").

- Push your knees out to the side and push your butt back (do not concentrate on sitting down but sitting back).

- Keep the back arched as you sit your butt completely on the box and pause, then come up.

- When sitting on the box, every muscle is kept tight (excluding the hip flexors). When the athlete releases, then contracts the hip flexors along with arching the upper back, the athlete will explode off the box, building great starting strength.

- Additionally, box squats teach the athlete to explode up using the hips, hams, and glutes. This is very important for any sport that requires explosive movements. This may not be your core lower body movement when prepping for a show, but it certainly can help bring up weaknesses in the off season or just periodically be cycled in your training plan.

Squats and Overall Development

Squats are the king when it comes to building muscle!

Remember, people with larger amounts of muscle mass have higher metabolic rates. The more muscle one has, the more calories one burns, even at rest.

Award-winning ISSA Certified Personal Trainer, George Baselice, added this on the subject of fat loss as it relates to squat:

> The squat challenges your cardiovascular system to an extent unequaled by any other weight training exercise. The reason being the hypoxia effect, in which oxygen intake or use is temporarily inadequate. This breathless state is a tremendous metabolic stimulator. Squats will build an armor-clad heart and lungs, like a high-performance engine.

In addition, numerous studies show lifting weights with the hypoxia effect increases the secretion of anabolic hormones along with sparking a hypertrophic response from training.

Build a base—it's time to start squatting!

Squatting Myths Dispelled

"Squats will give you a broad butt." First of all, my practical observation is that many folks squat without getting big butts. Wide, intermediate, or narrow, it doesn't really make that much difference.

When the hypertrophy of the gluteus maximus takes place, the glutes grow back, not out. The origin and insertion of the muscle is not at the hips. Again, think practically: Most guys who are lean and squat massive poundages have butts that go back, not out! There is no anecdotal or peer-reviewed information that suggests squatting widens the hips. This is a favorite of pure "bro science" practitioners; unfortunately, it is just a self-serving prophecy that eliminates a difficult movement.

"Squats are bad for the knees." Think of the SAID Principle (Specific Adaptations to Imposed Demands): Calluses build up on the hands when you routinely pick up heavily knurled pig iron.

The same concept applies to ligaments, tendons, and other connective tissues that thicken in response to the stress imposed upon the joints during weight training. Also, strengthening the muscles that move the knee joint improves its stability (a plethora of journal published peer-review studies confirm this), and there's some evidence that even the portion of the bone into which the tendons insert becomes stronger, further improving the joint's integrity.

This all goes out the window if you relax the muscles while in a rock-bottom position; that's just asking for trouble because the relaxed muscles allow the knee joint to separate slightly, placing the ligaments and cartilage under stress that may exceed their tensile strength.

While proper stress produces adaptation, overly stressful exercise can cause breakdown of bodily tissue. We are talking about full squats here; full squats allow the muscles of the posterior chain to aid in naturally stopping the movement and reversing the muscular action.

I am confident to say someone who has no preexisting conditions and does full squats with proper technique will have healthy, more stable knees.

"Smith Machine squat variations and leg presses are safer than free squats." Whether it's a Smith Machine squat or leg press, regardless of the design, the apparatus has a preset motor pattern determined by the manufacturer. This motor pattern may not be ideal for your individual body type. It is built for the average person, and odds are you are not "average"

and there may be no real adjustment for body structure. Very few people would fall into what the manufacturer considers an average person.

Consequently, you may condition postural and movement dysfunctions as well as lead the way to overuse injuries because of the fixed, restricted joint movement pattern. Studies have shown Smith Machines place over 40% more sheer forces on the knees than proportionate loads in the free squat.

The leg press has been shown to make athletes more prone to lower back problems, because at the bottom position they are very deep into flexion. The knees get close to the chest, and many times the back is raised off the pad. This is actually more common than you think, and instead of the leg press saving your spine, it leaves the spine very susceptible to large compressive forces. Because the leg press is built to optimize leverage and there is no stabilization involved, much more weight is used than with a squat, making the compressive forces in this unnatural position with heavier weights potentially much more dangerous.

World-renowned personal trainer Brian Dobson, owner of Metroflex Gym, says, "My daughter can leg press 800 pounds, yet she struggles to squat 115."

How is this possible? The answer is simple. The leg press requires no balance, as the lower back and hips are not stabilized by the core of the body.

This brings us to the point that when a machine eliminates the stability factor, the legs are able to lift poundage much greater than when trunk stability is a factor. Henceforth, the forces transmitted on leg muscles and joints are much greater than the body could naturally transmit during the free squat. This potentially puts the hips, lower back, and knees at much greater chance of injury because of the artificially heavy loads you are forced to handle for maximum muscle stimulation.

"Squats are bad for the heart." Many weight-training exercises restrict blood flow because of prolonged muscular contraction. The result is elevated blood pressure. The condition isn't dangerous, and it's temporary.

The heart, like every other muscle in the body, responds to stress by adapting to it. In time, the cardiovascular system is strengthened through weight training. This, of course, excludes those with preexisting heart conditions like extreme hypertension. For example, people suffering from coronary disease will find heavy squats more taxing than beneficial. If you are healthy, squatting can help you build a stronger, healthier heart.

"Squats are bad for the back." Dr. Robert Wolff, in his iconic book, *Bodybuilding 201,* points out research has shown that squats—often criticized on the basis they're "bad" for your back—could actually be doing your spine some good. In many modern health clubs, the popularity of exercise machines has left the squat rack relegated to a dark, dusty corner

in the back of the gym. However, this recent trial shows that squats (and other related exercises, such as the deadlift) could be the best way to maintain the strength of your spine as you get older.

A study published in the *International Journal of Sports Medicine* examined the back of the man holding the current world record for the squat. Despite being able to squat over 1,000 pounds, several scans revealed a remarkably healthy spine.

MRI scans revealed normal spinal alignment. There was no evidence of disc herniation.

In addition, there was no sign of compressive disc disease. More important, the scans also showed an extremely high level of "bone strength" (called bone mineral density) in the spine.

This is important, especially for women. According to some estimates, one out of every three women over the age of 65 will suffer a fracture of the spine. A reduced bone mineral density—which increases your risk of a fracture—is far more widespread than previously thought. Recent surveys show that almost 4 out of 10 women aged 50 or over have osteopenia, which is a mild bone mineral loss.

When calcium in your diet runs short, the body drains the calcium stored in your bones. This weakens them significantly. Some bones, especially those in the spine, can become so weak that just the weight of your body causes them to suddenly disintegrate, often into scattered fragments that can't be reassembled. Your spine can also become "compressed" during old age, forming what is often called "dowager's hump." This is the posture assumed by many older women as they appear to get shorter.

One last tip: When squatting with a heavy weight, make sure to avoid the popular recommendation to keep your back flat. According to Dr. Mel Siff, in his book *Facts and Fallacies of Fitness,* a flat back is "virtually impossible" for most normal people to achieve:

Keeping the back "flat" is common advice in the gymnasium training environment, yet its validity is rarely questioned. Actually, not only is a flat back devoid of any curvature virtually impossible for a normal person to achieve, but it also reduces the ability of the spine to absorb or distribute shock and stress effectively.

Although numerous factors affect the strength of your bones, training with heavy weights is one of the best ways to ensure you're still leading an active life right into old age.

Final Thoughts on Squatting

I think this poem by Dale Clark sums it up well:

Way down this road in a gym far away
A young man was once heard to say
"I've repped high, and I've repped low
No matter what I do my legs won't grow."

He tried leg extensions, leg curls, leg presses too
Trying to cheat these sissy workouts he'd do.
From the corner of the gym where the big men train
Through a cloud of chalk and the midst of pain

Where the big iron rides high and threatens lives
Where the noise is made with big forty-fives
A deep voice bellowed as he wrapped his knees
A very big man with legs like trees

Laughing as he snatched another plate from the stack
Chalking his hands and his monstrous back
Said "Boy stop lying and don't say you've forgotten.
Trouble with you is you ain't been squattin."

THE OVERHEAD PRESS

"Only military presses provide the compound distribution of stresses necessary for over-all shoulder width and thickness," Ronnie Coleman said in the May 2004 edition of *Flex* magazine.

The overhead press is performed by an athlete's resting the bar on the shoulders in the front; legs are locked and his back is straight. From the resting, or rack position, the bar is lifted until the elbows are fully extended over the head, with the head all the way through.

A common mistake is to not fully lock the weight out and push the weight in front you; by doing this, you completely rob the posterior portion of your shoulder, not to mention the peak contraction at the top of the movement.

While the overhead press is primarily a shoulder movement, it forces the entire body to work in concert. The athlete's legs and core stabilize the weight, while the shoulders and triceps press the weight up.

A good coaching cue is to remind the athlete to "squeeze your glutes." This will force the athlete to stay upright and not excessively lean back; this is the reason the movement has been dropped from competition; it is difficult to judge what is a legitimate overhead press and at what point it becomes a standing bench press. As bodybuilders, we try to safely maximize the growth of the shoulders; why it is important to stay upright is obvious.

For the most part, the overhead press works the entire shoulder, unlike the bench press, which works mostly the anterior deltoid. Specifically, overhead pressing allows free movement of the scapula, whereas in the bench press the scapula is retracted. Because of how the shoulder is worked in this lift, the overhead press can eliminate muscle imbalance issues and enhance overall shoulder health. When selecting exercises, it is important we think of not only potential muscle gains but also overall balance and health of the body.

The overhead press does have some variations. Two of the more popular ones are seated overhead press with a barbell, which has been a staple in the regimen of both Ronnie Coleman and Branch Warren; and seated overhead press with a dumbbell and the standing dumbbell press, which is performed like the standing press except that dumbbells are used.

Dumbbell military presses, seated or standing, offer some advantages. Dumbbells allow for each limb to move independently and are harder to stabilize than barbells.

Dumbbells allow the joints to follow their natural/desired movement pattern. The dumbbell military press can be performed seated or standing. By performing the dumbbell press unilaterally with one arm held in extension and the other dynamically pressing the weight, time under tension can be greatly increased without a major sacrifice in intensity.

Another unilateral variation is standing and pressing the weight unilaterally with one arm while bracing on a squat rack with the other; this will hit the muscle at a different angle and allow a greater range of motion to be achieved. This is also an effective way to overload the deltoids with "cheat" reps because of the relative simplicity of the movement compared to the bilateral push press. Plenty of variations of this old-time favorite can be used to build massive bowling-ball delts and increase physical prowess.

The majority of the most muscular and strongest men of all time have included the overhead press in their arsenal. If you do not have limiting pre-existing conditions, it would be wise to follow suit.

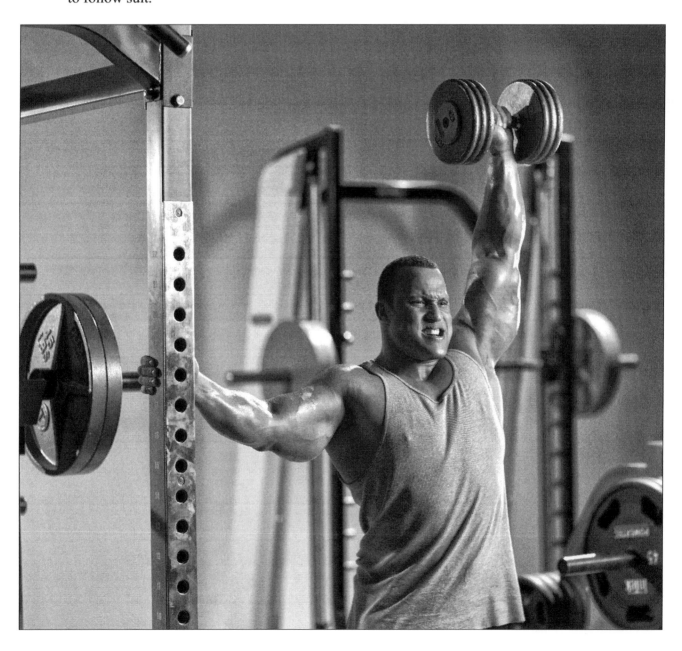

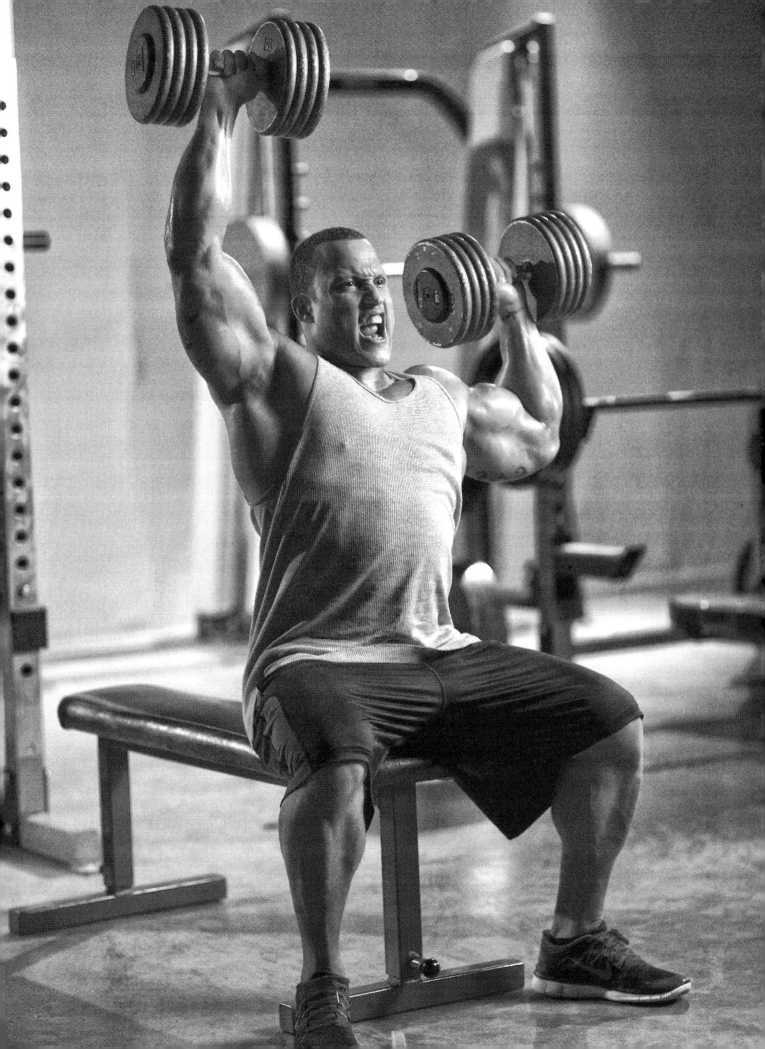

CHIN-UPS

Former World's Strongest Man winner and world record holder in powerlifting, Bill Kazmaier, once said, "A strong back equals a strong man." I will take that a step further and say a well-developed back equals a well-developed man.

Brian Dobson, ISSA Master Trainer, bodybuilding guru, owner and founder of Metroflex Gym, my dear friend and former training partner, and the man who introduced Ronnie Coleman to bodybuilding, has espoused on numerous occasions, "Chin-ups and deadlifts are the king when it comes to building the back."

Let's take a look at the first half of that equation and look at why this amazing exercise is being classified as a core lift.

Chin-ups will require you to lift your own bodyweight and, as you advance, additional weight should be used. Making this a closed-kinetic-chain exercise is generally more effective for adding muscle mass and building functional strength.

Chin-ups are very hard for many people, especially heavier people. Many folks new to strength training will not be able to perform even a single chin-up. With dependency on anabolics and shortcut training methods, unfortunately, many heavier bodybuilders will struggle to squeeze out even a few chin-ups.

That's a big mistake.

I keep saying chin-up, and many will wonder: Is there a difference between a chin-up and a pull-up? The answer is, yes. Pull-ups are harder than chin-ups. Pull-ups require your grip to be pronated (meaning you have an overhand grip with palms facing away from you). Both can play a vital role in your pursuit of physique and power.

When performing chin-ups, your grip is supinated (meaning it is underhand and your palms are facing you). Pull-ups focus more on the back muscles alone, while chin-ups hit the back and the biceps as well.

A large number of bodybuilders and gym rats alike whose biceps have reached behemoth proportions favor cheat curls over strict isolations and machines for biceps growth. This may be contrary to what you read in the health fitness section of your local newspaper.

Look no further than Arnold Schwarzenegger, the pioneer who broke the mold and implemented cheat curls in his training. Most of his peers felt he was crazy! Since then, whether it be Bill Kazmaier or Ronnie Coleman, cheat curls have played a role in helping to develop the biggest, strongest arms of all time.

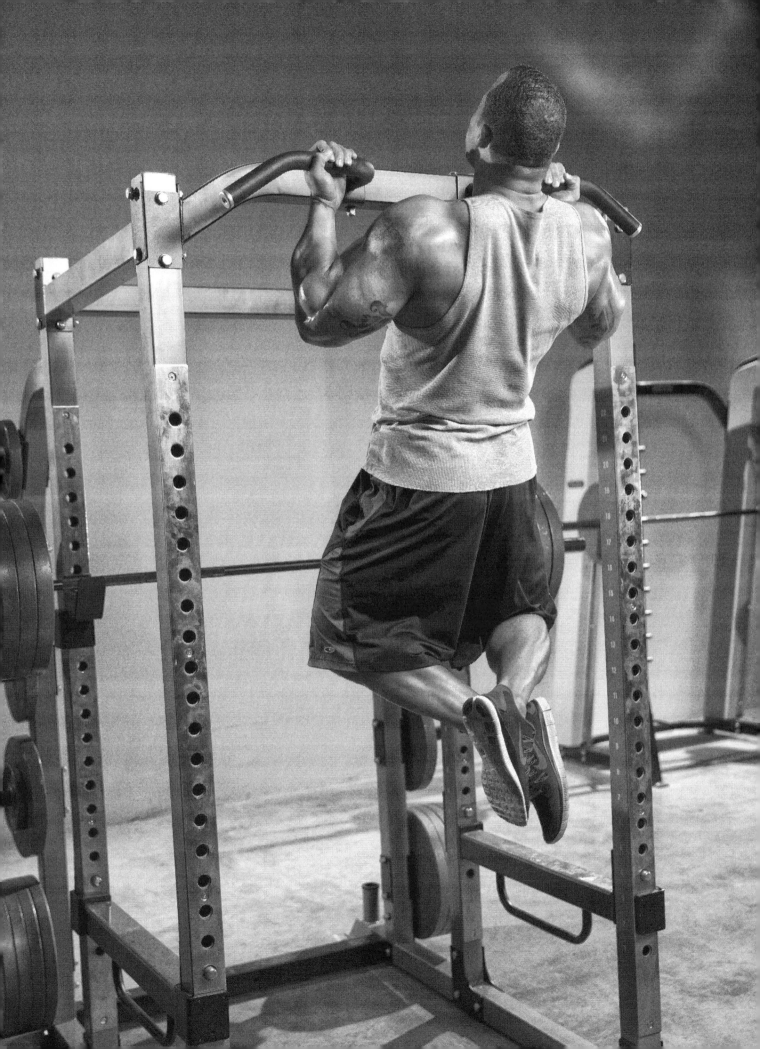

This is not taking a bizarre twist, though, as chin-ups and cheat curls have some similarities that are a catalyst for biceps growth.

While performing a chin-up, the back will assist you and the biceps are in flexion at the end of the movement. This provides a huge biceps overload at the top portion of the movement, like a heavy cheat curl.

Arnold was mocked because of his implementation of the cheat curl; however, one generation's heretic is another generation's hero. This discovery has helped many build huge biceps and is even considered an illustrious Weider Principle.

Is the cheat curl effective? *Absolutely.*

Is it dangerous? Well, it certainly can be.

Unlike the cheat curl, the chin-up is one of the safest ways to build your biceps. Think about it logically. Since we know compound movements build big muscles, increase inter-muscular coordination and intra-muscular coordination, and release the anabolic hormones, chin-ups will make your biceps grow.

Closed-kinetic-chain exercises are superior to open-kinetic-chain exercises for a few different reasons.

A closed-kinetic-chain movement essentially means during the exercise you move through gravity; an open-kinetic-chain exercise means the object you are lifting moves.

Think about a bench press and a push-up: During the push-up you move; during the bench press the bar moves.

Let's apply this to the cheat curl and the chin-up: During the cheat curl the bar moves; during the chin-up you move.

Closed-kinetic-chain movements are much safer on your body because they allow the individual's body structure to determine the movement pattern of the joints and the range of motion they operate. This in turn removes excessive stress off the joints and places it on the muscles, which should be doing the work, and then they have no choice but to grow.

On the Internet, some functional training extremists like to pontificate that to maximize biceps development, all you need to do is chin-ups. I believe this is false, but they certainly can aid in the quest for massive, muscular arms.

These are the two basic variations, but there are plenty of others.

Neutral-grip chin-ups are performed with a medium grip, but variations can be with hands wider or narrower. The shoulder is able to stabilize your body most effectively with a neutral

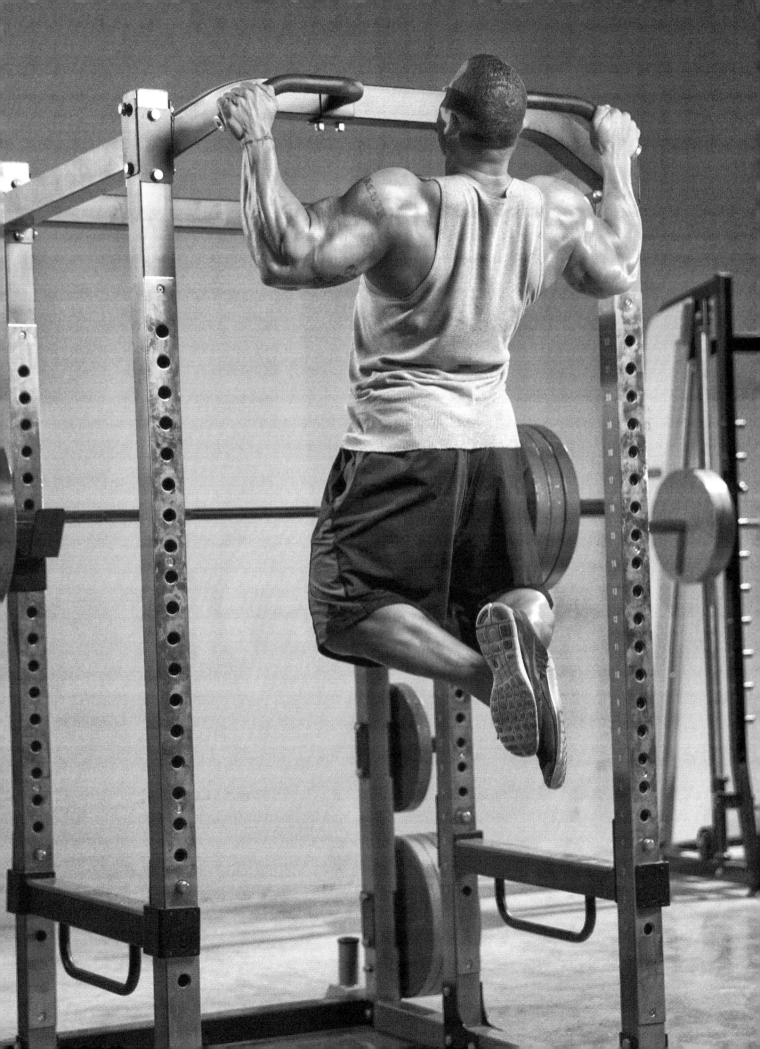

grip. This grip puts the elbows and shoulders in their most effective line of pull. This is the easiest chin-up variation, so additional loads can be used more quickly. The biceps are used much more with this grip than with traditional chin-ups.

Not only do chin-ups increase your limit strength, but they also take your grip strength to a whole new level. Your fingers, your hands and your forearms are all used when performing chin-ups. Since you have to stabilize your core in a chin-up, even the abdominals get a workout.

If you cannot do chin-ups, the most effective way to train them is through band-assisted chin-ups. Simply attach the jump stretch bands to the chin-up bar. Then, attach the band to your weight belt. Start from a dead hang and pull up. As you pull up, the bands will start to assist you.

Negatives can help an athlete become more efficient at handling his bodyweight. These are done by having the athlete perform only the negative (eccentric portion) of the pull. These are also a great way to extend sets past failure: When you can no longer perform the positive portion of the rep, you can jump above the bar and slowly lower yourself through the negative portion of the rep.

To do this, the athlete jumps up, then lowers his bodyweight with no assistance for a specified amount of time. Partner-assisted chin-ups are another helpful modality in enabling an athlete to develop the strength to do a chin-up. These are done like a normal chin-up, but with partner assistance.

As an athlete advances, he can do the negative without assistance. The only drawback to partner assisted chin-ups is the lack of quantitative data on the concentric (upward) phase of the movement. It is impossible to know with accuracy how much a partner is helping. This can be troublesome in planning/tracking workouts.

Lat pull-downs are not as effective a means to develop the strength to do a chin-up. Chin-ups require you to stabilize your bodyweight. Lat pull-downs are done on a machine. Since we are focusing on limit strength, we know that free movements, particularly closed-kinetic-chain ones, are superior to machine-regulated ones.

Lat pull-downs are an open-kinetic-chain movement. On the other hand, chin-ups are a closed-kinetic-chain movement; the latter are generally superior for muscle building, strength, and functionality.

Additionally, when performing lat pull-downs, the concentric portion of the lift is downward from the arms extended to the chest; this is the opposite of a deadlift, bench press, military press, or squat. Any self-respecting gym rat wants to be strong in the aforementioned core movements; chin-ups offer superior transference to them.

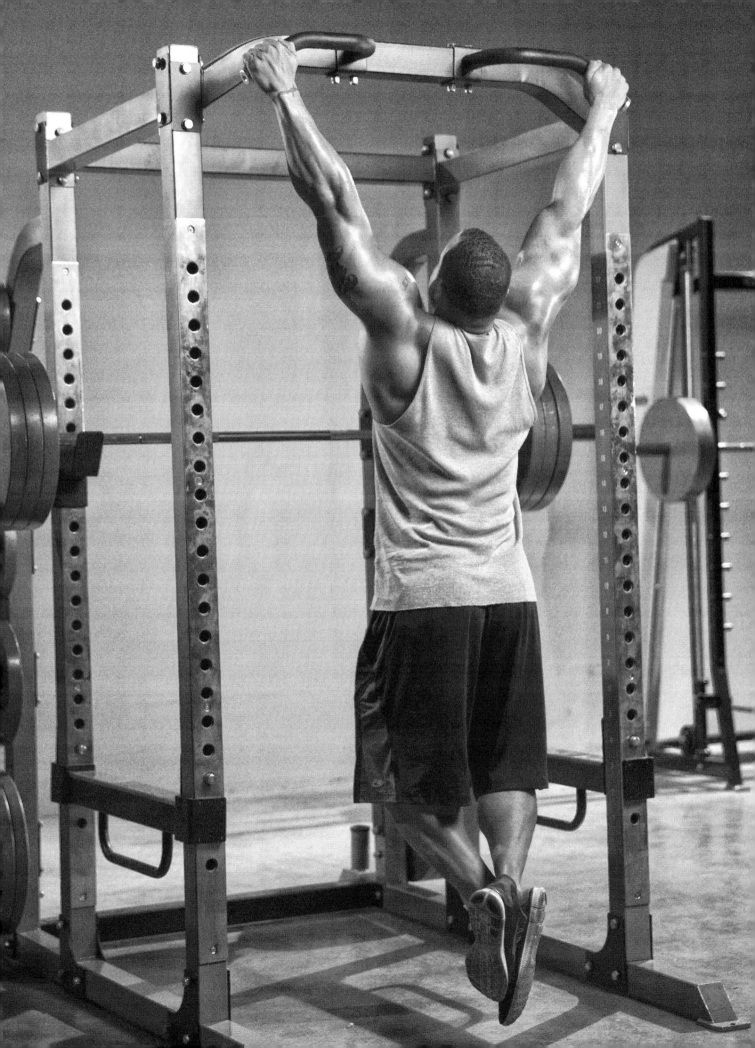

Some points to ponder when doing a chin-up:

- Always use a full range of motion.
- Look up on the way up.
- Bend your legs and cross your feet, effectively squeezing your glutes.
- Keep your chest up.
- Drive up with your elbows facing the floor.

THE BENCH PRESS

I have a soft spot in my heart for the bench press. I was the youngest person to bench press 600 pounds raw and currently train the two top bench pressers in the world, Jeremy Hoornstra and Al Davis.

Here are some tips that have helped my clients and me develop big bench presses:

1. *Practice compensatory acceleration training (CAT).* CAT is lifting your submaximal weight with maximal force. By building explosive power in the bench press, you blast through sticking points. Lifting the weight with the intention of being explosive will make the weight feel lighter. Need proof? Walk over to the dumbbell rack, pick up a 50-pound dumbbell quickly, and then lift it slowly. The weight will feel lighter when picked up quickly. You can't intentionally lift a maximal weight slowly.

2. *Implement dead benches into your routine.* A dead bench is done in a power rack. The weight starts at chest level and is pressed up as explosively as possible. You will not be able to lift as much weight this way because of the absence of elastic-like energy stored on the negative portion of the lift. Because this lift is concentric (upward phase) only, you build tremendous starting strength. Bench pressing big weight begins with great starting strength off the chest. Build it with dead benches!

3. *Do more sets with fewer reps when training for a one-rep max.* Let's look at two scenarios: In Workout A, you do 8 sets of 3 reps; in Workout B, you do 3 sets of 8 reps. In both workouts, you completed 24 repetitions; however, in Workout A, you had 8 first reps, whereas, in Workout B, you had only 3 first reps. Since you are training for a one-rep max, first reps are important.

4. *Work your arms.* Very few men with spaghetti arms bench huge weights. Obviously, the triceps are crucial to lock the weight out and can be built through close-grip bench, board presses, various extensions, and a plethora of

other exercises. However, the biceps help stabilize heavy weights, and strong forearms help you squeeze the bar tight. This will make the weight feel lighter in your hand. The old adage, "Curls are for girls," is not true when it comes to the bench press.

5. ***Visualize your success.*** Your central nervous system cannot tell the difference between a real and an imagined experience. Set some time aside every day to visualize yourself blasting maximal weights. Go to the gym, load your goal weight on the bar, and stare at it; see yourself lifting it. The more vivid the experience, the more real it is. When you eventually attempt the weight, you will only be going through the motions, because you have done it over and over in your head.

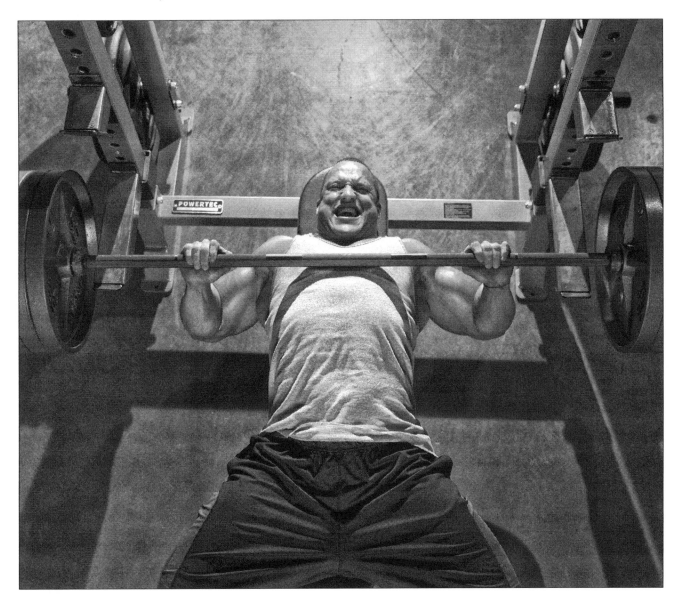

Former powerlifting world champion and renowned trainer, Rickey Dale Crain, once said, "The bench press is the best basic upper body lift, and that is, it works more muscle groups than any other upper body lifts."

The bench press has been hailed by some as the holy grail of lifting, and other chest movements mocked as a complete waste of time. Arnold Schwarzenegger, Doug Young, Ronnie Coleman, and Bill Kazmaier all had the bench press at the core of their chest routine.

In recent times, there has been sort of an anti-bench-press renaissance among strength and conditioning professionals. Usually, this ruckus is initiated by a "strength" coach who lacks an impressive physical stature or a practical weight training background and is looking more for an ego-defense mechanism.

Because of insecurities, these folks are scared of the movement, so they avoid it and want everyone else to follow suit. These guys need to check their egos at the door. Their responsibility is to get clients results, not protect their egos and hide behind a premise of "functionality." The bench press is the king when it comes to adding slabs of meat to the upper body.

Remember, the bench press allows for the heaviest weight of any exercises to be handled, and it is a true strength builder. The bench press is a compound, multi-joint exercise that can be beneficial to most bodybuilders.

Some things to remember when bench pressing:

- Your grip width for a regular bench press grip should be slightly wider than shoulder width.
- You can bench with your thumb wrapped or not wrapped around the bar. If you choose to not wrap it around the bar, use excellent form to make sure the bar doesn't move away from your grip during the movement.
- The bar should be close to your wrist and palms, in your hands, not by the fingers (this would be a recipe for severe wrist pain).
- When gripping the bar, the athlete should make sure to squeeze the bar.
- Tighten your upper back before you lift the weight out of the rack. This gives you a solid base from which to perform the press. If you do not keep your chest up, you enhance your chance of shoulder injury and lose power. You also lose the benefit of the peak contraction at the top of the movement.
- You must maintain this chest position through the entirety of the lift.
- Use a full range of motion for the majority of your training. The pectorals are the prime movers for the bottom portion of the movement; and by missing the peak contraction at the lockout of the movement, you rob yourself of full chest development.

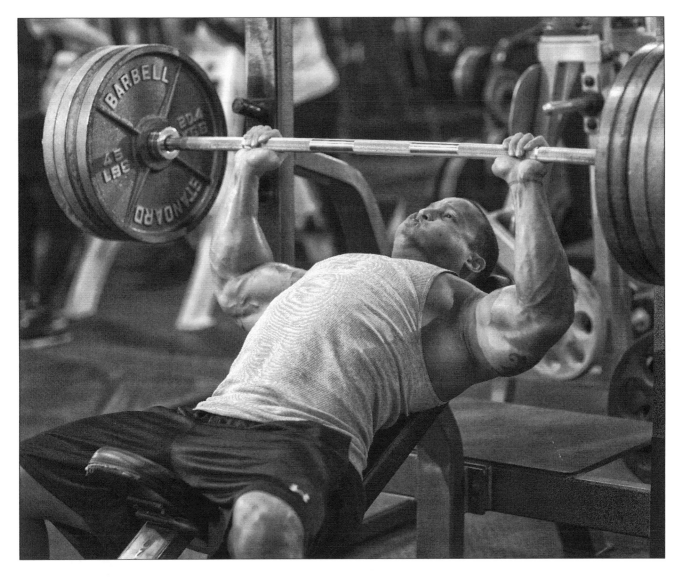

Bench Press Variations for the Bodybuilder

Two of the more popular variations of the bench press are these:

The incline bench press. This movement is used by bodybuilders to maximize the development of the upper (clavicular) portion of the chest. This is not just "bro science," as EMG studies have actually shown that the upper pectorals have higher electrical activity than on a barbell bench press.

Generally, the most effective angle is 15 degrees all the way up to 40–45 degrees; below this, the emphasis will shift more toward the lower portion of the chest, and above this the work will move more to the anterior deltoids. Dumbbells can be used for this movement as well. This is a very effective movement for building limit strength and, of course, developing a massive chest.

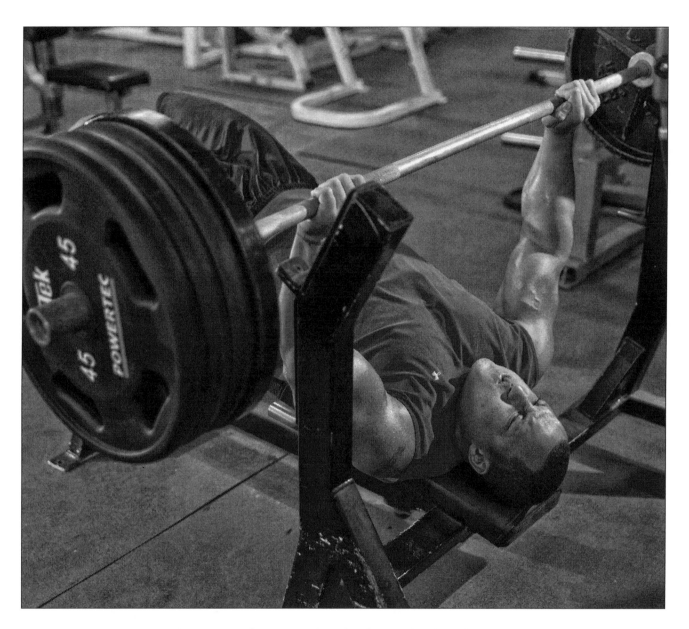

The decline bench press. Declines are a favorite for overloading the lower (sternal) portion of the chest. Like the incline or the flat bench, dumbbells can be used. Declines seem to be most effective at an angle of 20–25 degrees. Going below this angle will bring the lats too much into play, and above this the movement will start to engage the clavicular portion of the chest more than desired. Many bodybuilders will be able to lift more weight on this movement than even a flat bench press, providing an amazing overload.

Remember that the pectoral muscles perform two primary functions: flexion and adduction of your upper arm. Both of these happen during the upward phase of a decline bench. This is why six-time Mr. Olympia, Dorian Yates, feels the decline bench is superior bodybuilding for chest development.

Final Thoughts on the Bench Press

Plenty of other bench press variations are very effective. Look at some of the ones that powerlifters, our brothers in iron, use: neutral grip bench press, close grip bench presses, wide grip bench press, floor presses, and board presses. These are just the tip of the iceberg.

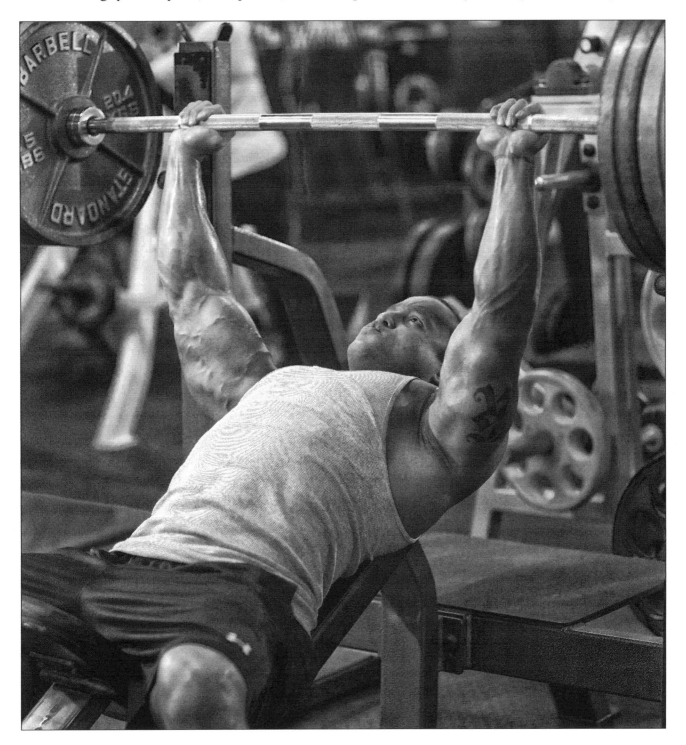

THE DEADLIFT

It is safe to assume the deadlift is the oldest strength-training maneuver in existence. There's no real documentation to back this up, but it makes perfect sense when you think about it. Bench presses and squats took ingenuity on the part of our iron-game predecessors. But there is nothing more primordial than picking up an object and putting it down. Deadlift training, technique, and programming have been refined, but the main objective remains the same: You pick up heavy pig iron, you put it down, and you grow.

Ronnie Coleman has the largest back of all time; big enough for eight Mr. Olympia titles. It is important to pay attention to how he built it. Brian Dobson, MFS, and Coleman's longtime trainer, attributes Big Ron's massive back to one factor that's remained constant in his training programs through the years: "Deadlifts," says Dobson, "are the king."

Deadlifting forces you to use virtually every muscle in your body to take the bar from the floor to waist height. In the chain of muscles involved in this process, nothing is left behind, and everything kicks in eventually.

"Everything" starts with your lower back.

Nothing builds your spinal erectors like the repetitive action of bearing and moving a massive load. The deadlift isn't just a lower-back exercise, though. As you move through your range of motion and transition from the lower part of the lift to the upper lockout phase, your lats, traps, and other upper-back muscles take over.

At the top of the movement, you're holding a very heavy weight in a dead-hang position—which places immense pressure on your traps. This is a highly efficient combination of movements for building thickness in your upper back and shoulders.

In the bottom position, proper deadlift technique entails pushing through your heels to move the bar out of a static position. By focusing on this leg drive, you're applying a tremendous amount of force to your quads, hamstrings, and calves. Dropping your butt and pushing through your heels with every rep will add mass throughout your lower body.

At the top of the deadlift, when you lock out your hips, your glutes act as the movement's agonist—its prime mover—while your hamstrings are targeted as the synergists, or assisters. When it comes to developing your glutes and hamstrings through the application of force, there's no better exercise than the deadlift. While this is not our primary focus as a bodybuilder, it's a great byproduct.

The benefits aren't limited to your lower body.

Your arms come into play throughout your range of motion. When you're trying to both hang onto a heavy load and move it upward, all the muscles in your arms are forced to

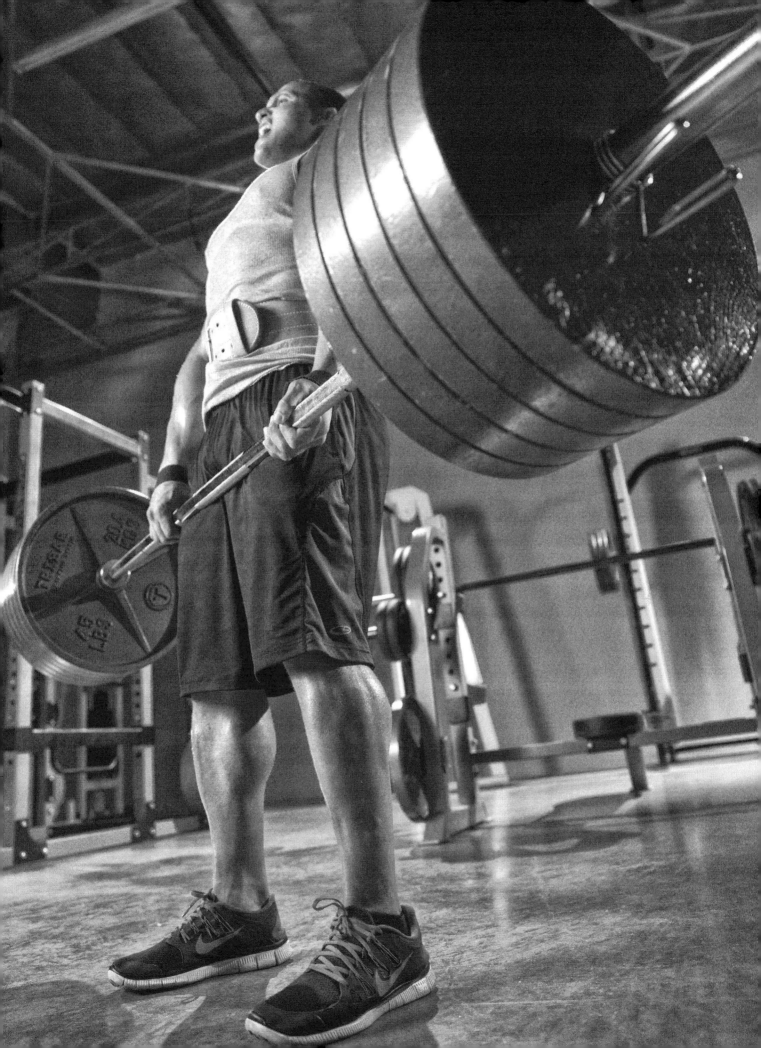

contract, and enormous amounts of grip strength are required to hold onto a heavy deadlift without straps; this is a catalyst for forearm hypertrophy.

If grip is the limiting factor on the deadlift, wear straps. After all, we are using deadlifts to add mass and build the back, not for grip strength and forearm development.

Furthermore, straps will allow you to perform deadlifts without a mixed grip (meaning one hand is pronated and one supinated); a pronated grip can be used.

The advantage to this is a more efficient lockout because the hips are in a more efficient biomechanical position to lock the weight out. It also eliminates the possibility of asymmetrical development. The concentration can be on the muscles being worked and exercise technique, but, most importantly, the chance of a biceps tear is drastically reduced. Biceps tears are one of the most common serious injuries developed from the deadlift.

Some reminders for proper deadlift technique:

- Push through your heels.
- The middle of the foot should be directly under the bar; the shins must be touching the bar.
- The back is in extension; don't round.
- The shoulder blades should be directly over the bar.
- The elbows must remain in full extension throughout the entirety of the movement.
- Lower the bar in the opposite way the bar was lifted, in terms of hip and knee angles.

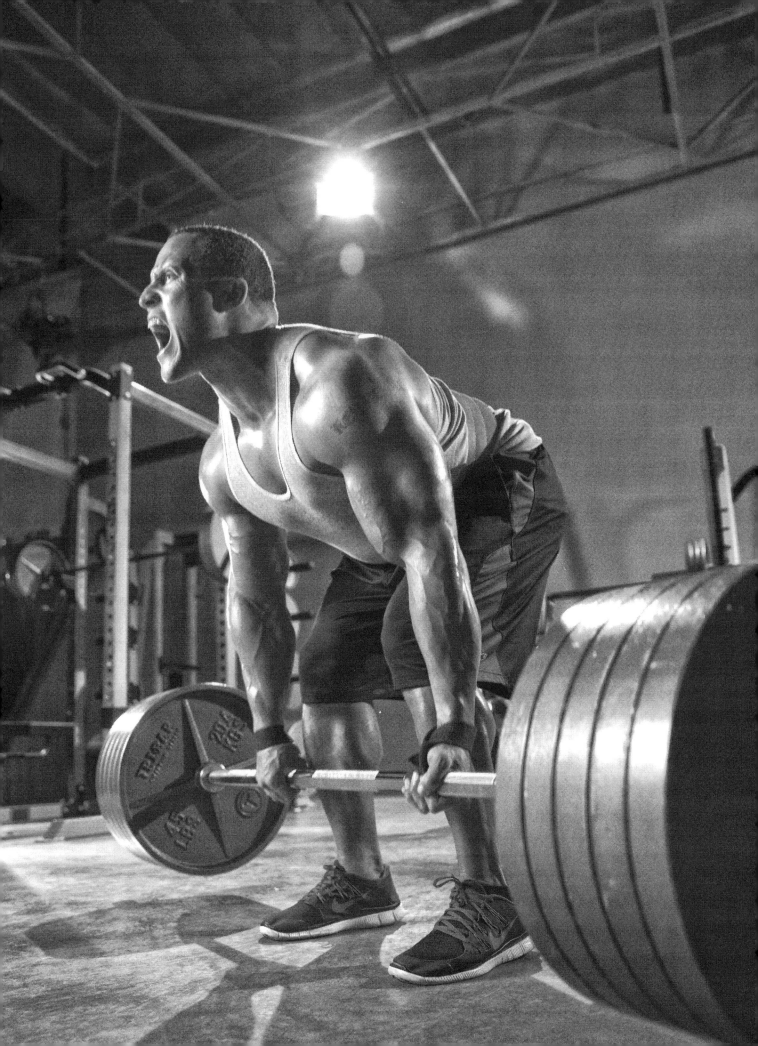

Partial Deadlifts

Partial deadlifts can be performed in a power rack or off of boxes. If you have access to boxes, this is a more effective variation because the flex of the bar is more similar to a traditional deadlift, as the plates rest on boxes like they do on the floor. This provides a similar feeling of bar flex at the commencement of the movement.

In a rack, the bar rests on the pins, so the feeling is much different at the start. Additionally, you can lift more weight in a partial deadlift off of a box. Generally, perform partial deadlifts at knee level and as much as 2–3 inches below and as high as 2–3 inches above.

Sometimes a partial deadlift will hit a sticking point, so even though you are lifting the weight less distance, you will not be able to handle as much weight as a full-range-of-motion deadlift.

This is important, even for the bodybuilder, because a glaring weakness will stall overall progress. If you are going for the overload effect, obviously you will need to do the partial deadlift from a point where you have strong leverage.

Wear straps for this movement; grip training is not our primary purpose. Perform the lift by taking a hip- to shoulder-width stance. Bend your knees slightly, keep your back flat, and make sure your lower back is tightly arched. With arms in full extension throughout the entire movement, extend your hips and stand upright. Accentuate the lockout and hold this position for 1–2 seconds at the top to maximize muscular development.

Partial deadlifts allow us to attack weaknesses and provide a huge overload; hoisting massive weights equals massive development. This movement, in my opinion, is one of the most underrated for upper back development and helpful in building your limit-strength base.

Final Thoughts on the Deadlift

The deadlift is the ultimate back builder, but deadlifts also work virtually every muscle in your body. Because of the amount of motor units recruited, deadlifting (like squatting) is a catalyst for muscle growth.

Like the squat, the deadlift produces a very favorable spike in the natural production of growth hormone and testosterone production. If your goal is to lose fat, your post-oxygen debt will be larger because of all of the muscle mass recruited (meaning your metabolic rate is greatly increased). Therefore, whether you are cutting or bulking, the deadlift can be a great aid in your arsenal.

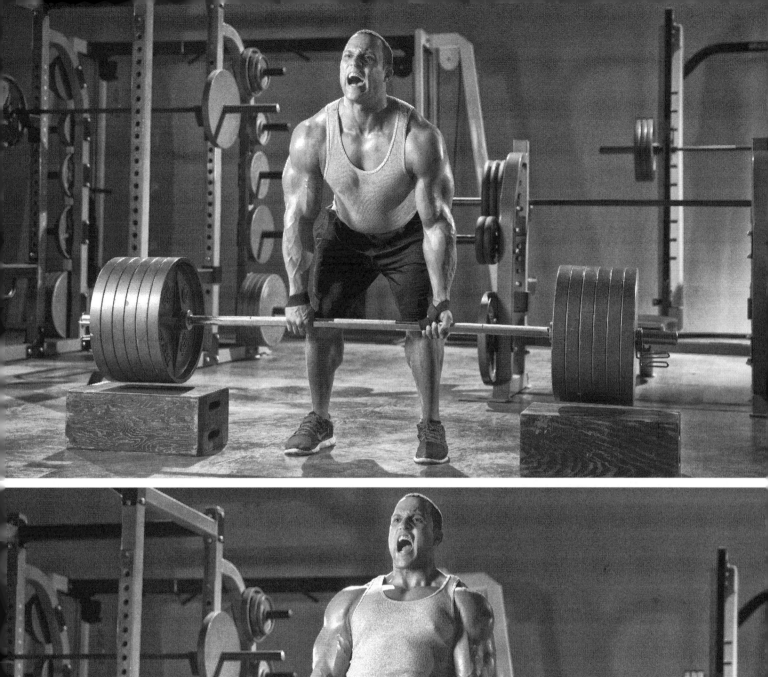
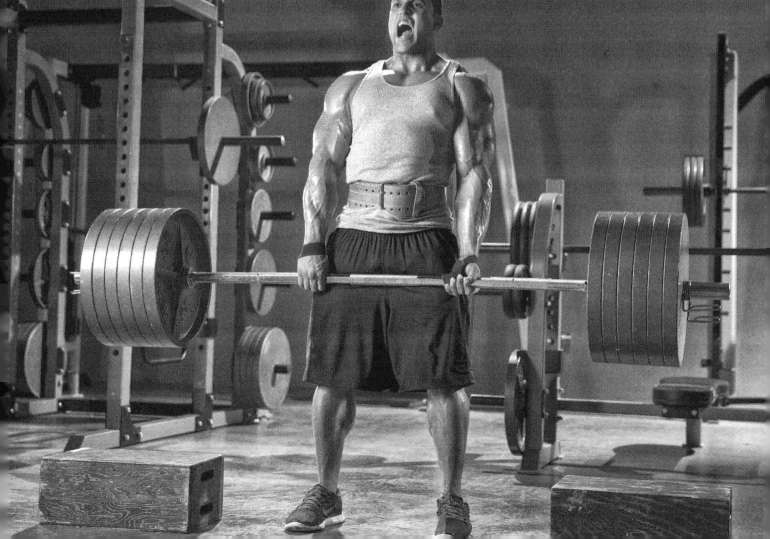

BAR DIPS

Bar dips are called by many the upper body squat. The reason is the massive amount of muscle they can pack on the upper body. Once an athlete is able to master his body weight on this exercise, it is not time to ditch because the intensity is too low—it's time to add weight. This can be done simply with a weighted dip belt that can cost as little as $20.

Weighted dips were a staple muscle-building and strength-training movement before modern machines and gimmicks. Many top-level physique athletes swear by this movement for building the sternal (lower) portion of the pecs.

Here are some good reasons to include weighted dips in your training program:

- When performing dips with a more upright posture, the stress is more on the triceps.

- Dips with a forward lean and the chin tucked toward the chest while getting a good, deep stretch make this arguably the best chest builder on the planet.

- Weighted dips force you to handle your bodyweight plus an additional load. This means it is a closed-kinetic-chain movement, which is generally safer and more effective.

- Weighted dips force you to use your upper body and core to stabilize the load; unlike push-ups, your feet are not on the ground.

- Do a Google search on weighted dips for muscle hypertrophy. Many of the results will refer to this exercise as the "king" for the chest and the triceps. How many exercises can claim this kind of monopoly on two different muscle groups?

- Dips build strength in functional activities and in strength tests. Pat Casey, the first man to bench press 600 pounds, had weighted dips at the core of his program. Want to bench big? Try dips! Not to mention they help the overhead press. Dips helped me win the overhead press with ease at the Atlantis Strongest Man in America Contest.

- Athletes with shoulder or elbow injuries may find dips to be a good substitute for bench pressing.

- Dips have been the staple of many great physique athletes. I have personally witnessed Branch Warren and Ronnie Coleman do dips on many occasions.

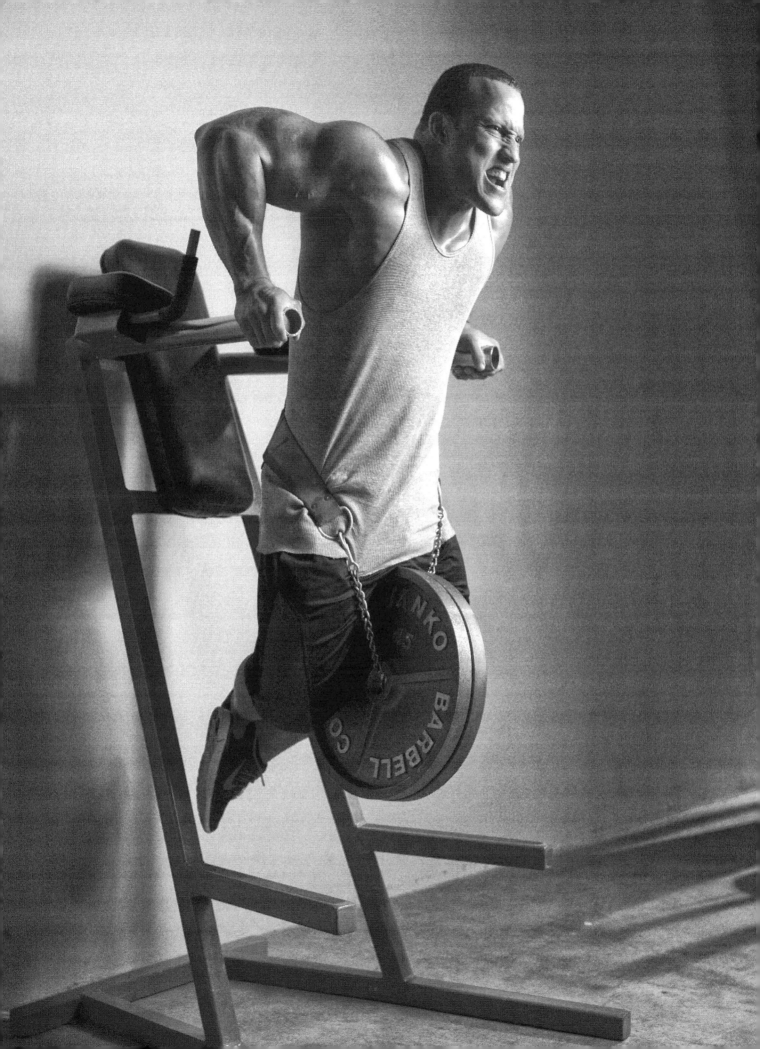

HORMONAL RESPONSE TO HEAVY CORE LIFTS

The more muscle fibers that are used during an exercise, the greater the hormonal and remodeling response will be. Only the muscle fibers that are used during the resistance training are subject to adaptation.

To increase the concentration of serum testosterone, remember these principles:

- Use heavy weights (greater than 85% of one-rep max)

- Use moderate to high volume, meaning multiple exercises or multiple sets and short rest intervals.

- Increase growth hormone levels by performing higher repetitions (in the 10-rep range) and using short rest periods between sets.

- Optimization of the response of adrenal hormones to resistance training is done by using high volume, large muscle groups, and very brief rest periods.

- Optimizing your hormonal response to exercise will keep you anabolic and increase your strength, and that's the goal of the powerbuilder.

A FEW LAST WORDS

Heavy core lifts may prevent injuries because they stimulate new bone growth, so follow these guidelines when trying to stimulate bone growth:

- 3–6 sets with less than 10 repetitions.

- Rest period 1–4 minutes using a typical periodization scheme designed to increase muscle hypertrophy and strength.

- The exercises should be compound movements. (All of the previous exercises discussed would fall into this category.)

The body will adapt differently to various weight training programs. If the goal is an increase in muscle size (hypertrophy), a moderate load is called for (65%–80% of your one-repetition max), rest periods should be short (approximately 60–90 seconds), and repetitions should be in the 6–15 range. The optimal number of reps for muscle hypertrophy will vary with the individual.

Other factors (besides genetics, nutrition, and supplementation) that influence hypertrophic response to resistance training are time under tension, amount of weights used, range of motion and, of course, exercise selection.

If your goal is strength, you will need to use more than 85% of your one-rep max, repetitions will be 5 or less, and a full recovery of 2–5 minutes will be taken.

If you are a bodybuilder, your goal is to build strength, size, and symmetry. Remember that exercise selection, rest intervals, and rep ranges will cover a wide spectrum.

Building size and strength takes time, so be patient. The gains will come. It is done best with core lifts as the foundation of your training program.

If I had to choose between core lift training and single-joint isolation lift training, the choice would be simple. The core lifts are the way to go.

Look at all of the great bodybuilders who started as powerlifters: Ronnie Coleman, Arnold Schwarzenegger, Franco Columbo, Branch Warren, Johnnie Jackson, Ben White—and the list goes on. All of them have or had dense, grainy, shredded muscle. This was accomplished because of their limit-strength base.

Even if you decide to become chemically enhanced, it is important to build a great drug-free base. The reasons are simple: You will be able to maintain your gains much better after you cease the use of anabolics; and these lifts develop tendons and ligament, something steroids cannot do.

Heredity may have dealt you the cards, but training plays the hand.

You cannot shoot a cannon out of canoe… you need a base, so build it!

SOURCES

Andrews, J. G., J. G. Hay, and C. L. Vaughan. "Knee Shear Forces During a Squat Exercise Using a Barbell and a Weight Machine." *Biomechanics VIII*, ed. B. Hideji Matsui and Kando Kobayashi, 923–27. Champaign, IL: Human Kinetics, 1983.

Baechle, Thomas R., and Roger W. Earle (Eds.). *Essentials of Strength Training and Conditioning,* 2nd ed. Champaign, IL: National Strength & Conditioning Association, 2000.

Bryant, Josh. "Bridge the Gap: Sprint-Resisted Training." *EliteFTS* (30 July 2009). http://articles.elitefts.com/training-articles/sports-training/bridge-the-gap-sprint-resisted-training/.

Bryant, Josh. "5 Front Squat Advantages." *Elite FTS* (13 August 2010). http://articles.elitefts.com/training-articles/5-front-squat-advantages/.

Bryant, Josh. "Squats: Superior to Leg Presses for Muscle Hypertrophy and Athletic Prowess." *SB Coaches College* (21 May 2010). http://www.sbcoachescollege.com/?s=squats%3A+superior+to+leg+presses.

Cantor, Myles. "The Ten Unique Benefits of Deadlifting." Posted excerpt of interview with Eric Cressey. *Mark Fu's Barbarian Blog* (30 August 2007). www.mkonen.com/bblog/people/the-ten-unique-benefits-of-deadlifting/.

Coleman, Ronnie. "Title in Title Case." *Flex* 22, no. 3 (May 2004): 354.

Dickerman, R. D., R. Pertusi, and G. H. Smith. "The Upper Range of Lumbar Spine Bone Mineral Density? An Examination of the Current World Record Holder in the Squat Lift." *International Journal of Sports Medicine* 21, (2002): 469–70.

Glass, S. C., and T. Armstrong. "Electromyographical Activity of the Pectoralis Muscle During Incline and Decline Bench Presses." *Journal of Strength & Conditioning Research* 11, no. 3 (1997): 163–67.

Hatfield, Frederick C. "I May Not Know Diddley… But I Know Squat!" *Dr. Squat* (n.d.). http://drsquat.com/content/knowledge-base/i-may-not-know-diddley-i-know-squat.

Hodge, Glenn. *Comparison of Muscle Fiber Activation During the Front Squat and Back Squat Exercises.* www.uta.edu. (Stand-alone web article.)

Life Chiropractic College West. http://www.lifewest.edu/courses/syllabi/uppercrossedsyndrome.pdf. (Stand-alone web article.)

McBride, J. M., D. Blow, T. J. Kirby, T. L. Haines, A. M. Dayne, and N. T. Triplett. "Relationship Between Maximal Squat Strength and Five, Ten, and Forty Yard Sprint Times." *Journal of Strength & Conditioning Research* 23, no. 6 (2009): 1633–36.

Mehdi. "How to Do Pull-ups and Chin-ups with Proper Technique." *Stronglifts.com* (1 October 2007). http://stronglifts.com/how-to-do-pull-ups-and-chin-ups-with-proper-technique/.

Morris, S. "Top Nine 'Get Faster for Football' Exercises." *EliteFTS* (10 February 2011). http://articles.elitefts.com/training-articles/top-nine-get-faster-for-football-exercises/.

Poliquin, Charles. "What Is a Strong Front Squat?" *Poliquin Live* (26 April 2011). http://www.charlespoliquin.com/Blog/tabid/130/EntryId/360/What-is-a-strong-front-squat.aspx.

Santorno, Nicole. "Front Squat or Back Squat: Which Is Better?" *The Journal of Physical Education, Recreation & Dance* 81, no. 2 (2010): 9.

Siff, Mel C. *Supertraining.* Denver: Supertraining Institute, 2003.

Simmons, Louie. "Box Squatting." *Powerlifting USA,* (1998, March–April). http://www.westside-barbell.com/westside-articles/PDF.Files/05PDF/BOX%20SQUATTING%20BENEFITS.pdf.

Tate, Dave. "Squatting from Head to Toe." *EliteFTS* (1 January 2006). http://www.elitefts.com.

Weis, Dennis. "Hip Belt Squats The Anabolic Equalizer." *T Nation* (date). 4 Sept. 2010. http://www.t-nation.com.

Wolff, Robert. *Bodybuilding 201: Everything You Need to Know to Take your Body to the Next Level*. Chicago: Contemporary Books, 2004.

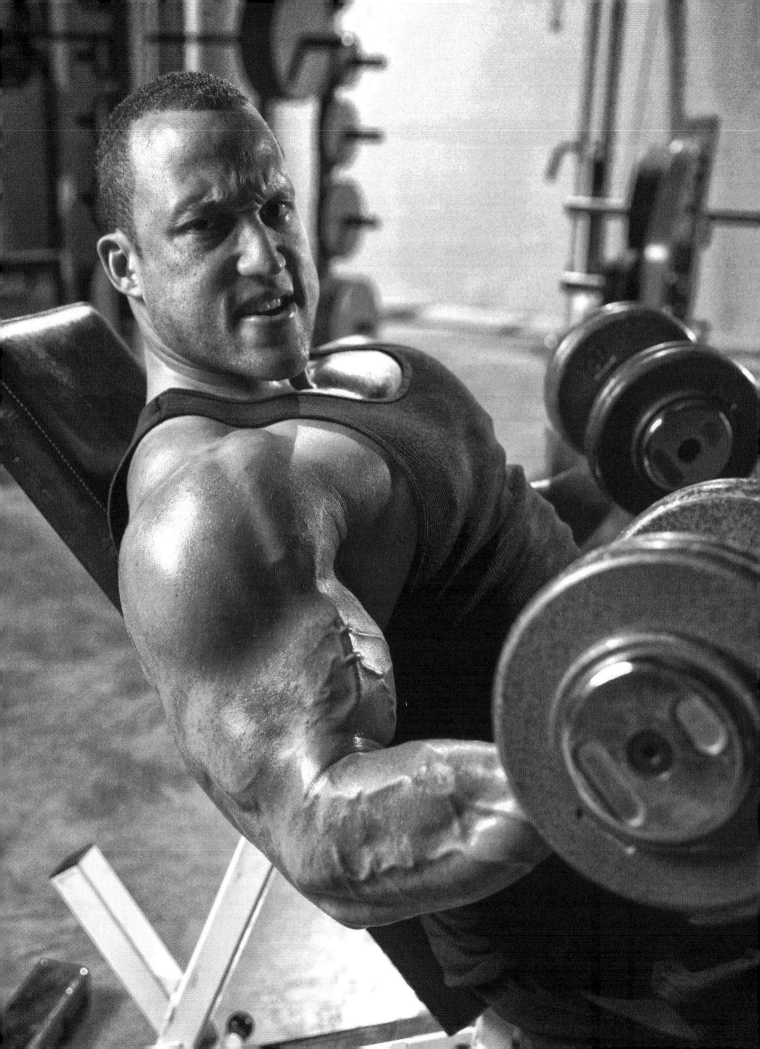

CHAPTER 4.

Periodization

INTRODUCTION

"Periodization is the latest and greatest '12 weeks to mass' training system!"

Not quite.

Periodization.

Nothing fancy. It simply refers to how one's training is broken down into discrete time periods called macrocycles, mesocycles, and microcycles. Periodization is purpose-driven training. It is essentially systematically cycling volume, methods, and intensity toward one's goals.

A BRIEF HISTORY OF PERIODIZATION

The concept of breaking training down into discrete periods of focus is not a new concept and is not solely a practice of athletes.

Siff and Verkhoshansky in their 1996 book, *Supertraining,* noted that ancient civilizations, such as the Chinese, Greeks, and Romans, understood the need for proper physical preparation for warfare. They realized that you simply couldn't give a soldier his weapon and start to teach fighting techniques. The first thing they needed was to be whipped into shape.

This same concept applies to your physique. Before you can really focus on developing individual muscles with single-joint movements, you need to build your limit-strength base.

As for athletic training, the ancient Greek Olympians spent time in preparatory training for up to 10 months during each year, even in non-Olympic years.

In a textbook written during the Russian revolution, Kotov (1917) advised that training should be divided into general, preparatory, and specific training stages. Several Russian texts were written after this, emphasizing such training in track and field, skiing, gymnastics, boxing, water polo, and swimming.

Think about great bodybuilders of the past who focused on strength and size in the off season, then fat loss and symmetry as a contest approached.

By cyclically attacking these goals and changing training methods and modalities as objectives were sequentially accomplished, this was periodization in action. Just think about it logically. Would a bodybuilder train the same way for a show four weeks out as he would four months out?

TYPES OF PERIODIZATION

Linear periodization is also called classic or Western periodization. The basic premise of this type of periodization is that the training cycle starts with low intensity and high volume; progressively the intensity increases, and subsequently the volume decreases. As reps decrease, the weight used (intensity) increases in each successive mesocycle generally lasting 3–4 weeks.

For example, Cycle One may consist of 15 reps, Cycle Two 10 reps, Cycle Three 10 reps, Cycle Four 6 reps, and so on. Intensity and volume are cycled linearly. While more effective methods of periodization now exist, there is no denying that this approach, which many now consider antiquated, has produced many champions; in powerlifting, Ed Coan and Bill Kazmaier both used this approach, and many top lifters still use it today.

Reverse Linear Periodization

This is classical periodization in reverse. Maximum intensity and low volume are at the commencement of the training cycle; then, as the training cycle progresses, volume is increased and intensity is reduced. Bodybuilders use this approach many times, increasing reps and decreasing weight as a show approaches. From a foundational point of view, this approach is logical; your limit strength is your foundation, and it is the first thing addressed.

Undulating Periodization

This is basically a non-linear model of periodization. The key is to manipulate training variables often by frequently adjusting loading parameters. This can be done workout by workout, daily, or weekly. Undulating periodization means training volume and overall intensity are increased or decreased constantly. Generally, this model is more effective for the bodybuilder whose main objective is to provide overload to the muscle, with variables constantly changing by default.

Some studies show undulating periodization is significantly more effective than classical periodization, whereas others show the systems to be fairly equal. The problem is, most of these studies are performed on untrained athletes, not bodybuilders.

Flexible Nonlinear Periodization

This is like the undulating training model but allows changes in training based upon the readiness of an athlete, which is based on specific tests done pre-workout. Lots of bodybuilders do a variation, essentially auto regulation; this means when they feel good they increase intensity, and when they do not feel good they decrease it.

Block Periodization

Popularized by Vladimir Issurin, block periodization could be called "focused training." This is where you give one quality in training special emphasis. Using specific exercises that focus on the specific quality you seek, in a conjugate sequence, you maintain your other qualities and then rotate your emphasis and continue maintenance. This is antithetic of what you see at most commercial gyms, where people concurrently train for multiple goals and generally fail miserably.

For the bodybuilder looking to bring up his arms specifically, he would still train the rest of his body but increase frequency of arm workouts from once a week to maybe 3–4 times. For the bodybuilder looking to increase strength, his emphasis might be to decrease reps and increase intensity on core lifts, yet he would not eliminate single-joint movements.

Here are Issurin's own words on block periodization:

> Its general idea proposes the sequencing of specialized training cycles (i.e., blocks, which contain highly concentrated workloads directed to a minimal number of targeted abilities).

> Unlike the traditional model, in which the simultaneous development of many athletic abilities predominates, block-periodized training presupposes the consecutive development of reasonably selected target abilities. The content of block-periodized training is set down in its general principles, a taxonomy of mesocycle blocks, and guidelines for compiling an annual plan.

A study in the June 2012 edition of the *International Journal of Physiology*, titled "Strength Gains: Block Versus Daily Undulating Periodization Weight Training Among Track and Field Athletes," showed greater strength gains over the course of a year when comparing the block method of periodization to what was considered the superior undulating method. This is important because these are trained athletes.

ABC BODYBUILDING PERIODIZATION MODEL

In an excellent article titled "Finding the Ideal Training Split," Fred Hatfield, Ph.D., came up with numerous variables pertaining to recovery for training splits.

Some of these variables included tolerance to pain, level of "psych," and amount of rest between workouts. Hatfield also determined that the "slow gainer" and the "fast gainer" have different recovery periods.

A "slow gainer" typically can complete 15–20 reps at 80% of his one-rep max. A "fast gainer" can complete only 4–6 reps at 80% of his one-rep max. The athlete should perform this "test" on several muscle groups, as each muscle group has a different tolerance to exercise.

Table 4.1, extrapolated from Hatfield's article, will help you determine which type of gainer you are.

Table 4.1. What Type of Gainer Are You?

REPS PERFORMED WITH 80% MAX	STANDARD DEVIATION FROM MEAN	TOLERANCE LEVEL	ABILITY TO MAKE GAINS
4 or less	−3	Very, very low	Fast Gainer (20%–25% of total population)
4–6	−2	Very low	
6–10	−1	Low	
10–13	Mean	Average	Average Gainer (50–60% of total population)
13–17	+1	High	Slow Gainer (20–25% of total population)
17–21	+2	Very high	
21 or more	+3	Very, very high	

Once you have determined the category pertaining to you, the adequate amount of recovery can be determined. Hatfield recommended a different workout with different prescribed levels of intensity: An A workout was a low intensity workout, a B workout was a moderate level of intensity, and a C workout was a high intensity workout. Dividing workouts according to intensity levels allows the right levels of fatigue to be accumulated, which ensures that optimal levels of fitness are developed.

Typically, a slow gainer will need 3–5 days of recovery, depending on which muscle group has been worked. Abdominal, calf, and forearm work will need 3 days of recovery; larger muscle groups, like the legs and lower back, will need 5.

The fast gainer will need 5–7 days of recovery. Rest the abdominals, calves, and forearms 5 days; the lower back and legs will need to be rested 7 days.

A common objection is that many exercises, particularly compounds, work numerous body parts. Look at a bar dip. If you lean forward with your chin tucked to chest, the emphasis shifts to the chest. If you have a more upright posture, the triceps become the prime mover. You can shift emphasis, but you cannot eliminate contributions by assisting muscles, not to mention the major contribution of the anterior deltoids.

Hatfield offers a solution: By dividing your split around the compound movement being performed in the particular training session, you won't have to try to totally isolate one muscle. Hatfield spoke of movement-based programs prior to their becoming popular; he was ahead of his time in this regard.

In a personal communication with Dr. Hatfield, I learned this is the system he used while training eight-time Mr. Olympia, Lee Haney. Regardless of how you train, intensity and volume must be managed to optimize results; thankfully, pioneers like Hatfield took this knowledge from the lab to the gym.

THE NEED FOR PERIODIZATION

"Through scientific research and training practice, periodized training proved to be more effective than non-periodized in trained subjects," concluded Vladimir Ilić and Igor Ranisavljević from the Faculty of Sports and Physical Education, Belgrade, Serbia, in their scientific review published for the University Banja Luka, Faculty of Physical Education & Sports, in November 2010.

But is periodization necessary to look the best on stage?

If so, why?

And why not just train hard all the time and just diet as a show approaches year round?

These are seemingly logical questions, so let's have a look at what noted sports scientists have to say.

> The needs for different phases of training were indicated by physiology since the development and perfection of neuro-muscular and cardio-respiratory functions, to mention just a few, are achieved progressively over a long period of time. One

also has to consider the athlete's physiological and psychological potential, and that athletic shape cannot be maintained throughout the year at a high level.

—Tudor O. Bompa
(*Theory and Methodology of Training,* 1983)

If a bodybuilder tries to stay in contest shape year round, he will inhibit his ability to pack on muscle mass. Because he is seemingly eating a perfect diet year round, it will be nearly impossible to diet down any further for a contest.

REVIEW OF THE SEVEN GRANDDADDY LAWS

The Law of Individual Differences

This law states that not everyone can train in the same manner. It is relevant to periodization when you consider the fact that the athlete's individual differences will change with training. Each person will become an entirely different individual after a year of proper training. Certainly, a beginner will not keep the same physical and psychological characteristics after training—that person will literally become a different individual in that he will be stronger and faster, recover more quickly, and have a different perspective on training than when he began. Everyone reacts differently to certain exercises, amounts of volume, rest periods, rep ranges, cardio prescriptions, etc.

The Laws of Overcompensation and Overload

Simply put, training must progressively increase in intensity over a period of time. Using the same reps, sets, frequency, training loads and methods of training time after time will not result in increases in performance or muscle mass. This applies even to the advanced bodybuilder; usually, if the same bodybuilder does the same workout over and over again yet makes some progress, it is a change in nutritional strategy and enhanced pharmacology.

The SAID Principle and the Law of Specificity

SAID stands for *specific adaptation to imposed demand.* The body will adapt in a highly specific manner to the stress it receives. Simply put, if you want to get big, you have to train and eat big. If you want to be a bodybuilder, train to maximize muscle mass and minimize body fat. If you want to be a jockey, a different strategy is required.

The GAS Principle and the Law of Use/Disuse

GAS stands for *general adaptation syndrome.* Periods of high intensity must be followed by periods of low intensity. If you complete only one hard workout, adaptation for larger muscles may take weeks; too long *not* to train! Therefore, there must be frequent periods of low intensity between periods of high intensity. We like to call this *a deload.* This period of lower intensity generally needs to be less than 70% of total volume and intensity. If you were in a state of overreaching, this deload period can invoke supercompensation and maximum hypertrophy, and strength gains will take place during this time.

FITNESS FATIGUE MODEL

The GAS Principle is a single factor model of training that describes your body's short-term and long-term reactions to stress. This principle is the foundation for periodization. This means if a stress (training stimulus) is great enough, fitness decreases for a time and then "supercompensates" to its original state, then beyond. Fitness and fatigue are variables that determine adaptations to training.

The Fitness Fatigue model is not replacing GAS, it is expanding on it. GAS is a one-factor training model, whereas the Fitness Fatigue is a two-factor model of training. GAS is just too simplistic to explain the effects of training. The Fitness Fatigue model looks at the long-term aftereffect from training stimuli. The aftereffect will cause an increase in specific fitness, such as increased thigh mass from a heavy training cycle of squats. The gain in mass is the fitness component. The fatigue effect is the short-term aftereffect from training stressors; multiple sets of heavy squats will cause fatigue.

Significant delayed onset of muscle soreness (DOMS) is one example of fatigue. Fabled Sprints Coach, the late Charlie Francis, at his seminars used to say that the CNS is like a cup of tea that you must never let overflow. Every stressor, whether it's personal problems, interval training, weight training, or lack of sleep, adds tea (in this case fatigue) to your cup. If the cup of tea (fatigue) does not overflow but is adequately stressed, supercompensation (fitness) takes place.

When it comes to weight training, volume is a product of poundage lifted times repetitions times sets. Take a look at a bodybuilder with a maximum bench press of 400 pounds performing three different workouts on the bench press: If he does 300 pounds x 3 x 8 sets, more neural adaptations will take place; if he does 300 pounds x 8 x 3 sets, more hypertrophic response will be induced; if he does 100 pounds x 24 reps x 3 sets, this will be more like an active recovery response.

A flushing workout can immediately increase fitness, without the onset of fatigue. All three of these set-and-rep schemes will produce a totally different response hormonally and neuromuscular wise, along with inducing fatigue and gaining fitness during supercompensation, yet each workout is 7,200 pounds of total volume.

The GAS Principle looks at total work as the sole variable to influence fitness response from training, where the Fitness Fatigue model expands on this simplistic outlook by taking into account not only total volume but the intensity/magnitude of training stimuli. Remember, squatting 1,000 pounds for a single is different from squatting 100 pounds for 10 reps, even though total volume is the same.

Each individual training variable is independent of the others, but their total summation will equate to total fatigue produced and total specific fitness gained. If too much fatigue is accumulated, over time a snowball effect will take place. Initially, this will be overreaching, which may in fact be your immediate desired result, so fitness gained can take place on a period of deloading; but if this goes beyond overreaching to the point of overtraining, it can take months to recover.

A classic example of this situation is when a bodybuilder is severely overreaching and switches to an extremely low volume program like the Heavy Duty Training System. Initially he will gain size, because supercompensation is taking place by a de facto deload. These gains will not continue with insignificant stimulation, once supercompensation has manifested itself.

Periods of significant fatigue followed by significant recovery produce significant results! Different training methods and stimuli trigger different responses. This is especially true for advanced bodybuilders; beginners are developing a general fitness base and will respond well to most training stimuli.

If you are training for maximal strength, you will not get your best results if you're concurrently attempting to train for maximal endurance capacity. No one has ever run a 5-minute mile and bench-pressed 500 pounds raw! Training needs to be purpose-driven and focused on specific goals so specific fitness and fatigue adaptations don't fight against one another; instead, they concurrently merge for your bodybuilding success.

Before a major contest in track and other sports, athletes taper off training volume to peak at the contest. This idea is the delayed training effect and, in a way, is the whole premise behind the Fitness Fatigue model.

After stressful training, a period of lower volume and less intensity (deload) is required for optimal performance. Remember, the same applies to you, the bodybuilder: To gain the positive fitness effects after a period of stressful overreaching, a deload is called for to eliminate fatigue aftereffects and for you to get the gains you deserve from hard training.

In 1995, in his book, *Science and Practice of Strength Training,* Vladimir Zatsiorsky stated that in a workout of average intensity, the fitness effect endures roughly three times longer than the fatigue effect. That means, if the fatigue aspect from a training session dissipated after 2 days, fitness gains will persist for 6 days.

AVOIDING OVERTRAINING AND OVERREACHING

The problem is not training too much; in fact, athletes can handle much more training than they or their coaches believe is possible. But, simply put, if athletes are "overtrained," they

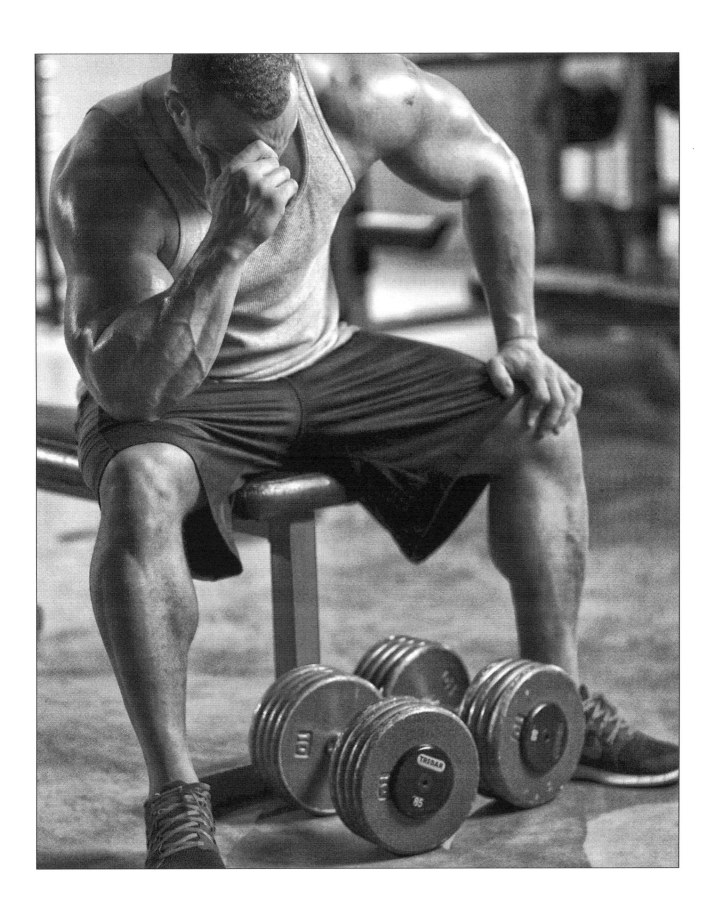

haven't recovered efficiently. In a sense, they haven't "overtrained," they have "under-recovered." Overtraining is serious and can sometimes take months to recover from.

At this point, an adverse hormonal response has taken place, and signs like decreased motivation, sex drive, depression, decreased appetite, and insomnia have already started to manifest themselves, and a large decrease in performance is taking place.

As overreaching is sometimes a desirable state, it is a much shorter and less severe state of overtraining. Many times, you can recover from this in just a few days. Many periodized training programs purposely invoke phases of overreaching to provide variety of the training stimulus and to maximize the supercompensation effect during the periods of less intensity.

Another strategy you can use is to alternate between periods of incomplete recovery (overreaching) and periods of complete recovery. Periods of increased loading are alternated with periods of decreased loading, which enhances recovery and helps to prevent adaptation to training programs.

One mesocycle might be an intense 6-day-a-week split for 3 weeks, followed by a deload week with a reduction of total/volume and intensity to 60%, followed by 3 weeks of a more moderate 4-day-a-week split.

If you train hard all the time, too often you will overtrain. However, periodizing your training (mixing periods of high and low intensity not only on a weekly basis, but overall) will result in your ability to recover and train harder more often—thus, *not* overtraining.

CREATING A PERIODIZED PROGRAM

The importance of a periodized program should be realized by now.

Let's explore how such training can be organized in a logical manner; it isn't as clear cut as it may seem.

There are many factors involved in creating an effective periodized program. They are:

Age- and Experience-Related Factors

Knowing that the Law of Individual Differences does exist, the age and experience level of the particular athlete must be taken into consideration, so remember these points:

- Younger athletes will recover more quickly than older ones.
- Younger athletes are also usually less experienced than older ones.
- Each athlete will change in experience level and recovery ability during training. Over a lifetime of training, the body will decrease in recovery ability,

but during that lifetime, it will also undergo certain training effects that allow for harder and more frequent training.

With these points in mind, younger bodybuilders with less competition experience will need a foundational regimen focused on core strength movements.

As athletes progress and mature, more bodybuilding-specific training will be needed, and the foundational period, while remaining important, can be shortened.

A novice bodybuilder could benefit from two full 12-week powerlifting cycles yearly, focused on gaining strength in core movements and adding size. But this would not be necessary for a Ronnie Coleman or a Jay Cutler in the twilight of his career.

However, this cannot be discounted from the seasoned pros. From 2007 to 2011, Johnnie Jackson's bodybuilding career appeared to be on a downward spiral, but in the fall of 2011, Johnnie did a foundational powerlifting cycle with me and ended up pulling 832 pounds raw in competition—one of the top deadlifts in the world.

Johnnie went on to win the FIBO Pro Show in Europe and place 2nd at the New York Pro. His physique has undergone a major metamorphosis in his return to the basics, and Johnnie is 41 years old! Remember, aging athletes may need more recovery time, and the individual differences may require more of a foundational period of training.

Macrocycles, Mesocycles, and Microcycles

These terms are used to describe the discrete breakdown of training goals and varying intensity levels.

Macrocycles. A macrocycle can be thought of as an entire training period. While it is generally thought of as a year, it is not always the case. For the national-level bodybuilder, this would be like preparation for the USA's in a hope to win a pro card.

The bodybuilder's yearly plan is important because it guides his training over a year. The objective of his preparation is to reach a peak level of performance in a methodical manner for a major show.

The preparatory phase consists primarily of foundational training compound movements but, of course, will include some single-joint movements. This could last as little as 8–12 weeks for the seasoned pro and literally a year plus for the undersized amateur.

Some top pros have taken more than a year after earning their pro card for serious foundational training; it has worked well for perennial Arnold Classic Champion Branch Warren, who at this writing is in contention for Mr. Olympia.

Those in the trenches refer to this as the off season, as during this phase bodybuilders are generally trying to add muscle mass and bring up weak points. Adding an inch to your arms is impossible in a state of reduced caloric intake, as the body is not in a caloric surplus anabolic environment.

The competitive phase of training has the objective of minimizing body fat and maximizing symmetry through nutritional strategies, low-intensity aerobic training and/or high-intensity interval training (HIIT), supplementation of fat burning agents, and a greater emphasis on single-joint movements without completely eliminating foundational movements.

The transitional phase of training is used primarily for biological regeneration via psychological rest and physical relaxation and biological regeneration, and it can be used to maintain general physical preparation. This phase generally lasts about a month, in some cases more. Ronnie Coleman was known to stretch this phase up to 4 months; while this was excessive, it certainly gave him the rest he needed to heal up and attack the iron with ferocity.

Mesocycles. A mesocycle is a periodical breakdown in a macrocycle. While the overall focus in a mesocycle is changed, it should be noted that mesocycles "blend" together. Foundational training does not end in the foundational period, nor does bodybuilding-specific training begin in the contest-prep phase. One quality may be more heavily emphasized over another in training, but the other is not eliminated from training.

A practical example would be a foundational period, in which compound movements would be a majority of the emphasis of weight-training movements; as the competitive phase approaches, specific single-joint movements may be an increased priority, but this does not mean eliminating compound movements—that is, if you want to be your best. An example of a mesocycle would be a 12-week prep for a show. This mesocycle could be composed of 3–4 microcyles lasting 3–4 weeks each.

Microcycles. A microcycle is described as one cycle in intensity. Recall that periods of high intensity must be followed by periods of low intensity before another period of high intensity can occur. For certain muscles, this could take as little as 5 days and as much as 3 weeks! Ken Lain, champion bench presser from the 1990s, said it took him 3 weeks to recover from a heavy bench press. (Granted, we are talking over 700 pounds.) While a microcycle is often thought of as "one week," this is not always the case. It can be as small as one workout.

Intensity Variables

Using the same reps, sets, frequency, training loads, and methods of training, time after time, will not help you get stronger or become more muscular; your muscles simply adapt, so you are no longer overloading them.

You should not have a "routine" if the identical method of training is used year in and year out. Regardless of where you are in your macrocycle, you will not continually make gains except with improved nutritional strategies and a heavy dose of pharmaceuticals.

What's the answer?

Besides switching the focus of training, intensity must be increased. If you do not progressively overload your training, you will not make gains. Increasing intensity is more complex than just piling more weight on the bar, although that is an effective way.

All intensity variables can be quantitatively tracked; this is why it is important to keep a training journal. Take a look at some effective ways to increase intensity:

1. Increasing training poundages. Increasing the amount of weight you use in a given exercise workout is the most obvious way to increase intensity. Heavy Metal superstar Henry Rollins, when writing about his passion for lifting weights, said, "Two hundred pounds is always 200 pounds, the iron never lies."

While simplistic, this is a concept many seem not to grasp. Since this is true, 210 pounds is 10 pounds more than 200 pounds; if you previously had used 200 pounds for your heaviest bench press set, now you have used 210 pounds and you have effectively overloaded your system in a way that can be tracked quantitatively.

Use more weight than you are accustomed to, and your body gets an overload. That why those who care only about how much they lift, yet routinely add more weight to the bar, assuming their form is not compromised, continually add muscle and get stronger.

This is the oldest, tried-and-true way to increase intensity, although it may be dismissed by many modern day gurus. It worked for Ronnie Coleman, the greatest bodybuilder of all time, and also one of the strongest men of all time.

A piece of advice here.

Look beyond 25s and 45s.

Many bodybuilders add weight to the bar using only 25- and 45-pound plates, and this is a mistake. For someone of the advanced strength level, a jump of 50 pounds (a 25-pound plate on each side of the bar) can take years. So incremental jumps must be small; even adding one-pound plates, you have still made gains.

If your gym also has 2.5-pound plates, 5-pound plates, and 10-pound plates, use them!

Charles Poliquin has stated that *a 10-pound gain in a major core lift generally equates to a 1-pound lean-tissue gain.*

If this doesn't convey to the bodybuilder the importance of getting stronger, nothing will.

2. Increasing total volume. Volume is weight times repetitions times sets. While this obviously increases intensity, the key is to increase volume within a given time frame. Performing 5 sets of 5 reps in the squat with 300 pounds, the total volume is 5 x 5 x 300 = 7,500 pounds. If you did 5 sets of 10, the volume doubles: 5 x 10 x 300 = 15,000.

Clearly, intensity has been increased, but the key to get the desired results is to perform this total volume in the same duration of time; if you did the 5 sets of 5 in 15 minutes, as you increase volume try to keep it in the same time frame so you can progressively add a rep to each set weekly and gradually intensify the workout without increasing the duration. In turn, this will not adversely affect the desired adaptations, and recovery and intensity variables can be compared on an apples-to-apples basis. Obviously, there are countless more examples.

3. Using bodybuilding methods. Use those that have been shown to increase intensity, such as drop sets, rest pauses, forced reps, negatives, and cheating. Even things like pre-exhaustion and superset/giant sets can intensify a workout in a major way.

Squatting 500 pounds fresh is a lot different from doing it after performing multiple sets of lunges, glute kickbacks, leg extensions, and leg curls to exhaustion. If you could do it fresh, now you do it after pre-exhaustion; you have increased intensity and made some gains.

The key to using these principles is to not overdo it, and to be able to track what you do. Quantitatively tracking a drop set can be tough; if you performed fewer reps on your heaviest set but more on your third drop than in the previous week, it is tough to quantitatively measure the training effect.

If you use pre-exhaustion, to what extent did you pre-exhaust? That is why you should be able to quantitatively track training, not in every way, but to ensure progress is being made.

4. Increasing sets. While this could be part of total volume, we will take a slightly more abstract view.

If you did 3 sets of 8 repetitions on the bench press with 250 pounds last week, and this week you are able to do 5 sets of 8 repetitions with the same weight, you have increased intensity and you have made progress. This method can be quantitatively tracked very easily.

5. Increasing repetitions. Last week, if you bench pressed 250 pounds for 8 repetitions and this week you do it for 10, congratulations—you have made progress! Intensity has increased in a way that is easily measurable.

6. Decreasing rest periods. Using the bench press workout of 250 pounds for 3 sets of 8 repetitions, if last week a 3-minute rest was taken between sets and this week a 2-minute rest is taken, let's look at the amazing increase in intensity.

250 pounds x 8 x 3 last week took 10 minutes to accomplish (total rest periods and lifting duration); this week it took only 7 minutes, a huge intensity boost.

7. *Increasing mechanical work/decreasing leverage.* This could also be called leverage manipulation or mechanical disadvantage. For instance, when performing a squat low bar with a wider-than-shoulder-width stance, you move the weight less than using a hip-width foot stance/high bar placement squat (Olympic squat); the range of motion on the powerlifting squat from bottom position to start position might be 16 inches, whereas on the Olympic squat it may be 22 inches.

Mechanical work is measured by the weight being used times the distance being covered. If you squat 350 pounds x 10 reps in the powerlifting squat, the total mechanical work performed for one set of squats is 350 x 10 x 16 = 56,000 pounds. (The 350 pounds is the weight on the bar, 10 is the number of repetitions, and 16 is the range of motion from bottom to completion; we are not factoring in the eccentric.)

Now let's look at the total amount of mechanical work performed for an Olympic squat using the same sets, reps, and weight: 350 x 10 x 22 = 77,000 pounds, which is quite an increase.

Not only is more mechanical work performed, but it is performed typically with a less powerful stance.

Intensity can also be increased as easily as adjusting the angle an incline press is performed, or adjusting the stance when doing a deadlift; mechanical work and leverage manipulation should not be overlooked by the bodybuilder looking to optimize his physique and attack muscles from different angles.

8. *Adding bands and chains.* Chapter 6 is dedicated to the benefits of using bands and chains. While strength sports and more traditional athletics have jumped on this bandwagon, bodybuilders are the last to climb on board. Bands and chains can help develop strength through sticking points and intensify a lift throughout its entire range of motion; and as leverage improves, so does resistance.

Numerous other ways exist to increase training intensity, and that is the goal of progressively overloading your training. It is much more complex than just adding weight to the bar; the key is to know the science of increasing intensity in your workouts but at the same time possess the creativity of an artist. The best trainers are able to synergistically blend the art and science of intensity variable manipulation.

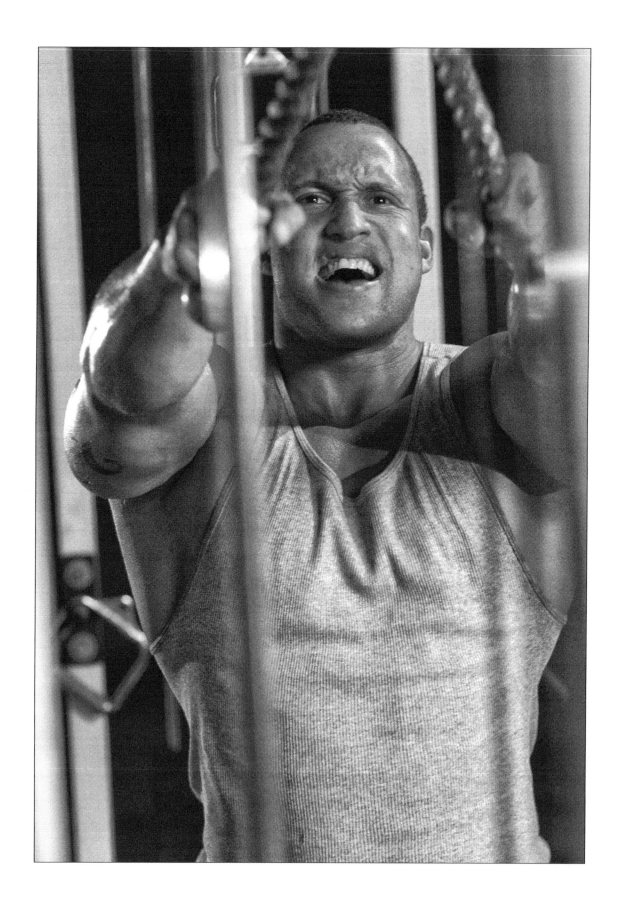

SEQUENCE OF TRAINING

A dilemma that often plagues the novice bodybuilder is "What should I do first?" All exercises are important, but which ones should be done first?

Because speed and explosive movements require much of the body's resources, they hold precedence in order of training. While this is generally not a concern for the bodybuilder, if Olympic movements or their variations are trained in the off season, keep this in mind: Because bigger muscles require more energy and effort than smaller muscles, they should be done first.

Multiple joint movements also require more energy and effort than smaller muscles, and they too should be done first. As is true for flexibility training, the rule is, it should never be done when the body isn't fully warmed up.

Training is not limited to the weight room. Medical, nutritional, and supplemental technologies must be applied at all times. During training, psychological techniques and therapeutic modalities must also be applied.

With these points in mind, here are some general guidelines for proper order of exercises, drills and flexibility training:

1. Psychological training (visualization, concentration, etc.)

2. Warm-up

3. Dynamic flexibility training

4. Explosive training (CAT) (if applicable)

5. Multiple-joint movements
   a. Squats
   b. Bench press
   c. Dips, overhead press, etc.

6. Single-joint movements (Isolation)
   a. Larger muscles
   b. Smaller muscles

Flexibility training (static stretching, SFMR)

Cool-down

Application of appropriate therapy (ice treatment, TENS, etc.)

FOUNDATIONAL TRAINING

The main purpose of foundational training is to strengthen your weaknesses, recover from any injuries, and develop a "foundation" of strength in all muscles, tendons, ligaments, and health and fitness. Usually, this involves training for limit strength, but it can also involve the most nonspecific components of fitness involved in bodybuilding. If you get out of breath walking up a flight of stairs, some cardiovascular training will need to be performed.

Because limit strength is not a major component of any sport other than powerlifting (although limit strength is important), it is usually the main focus of this period. Its importance cannot be over emphasized for you, the bodybuilder. The higher your one-repetition max on squat, the more weight you can do for a set of 10 on squats.

There are two ways to gain strength: (a) improving neural coordination (increasing neural coordination in the movement from more efficient motor-unit recruitment by way of the central nervous system) and (b) increasing cross-sectional muscle fiber areas.

Basically, this means 50% of the ways to get stronger are by way of gaining muscle mass. For this reason, I have provided a few examples of "powerlifter peaking cycles" as a basic plan for developing limit strength.

Percentages, if listed, are of one-repetition max at the beginning of the program.

Ed Coan's 300-Pound Bench Press Routine

If you bench press 180 pounds, multiply weights by 0.6 (180/300). Divide your goal max by 300 pounds for your weights.

Week, Weight, Sets, & Reps
Week 1:   190 x 2 x 10
Week 2:   190 x 2 x 10
Week 3:   200 x 2 x 8
Week 4:   210 x 2 x 8
Week 5:   220 x 2 x 5
Week 6:   230 x 2 x 5
Week 7:   240 x 2 x 5
Week 8:   250 x 2 x 3
Week 9:   260 x 2 x 3
Week 10:   270 x 2 x 2
Week 11:   290 x 2 x 2
Week 12:   300 x 1 x 1

Ken Lain's Bench Press Routine

This is for someone who wants to go from a 275-pound to a 325-pound bench press.

The Monday (heavy) & Thursday (light) assistance exercises
Flat dumbbell flyes: 4 sets x 10 reps
Weighted dips: 4 sets x 8–10 reps
Military press: 4 sets x 8–10 reps
Front lateral raise: 4 sets x 8–10 reps
Close-grip bench press: 4 sets x 8–10 reps
Triceps push-downs: 4 sets x 8–10 reps

The Tuesday (heavy) & Friday (light) assistance exercises
Lat pull-downs: 4 sets x 10 reps
Chin-ups: 4 sets of 10 reps (You can choose which one you'll do, but do either the lat pull-down or chins each Tuesday and Friday workout)
Dumbbell pull-over: 4 sets x 8–10 reps
Seated cable row: 4 sets of 8–10 reps
Bent-over barbell row: 4 sets of 8–10 reps (You can choose which one you'll do, but do either the seated cable row or bent-over barbell row each Tuesday and Friday workout)
Barbell curl: 4 sets x 8–10 reps
Dumbbell curl: 4 sets x 8–10 reps

For legs
Squats: Do 1–2 warm-up sets followed by 3 heavy sets of 5–8 reps
Leg extension: 5 sets x 12 reps
Leg curl: 4 sets x 10 reps
Seated calf raise: 5 sets x 12 reps

Ken said that on week 8 of his bench press program, he stops doing all assistance exercises and focuses his strength and energy solely on the bench press. On the days he doesn't train—Wednesday, Saturday, and Sunday—he'll minimize all other physical activity and give his body plenty of time to rest and recuperate. That also means getting at least 7 hours of sleep each night.

The Power Bench Program

Week 1

Monday (heavy workout)—Use @ 55% of target maximum weight (e.g., 325 pounds)

- Do 2–3 light warm-up sets
- 3 sets of 10 reps with 180 pounds
- Do heavy weight assistance exercises

Thursday (light workout)—Use @ 80% of weight used on Monday's workout

- Do 2–3 light warm-up sets
- 3 sets of 10 reps with 145 pounds

Week 2

Monday (heavy workout)—Use @ 60% of target maximum weight (e.g., 325 pounds)

- Do 2–3 light warm-up sets
- 3 sets of 9 reps with 195 pounds

Thursday (light workout)—Use @ 80% of weight used on Monday's workout

- Do 2–3 warm-up sets
- 3 sets of 9 reps with 155 pounds

Week 3

Monday (heavy workout)—Use @ 65% of target maximum weight (e.g., 325 pounds)

- Do 2–3 light warm-up sets
- 3 sets of 8 reps with 210 pounds

Thursday (light workout)—Use @ 80% of weight used on Monday's workout

- Do 2–3 warm-up sets
- 3 sets of 8 reps with 170 pounds

Week 4

Monday (heavy workout)—Use @ 70% of target maximum weight (e.g., 325 pounds)

- Do 2–3 light warm-up sets
- 3 sets of 7 reps with 225 pounds

Thursday (light workout)—Use @ 80% of weight used on Monday's workout

- Do 2–3 warm-up sets
- 3 sets of 7 reps with 180 pounds

Week 5

Monday (heavy workout)—Use @ 75% of target maximum weight (e.g., 325 pounds)

- Do 2–3 light warm-up sets
- 3 sets of 6 reps with 245 pounds

Thursday (light workout)—Use @ 80% of weight used on Monday's workout

- Do 2–3 warm-up sets
- 3 sets of 6 reps with 195 pounds

Week 6

Monday (heavy workout)—Use @ 80% of target maximum weight (e.g., 325 pounds)

- Do 2–3 light warm-up sets
- 3 sets of 5 reps with 260 pounds

Thursday (light workout)—Use @ 80% of weight used on Monday's workout

- Do 2–3 warm-up sets
- 3 sets of 5 reps with 210 pounds

Week 7

Monday (heavy workout)—Use @ 85% of target maximum weight (e.g., 325 pounds)

- Do 2–3 light warm-up sets
- 2 sets of 4 reps with 275 pounds

Thursday (light workout)—Use @ 80% of weight used on Monday's workout

- Do 2–3 warm-up sets
- 2 sets of 4 reps with 220 pounds

Week 8

Monday (heavy workout)—Use @ 90% of target maximum weight (e.g., 325 pounds)

- Do 2–3 light warm-up sets
- 2 sets of 3 reps with 290 pounds

Thursday (light workout)—Use @ 80% of weight used on Monday's workout

- Do 2–3 warm-up sets
- 2 sets of 3 reps with 230 pounds

Week 9

Monday (heavy workout)—Use @ 95% of target maximum weight (e.g., 325 pounds)

- Do 2–3 light warm-up sets
- 1 set of 2 reps with 310 pounds

Thursday (light workout)—Use @ 80% of weight used on Monday's workout

- Do 2–3 warm-up sets
- 1 set of 2 reps with 250 pounds

Week 10—The Day You Bench 325 pounds

Monday (heavy workout)—Use @100% of target maximum weight (e.g., 325 pounds)

- Do 2–3 light warm-up sets
- 1 rep with 275 pounds
- 1 rep with 310 pounds
- 1 rep with 325 pounds

After completing the 10-week program, give your body a week off from training. (Ken recommends up to 21 days to recover from an all-out training program and world record lift, so judge your body accordingly.) Following a rest break from training, do only regular workouts for one month before beginning your next 10-week program.)

Josh Bryant's 8-Week Routine for Deadlifts

Following is an 8-week routine I designed for my "Deadlift Encyclopedia" article in *Muscle & Fitness.*

Perform one day per week:

Week 1

Deadlift: 75% weight, 3 reps, 1 set
Deadlift: 60% weight, 6 reps, 3 sets (60-second rest interval between sets)
3-Inch deficit deadlifts: 65% weight, 5 reps, 2 sets
Bent over rows: 8 reps, 3 sets
Shrugs: 12 reps, 3 sets
Chin-ups: Max weight, 10 reps, 3 sets
Glute ham raises: 8 reps, 3 sets

Week 2

Deadlift: 80% weight, 3 reps, 1 set
Deadlift: 60% weight, 8 reps, 3 sets (60-second rest interval between sets)
3-Inch deficit deadlifts: 68% weight, 5 reps, 2 sets
Bent over rows: 7 reps, 3 sets
Shrugs: 12 reps, 3 sets
Chin-ups: Max weight, 7 reps, 3 sets
Glute ham raises: 8 reps, 3 sets

Week 3

Deadlift: 85% weight, 3 reps, 1 set
Deadlift: 70% weight, 6 reps, 3 sets (90-second rest interval between sets)
3-Inch deficit deadlifts: 75% weight, 4 reps, 2 sets
Bent over rows: 6 reps, 3 sets
Shrugs: 12 reps, 3 sets
Chin-ups: Max weight, 6 reps, 3 sets
Glute ham raises: 8 reps, 3 sets

Week 4

Deadlift: 60% weight, 1 rep, 6 sets
Lat pull-downs: 8 reps, 3 sets
Shrugs: Light weight, 12 reps, 3 sets
Glute ham raises: 6 reps, 2 sets

Week 5

Deadlift: 90% weight, 2 reps, 1 set
Deadlift: 75% weight, 2 reps, 4 sets (120-second rest interval between sets)
3-Inch deficit deadlifts: 80% weight, 3 reps, 3 sets
One armed row: 6 reps, 3 sets
Shrugs: 10 reps, 3 sets
Chin-ups: Max weight, 4 reps, 3 sets
Glute ham raises: 8 reps, 3 sets

Week 6

Deadlift: 95% weight, 2 reps, 1 set
Deadlift: 80% weight, 2 reps, 3 sets (120-second rest interval between sets)
3-Inch deficit deadlifts: 82.5% weight, 3 reps, 3 sets
One armed row: 6 reps, 3 sets
Shrugs: 10 reps, 3 sets
Chin-ups: Max weight, 3 reps, 3 sets
Glute ham raises: 7 reps, 3 sets

Week 7

Deadlift: 100% weight, 1 reps, 1 set
Deadlift: 85% weight, 2 reps, 3 sets (120-second rest interval between sets)
3-Inch deficit deadlifts: 88% weight, 1 rep, 3 sets
One armed row: 6 reps, 3 sets
Shrugs: 10 reps, 3 sets
Chin-ups: Max weight, 3 reps, 3 sets
Glute ham raises: 7 reps, 3 sets

Week 8

Repeat Week 4

Week 9

Test your new max!

Brad Gillingham's Deadlift Routine for Intermediate Lifters

This routine is designed for an intermediate lifter looking to maximize deadlift strength.

Brad Gillingham is a five-time IPF World Powerlifting Champion and a 12-time USAPL National Powerlifting Champion. Brad has set 12 IPF Masters world records with highlights that include an 881-pound deadlift at the 2010 IPF World Championships in Potchefstroom, South Africa, along with 2,300+ pound totals in numerous meets in single ply gear. As a masters lifter, Brad set an IPF Open world record in the new 120+ kg Class with a deadlift of 395 kg (870 pounds) at the 2011 IPF Pacific Invitational in Melbourne, Australia, on July 31, 2011. Brad recently broke this record at the 2011 IPF World Championships in Pilsen, Czech Republic, with a deadlift of 397.5 kg (876 pounds). Brad is member of numerous strength Halls of Fame ranging from the state to international level. Even more impressive, all of Brad's lifts were completed in drug-tested meets. Clearly, when Brad speaks, we listen!

Phase 1—conditioning and developing base strength

Weeks 1–4

> Power cleans—2 sets 5 reps
> Deadlift from floor—2 sets of 10 reps at 65%
> Power rack lockouts above knee
> Shrugs—3 sets 10 reps
> Bent Rows—3 sets 10 reps
> Seated rows and/or lat pull-downs—3 sets 10 reps

Phase 2—peak strength development phase

Weeks 1, 3, 5, 7, and 9

> Power cleans—2 sets 5 reps
> Power rack lockouts—2 notches (above knee—below knee)
> Shrugs—3 sets 10 reps
> Bent rows—3 sets 10 reps
> Seated rows and/or lat pull-downs—3 sets 10 reps
> **Week 2** (assistance work should remain the same for weeks 2, 4, 6, 8, and 10)
> Deadlift from floor—2 sets 5 reps at 75%
> Bent rows—3 sets 10 reps
> Seated rows and/or lat pull-downs—3 sets 10 reps

Week 4

> Deadlift from floor—2 sets 5 reps at 80%.

Week 6

> Deadlift from floor—2 sets 5 reps at 85%.

Week 8

> Deadlift from floor—2 sets 3 reps at 90%.

Week 10 (10 days from meet)

Deadlift from floor—2 sets 3 reps at 95%

Josh Bryant's 8-Week Squat Routine

Following is the routine I designed for *Muscle and Fitness.*

Perform one day per week:

Week 1

Squats: 80%, 3 reps, 6 sets
Dead squats (hip/knee angle same stance as deadlift): 1 rep, 3 sets
Front squats: 5 reps, 2 sets
Leg curls: 8 reps, 3 sets
Calf raises: 30 reps, 4 sets
Planks (hold 1 minute): 1 rep, 3 sets
Side bends bar on your back: 12 reps, 3 sets

Week 2

Squats: 83%, 3 reps, 5 sets
Dead squats (hip/knee angle same stance as deadlift): 1 rep, 3 sets
Front squats: 5 reps, 2 sets
Leg curls: 8 reps, 3 sets
Calf raises: 30 reps, 4 sets
Planks (hold 1 minute): 1 rep, 3 sets
Side bends bar on your back: 12 reps, 3 sets

Week 3

Squats: 86%, 3 reps, 4 sets
Dead squats (hip/knee angle same stance as deadlift): 1 rep, 3 sets
Front squats: 5 reps, 2 sets
Leg curls: 8 reps, 3 sets
Calf raises: 30 reps, 4 sets
Planks (hold 1 minute): 1 rep, 3 sets
Side bends bar on your back: 12 reps, 3 sets

Week 4

> Squats: 60%, 2 reps, 4 sets
> Light front squats: 6 reps, 2 sets
> Leg curls: 12 reps, 2 sets
> Planks (hold 1 minute): 6 reps, 2 sets

Week 5

> Squats: 91%, 2 reps, 5 sets
> Pause squats: 3 reps, 3 sets
> Front squats: 3 reps, 3 sets
> Leg curls: 12 reps, 3 sets
> Calf raises: 25 reps, 4 sets
> Planks (hold 1 minute): 1 rep, 3 sets
> Side bends bar on your back: 12 reps, 3 sets

Week 6

> Squats: 95%, 2 reps, 4 sets
> Pause squats: 3 reps, 3 sets
> Front squats: 3 reps, 3 sets
> Leg curls: 12 reps, 3 sets
> Calf raises: 25 reps, 4 sets
> Planks (hold 1 minute): 1 rep, 3 sets
> Side bends bar on your back: 12 reps, 3 sets

Week 7

> Squats: 100%, 2 reps, 3 sets
> Pause squats: 3 reps, 3 sets
> Front squats: 3 reps, 3 sets
> Leg curls: 12 reps, 3 sets
> Calf raises: 25 reps, 4 sets
> Planks (hold 1 minute): 1 rep, 3 sets
> Side bends bar on your back: 12 reps, 3 sets

Week 8

> Repeat Week 4

Week 9

> Max out!

Josh Bryant's 13-Week Squat Routine

Here is a squat routine I have used successfully to give my clients and myself gains of well over 10% in the squat.

Perform one day per week:

Week 1

> Squat: 80% x 3 reps
> Squats (CAT): 65% x 4 x 6 sets (rest 1 minute)
> Olympic pause squats: 5 x 2 sets
> Glute ham raises: 3 x 6 reps
> One leg squat: 3 x 6 reps
> Weighted abs: 6 sets

Week 2

> Squat: 85% x 3 reps
> Squats (CAT): 65% x 4 x 8 sets (rest 1 minute)
> Olympic pause squats: 5 x 2 sets
> Glute ham raises: 3 x 6 reps
> One leg squat: 3 x 6 reps
> Weighted abs: 6 sets

Week 3

> Squat: 88% x 3 reps
> Squats (CAT): 65% x 4 x 10 sets (rest 1 minute)
> Olympic pause squats: 5 x 2 sets
> Glute ham raises: 3 x 6 reps
> One leg squat: 3 x 6 reps
> Weighted abs: 6 sets

Week 4 Deload

Week 5

> Squat: 92% x 2 reps
> Squats (CAT): 75% x 3 x 4 sets (rest 2 minutes)
> Band resisted squats: 3 x 4 sets
> Glute ham raises: 3 x 6 reps
> One leg deadlift: 3 x 6 reps
> Weighted abs: 6 sets

Week 6

> Squat: 97% x 2 reps
> Squats (CAT): 75% x 3 x 5 sets (rest 2 minutes)
> Band resisted squats: 2 x 4 sets
> Glute ham raises: 3 x 6 reps
> One leg deadlift: 3 x 6 reps
> Weighted abs: 6 sets

Week 7

> Squat: 101% x 2 reps
> Squats (CAT): 75% x 3 x 6 sets (rest 2 minutes)
> Band resisted squats: 1 x 3 sets
> Glute ham raises: 3 x 6 reps
> One leg deadlift: 3 x 6 reps
> Weighted abs: 6 sets

Week 8 Deload

Week 9

> Squat: 95% x 1 rep, 105% x 1 rep
> Squats (CAT): 80% x 2 x 6 sets (rest 2.5 minutes)
> Pause squats chains: 5 x 2 sets
> Glute ham raises: 3 x 6 reps
> One leg press: 3 x 6 reps
> Weighted abs: 6 sets

Week 10

> Squat: 98% x 1 rep, 109% x 1 rep
> Squats (CAT): 84% x 2 x 5 sets (rest 2.5 minutes)
> Pause squats chains: 4 x 2 sets
> Glute ham raises: 3 x 6 reps
> One leg press: 3 x 6 reps
> Weighted abs: 6 sets

Week 11

> Squat: 101% x 1 rep, 113% x 1 rep
> Squats (CAT): 88% x 2 x 4 sets (rest 2.5 minutes)
> Pause squats chains: 3 x 2 sets
> Glute ham raises: 3 x 6 reps
> One leg press: 3 x 6 reps
> Weighted abs: 6 sets

Week 12

Deload

Week 13

Max out!

IMPORTANT NOTES FOR YEAR-ROUND TRAINING

Athletes should begin all workouts with a general warm-up, such as 5–10 minutes on the bike, treadmill, or elliptical.

After warming up, athletes should always do dynamic stretches prior to lifting. For a warm-up routine, please see Chapter 12, Stretching. One study entitled "Four-Week Dynamic Stretching Warm-up Intervention Elicits Longer-Term Performance Benefits," published in the *Strength and Conditioning Journal* in 2008, showed that incorporation of 4 weeks of dynamic stretching increased power, strength, muscular endurance, anaerobic capacity, and agility performance enhancements in collegiate wrestlers. All of these qualities will help you, the bodybuilder.

A FEW LAST WORDS

Optimizing recovery, maximizing gains, and peaking at the right time come down to one thing: periodization.

The smart bodybuilder will use exercises, methods, and routines that have been empirically tested and proven to give excellent results and science—the superiority of the science of periodization—to build a champion physique.

SOURCES

Buford, T. W., S. J. Rossi, D. B. Smith, and A. J. Warren. "A Comparison of Periodization Models During Nine Weeks of Equated Volume and Intensity for Strength." *Journal of Strength & Conditioning Research* 21, no. 4 (2007): 1245–50.

Fleck, Steven J. "Non-Linear Periodization for General Fitness and Athletes." *Journal of Human Kinetics, Special Issue* (2011): 41–45. DOI: 10.2478/v10078-011-0057-2.

Fry, A. C., and W. J. Kraemer. "Resistance Exercise Overtraining and Overreaching. Neuroendocrine Responses." *Sports Medicine* 23, no. 2 (1997): 106–29. *National Center for Biotechnology Information.* http://www.ncbi.nlm.nih.gov/pubmed/9068095.

Hatfield, Frederick. *Specialist in Sports Conditioning*. Santa Barbara, CA: International Sports Sciences Association, 2001. (Unpublished manuscript.)

Herman, Sonja L., and Derek T. Smith. "Four-Week Dynamic Stretching Warm-up Intervention Elicits Longer-Term Performance Benefits." *Journal of Strength & Conditioning Research* 22, no. 4 (2008): 1286–97.

Issurin, Vladimir B. "New Horizons for the Methodology and Physiology of Training Periodization." *Sports Medicine* 40, no. 3 (2010): 189. (English abstract available.)

Kok, L. Y., P. W. Hamer, and D. J. Bishop. "Enhancing Muscular Qualities in Untrained Women: Linear Versus Undulating Periodization." *Medicine and Science in Sports and Exercise* 41, no. 9 (2009): 1797–807.

Kraemer, William J., and Steven J. Fleck. *Optimizing Strength Training: Designing Nonlinear Periodization Workouts*. Champaign, IL: Human Kinetics Publishing, 2007.

Painter, K. B., G. G. Haff, M. W. Ramsey, J. McBride, T. Triplett, W. A. Sands, H. S. Lamont, M. E. Stone, and M[ichael]. H. Stone. "Strength Gains: Block Versus Daily Undulating Periodization Weight Training Among Track and Field Athletes." *International Journal of Sports Physiology & Performance* 7, no. 2 (2012): 161–69.

Proceedings of the Faculty of Physical Education, University of Banja Luka, no. 2 (November 2010), 304.

Rhea, M. R., S. D. Ball, W. T. Phillips, and L. N. Burkett. "A Comparison of Linear and Daily Undulating Periodized Programs with Equated Volume and Intensity for Strength." *Journal of Strength & Conditioning Research* 16 (2002): 250–55.

Siff, Mel, and Yuri Verkhoshansky. *Supertraining*. Pittsburgh, PA: Sports Support Syndicate, 1996.

Wolff, Robert. *Bodybuilding 201: Everything You Need to Know to Take Your Body to the Next Level*. New York: Contemporary Books, 2003.

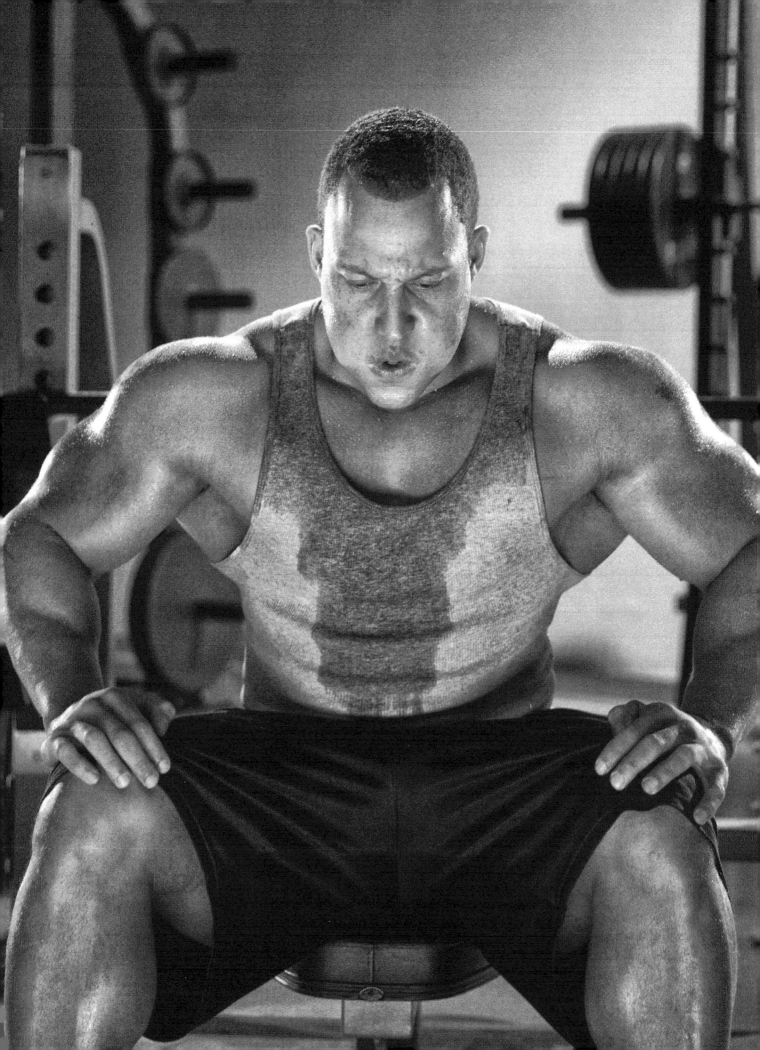

CHAPTER 5.

Bringing Up Symmetry and Attacking Weaknesses

Massive, lean and symmetrical muscle is all you want. For most bodybuilders, especially the novice, this can be accomplished simply by eating a clean diet and training heavy core lifts. However, as you evolve more and more, you're going to find that advanced techniques will be needed to keep the gains coming.

MUSCLE SHAPING

Intense strength training and proper nutrition cause muscles to grow larger. But with a cessation of training and/or a caloric deficit, muscles can atrophy or decrease in size.

After a muscle has been enlarged, can you control how it is shaped? Will exercise selection, volume, rep speed, and a mind-muscle connection literally cause a morphological change in muscle shape?

A majority of bodybuilders feel they can shape their muscles to some degree. Popularized by muscle magazines, terms like "mass exercises" are basic compound movements, and "shaping exercises" are generally a single-joint movement performed in a peak contraction style. Others argue the opposite, with a stick-to-the-basics approach.

Who's right?

Training with maximal intensity and low repetitions in the 1–5 rep range with greater than 85% of a one-repetition max causes myofibrillar hypertrophy.

On the other hand, sarcoplasmic hypertrophy is an increase in the volume of the non-contractile muscle cell fluid, sarcoplasm. This fluid accounts for 25%–30% of the muscle's size. Even though the muscle increased in size, the density of muscle fibers per unit decreased, resulting in no increase in muscular strength.

Sarcoplasmic hypertrophy is induced through higher repetition ranges and a greater amount of volume. Powerlifters with minimal body fat have a much different look and appear to have a different shape than bodybuilders with a similar percentage of body fat, although they weigh the same.

Genetics obviously are a major determinant in the aesthetics of a muscle. However, because the bodybuilder and powerlifter train differently, muscle can potentially look like a different shape, partly because the powerlifter's physique is largely the product of low rep training and increases in the contractile element of the muscle.

The bodybuilder who has fully developed a muscle will have up to 30% of his muscle developed from the non-contractile element. Another person with the same percentage of body fat and the same bodyweight could appear to have a different shape to the muscle as a result of training. Muscle shaping is not taking place; one is a maximally developed muscle, the other is not.

STRESSING DIFFERENT MUSCLE PARTS

The "Bro Science" crowd is convinced twisting your arm a certain way will develop a certain portion of the muscle, and the functional training crowd is convinced muscles get bigger and smaller only, and that diet is the only reason powerlifters and bodybuilders are built differently.

The "Bro Science" crowd is actually closer to reality on this one.

For decades, science has known that certain heads of muscles function differently from one another, examples being the pectoralis major and the deltoids. Top exercise science researcher, Bret Contreras (http://bretcontreras.com/), did a series of EMG studies that tested the electrical activity of muscle during exercise. Bret, unlike most researchers, is an avid bodybuilding fan and trains very seriously.

In e-mail correspondence he reiterated, "You can trust my form was great in these experiments and the data is good." Bret's work confirmed bodybuilders are correct, that various exercises can stress different parts of muscles. He said, "My research indicates that muscle fibers within a muscle can function differently from one another even if they don't have separate heads. For example, during my research I noted that the upper rectus abdominis and lower rectus abdominis function differently. I suspect this is true of all muscles." This would make sense because Contreras went on to point out that varying muscles many times have different points of attachments, numerous motor units and sometimes varying nerve suppliers.

This has huge implications for the bodybuilder.

That's why just sticking to the basics you cannot maximally develop a muscle. Ergo, the problem with high-intensity training and the lack of exercise selection. Implementing various exercises that attack the muscles at various angles, different cadences, rep ranges, and volume prescriptions is the only way to maximally develop a muscle.

When all elements of a muscle are fully developed and body fat is minimized, a muscle will appear different than when there is excess body fat and partial development. For 12 weeks straight performing 10 sets of 10 reps lateral raises or 10 sets of 10 reps front raises, both will produce a different effect on deltoid musculature than performing 10 sets of 10 reps in the overhead press. This is because of greater emphasis on selective fiber recruitment in exercise selection.

Even exercise technique plays a role in development of muscle: Performing dips with a forward lean and elbows out will place more stress on the pecs than a more upright posture.

Fred Hatfield said 30 years ago:

> In the final analysis, after a muscle has been developed to its maximum, the shape of a muscle is genetically predetermined. Bodybuilders who have succeeded in developing all of the components of all the muscle cells in the biceps, for example, can only hope that the good Lord, in His infinite wisdom, gave him the genes necessary for the biceps to be well formed aesthetically.

Hatfield was right, but few bodybuilders are close to maximum development!

ISOLATION EXERCISES

Muscles and joints work together synergistically to perform movement patterns and produce force; muscles are not designed to work in isolation.

Take a look at the leg extension: Real-life movement patterns do not isolate the quads and remove contributions of other lower body muscles. This is the functional trainer's argument against the implementation of isolation exercises. From a functional-movement standpoint, the argument seems logical.

But from a muscular-overload standpoint, the functional trainer solidifies the bodybuilder's need for isolation exercises. Muscles do not work in isolation; by forcing them to do so with single-joint movements, overload is taking place, folks. Overload is what we are after in training.

The average guy on the street can produce a respectable imposing physique with primarily core lifts only. The bodybuilder is in a different situation.

Bodybuilders need unnatural development in certain areas that will take more than overloading natural movements. The medial or side delts, with presses alone, will generally not develop the "capped" look.

Arm development is huge in bodybuilding; and regardless of what you read on the Internet, at some point it will take more than heavy presses and chin-ups to maximally develop arm musculature.

Quadriceps, the sweep, or "vastus lateralis," is tough to develop with squats alone; leg extensions will provide a huge overload to "unnaturally" overload this area.

Olympic lifters perform many deep high bar squats and front squats in training and many times have the vastus medialis or "tear drop" development bodybuilders are after, yet they lack the sweep of a bodybuilder. This is because Olympic lifters never go near a leg extension machine; deep Olympic squats sufficiently overload the vastus medialis. Some body parts need supernatural development that can only be accomplished with unnatural isolation techniques.

Check your ego at the door when performing isolation exercises. Complete isolation is impossible, but do your best; synergist and stabilizer muscles may be somewhat involved, but make an effort to place the load on the appropriate muscles.

This is done with muscle intention, which means purposeful contraction of the muscles being worked. Involving your ego by using copious amounts of weight will quickly turn the movement into a pseudo-compound movement; by lifting excessive weights placed on a single joint, the movement can become unsafe.

When performing a core movement, the weakest muscle group will limit the amount of weight that can be lifted. Picture this scenario: Your lower back is strong enough to deadlift 500 pounds, but your glutes lack the strength to lock the weight out. What's the end result?

Best case scenario, a missed lift; worst case is an injured hamstring caused by synergistic dominance. In other words, your hamstrings, which should be assisting your glutes in locking the weight out, take over because of the glutes' deficiency, and injury results. Isolation exercises can even help bring up the strength of a lagging muscle group that is not getting enough work because of overcompensation movement patterns.

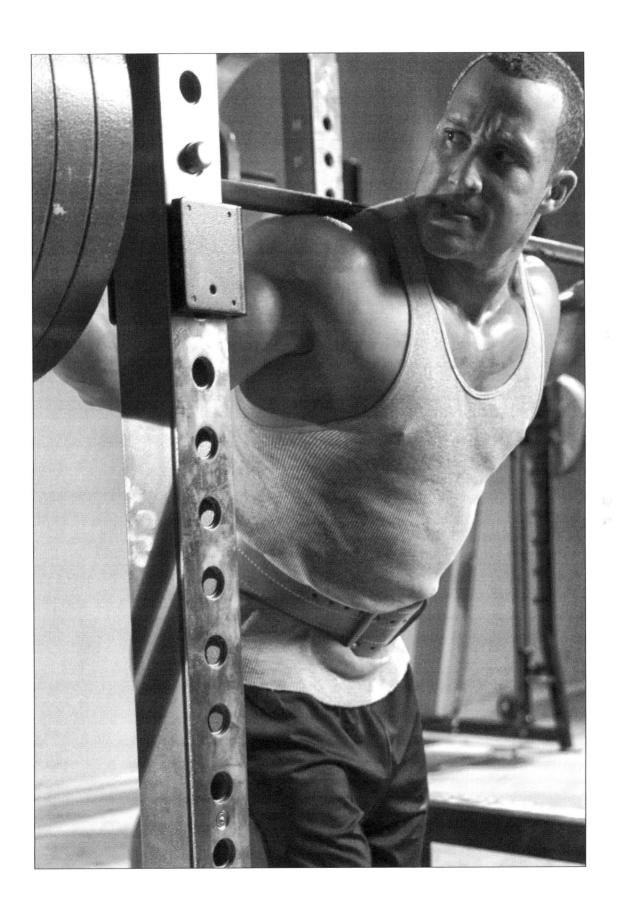

Isolation exercises should be used year round. In the off season, two-thirds of movements may be compound and a third might be isolation. As a contest approaches and you want muscles to really pop out and look defined, the percentage may reverse itself. When adding mass, generally, you are also targeting specific areas, this being done with isolation exercises.

IMPROVING SYMMETRY AND LAGGING BODY PARTS

You are big, you are ripped, but symmetry is lacking; one arm may be smaller than the other, or a muscle group might be lagging. Have no fear, friends!

Let's look at some strategies to eliminate this haphazard problem.

Unilateral exercise research has conclusively shown that unilateral resistance training (one limb at a time) forces your body to recruit more muscle fibers than bilateral resistance training. It requires much more effort for one limb, working by itself, to move a weight from one point to another, than for two limbs working collaboratively to move the weight the same distance.

The sum of the force that two independent limbs are capable of producing being together is less than adding the maximum force together one limb can produce. This is known as the bilateral deficit. Exceptions are highly trained powerlifters and Olympic lifters whose sport is to lift maximal weights bilaterally. Unilateral training takes advantage of the bilateral deficit.

How many people have one limb that is weaker than its respective counterpart?

Most people fall into this category.

Performing an exercise unilaterally many times is a great way not only to identify a specific weakness or imbalance but to stop it dead in its tracks! If you are doing an exercise using only your left arm, your right arm cannot overcompensate and assist in balancing the weight and/or helping the lift. If your left arm is lagging behind your right arm in development, this must sound intriguing, to say the least.

One great strategy to bring up that left arm is to perform exercises unilaterally.

Let's say we are focusing on the triceps: Overhead dumbbell triceps extension is the exercise of choice. Pick a weight at which you can do 10–15 repetitions with the left arm, do this weight to momentary muscular failure, and match the same amount of reps on the right arm (strong arm). Although the volume is the same on both arms, the intensity—the most important ingredient to growth—is maximally stressed on the weaker arm. This will help bring balance, but not at the expense of weakening and atrophying the arm, like more traditional strategies do.

If you completely ignore the good side, generally the result is two bad sides. The same strategy can be used for other body parts: For the quadriceps use one leg extensions, for hamstrings use one leg curls, and so on.

Unilateral exercise variations can also be great for increasing metabolic stress on muscle by increased time under tension (TUT), pressing exercises for instance. Instead of performing a traditional incline dumbbell bench press, perform each arm independently. As you press with one arm, hold the other arm in extension; as you hold the non-pressing arm isometrically in extension, focus on contracting that pec; the other will take care of itself by lifting the weight. You can use close to the same amount of weight this way, potentially identify and eliminate imbalances, and literally double your time under tension. Very exciting!

INCREASED FREQUENCY

The dark ages are over, although many still prescribe to the notion that a muscle group can only be worked one day a week and there is no other way.

"Comparison of 1 Day and 3 Days per Week of Equal-Volume Resistance Training in Experienced Subjects" was a landmark study published in the *Journal of Strength and Conditioning Research* in the year 2000.

The study compared 1 day versus 3 days of weight training weekly, with the training volume the same. There were two control groups: Group 1 lifted 1 day per week for 3 sets to failure (1DAY) and Group 2 lifted 3 days per week of 1 set to failure (3DAY). The 1DAY group achieved only 62% of the one-rep max increases of the 3DAY group in both upper-body and lower-body lifts! Muscle mass increases were greater in the 3DAY group. This study showed that a higher frequency of resistance training increased better strength and mass gains.

For a lagging muscle group, the answer can be increased frequency. This can be 2–3 extra sessions a week focused on the lagging body part; these sessions are submaximal; your muscles will recover. My concern is your central nervous system and joints, so be careful.

Let's say your lats are behind in development. If this is your current split—

Monday: Chest
Tuesday: Arms
Thursday: Back
Friday: Shoulders
Saturday: Legs

—then Monday/Saturday, in a separate session or mixed in your workout (if you cannot train twice a day), do lat pull-downs with cables on your knees (3 sets of 12 reps @ 70% intensity), straight arm pull-downs (3 sets of 12 reps @ 70% intensity), and wide grip chin-ups (3 sets of 8 reps @ 70% intensity). These extra sessions would be with submaximal intensity, no accommodated resistance or any type of eccentric overloading.

Over the course of 12 weeks, instead of working your back 12 times, you have done it 36. In the process, you have not fatigued your CNS or sacrificed other workouts because of the low intensity. The idea, as Lee Haney once said, is "stimulate, don't annihilate."

Many professors will say that it takes about 48 hours for a muscle to recover from an intense workout. This is a very simplistic notion; doing a German volume squat routine will take much longer. Sneaking in a few extra sets of submaximal lat pull-downs will take less. Think about it; does it take 48 hours to recover if you walk to get your mail? Of course not. Recovery is relative. Consider giving submaximal high frequency training a shot, to bring up a lagging body part.

Electromyostimulation (EMS) was a staple in the regimen of the Soviet Sports Machine. EMS incorporates the use of electrical current to activate skeletal muscle and initiate contraction. In clinical/rehabilitative settings, EMS is commonly used. The beneficial effects of EMS in today's world are pretty much universally accepted. What about to the healthy bodybuilder looking to bring up a lagging muscle group?

In the book *Supertraining,* Mel Siff, who has studied EMS extensively, offered these four uses for EMS to the strength and conditioning communities: (a) the invoking of physical stress to induce supercompensation (this could be increased strength, muscles mass, or explosive power), (b) restoration after injury or training, (c) neuromuscular stimulation for movement patterning, and (d) general endocrine restoration after intense exercise or injury. The recuperative benefits are covered in Chapter 11; muscle hypertrophy sounds intriguing.

Fred Hatfield has suggested applying electrostimulation to the muscle you are trying to bring up because your individual muscle cells each have their own excitation threshold, the level at which they're stimulated to contract. Some are easily stimulated with as little as a couple of millivolts of "juice" from your central nervous system. Others, especially the high-threshold motor units, need as much as 15–20 millivolts of electrical current in order to stimulate them to respond contractively.

EMS recruits fast-twitch muscle fibers first, counter to the size principle. Theoretically, then, EMS will be more beneficial in bringing up a primarily fast-twitch muscle group like the triceps, over a slower-twitch dominant one like the soleus. The idea is this: If a muscle group is lagging behind, it's important to get maximum excitatory stimulation in order to force previously unreached muscle fibers to contract. By doing this, a lagging muscle can potentially be brought up or create proportion between limbs.

What do studies say?

A 2005 French study whose results were republished in English by the American College of Sports Medicine in its *Medicine & Science in Sports & Exercise* journal, set out to investigate the effects of 4 and 8 weeks of electromyostimulation (EMS) training on both muscular and neural adaptations of the quadriceps. The results were astounding: A 27% increase was seen in strength of the quadriceps, and the size increased by 6%. This was without pounding the pig iron, just EMS. Studies on advanced bodybuilders are lacking, but to maximize your development, it is important to be aware of the tools at your disposal.

WORKING ORIGIN AND INSERTION

A muscle has an origin and insertion. The origin is the part that does not move, whereas the insertion is the part that does move. To fully develop a muscle, you need to attack both muscle functions. One way is to select exercises that do both. Charles Poliquin has proposed origin/insertion supersets. For the biceps, the example Poliquin cited was close grip chin-ups supersetted with incline dumbbell bicep curls.

Here is how it works doing chin-ups: The insertion is at the shoulder and the elbows are fixed origin. The opposite happens with incline curls. Even if you're not doing supersets, this is something that needs to be taken into account. Triceps could be done with upright dips and standing French presses. For quadriceps, a good combination is front squats and leg extensions.

For the chest, a push-up and dumbbell bench press could be used because with a push-up, the arms remain stationary and the torso moves; with a dumbbell bench press the opposite takes place. For the back, the same could be done with a lat pull-down and a chin-up variation with a pronated grip. (Although the terms *chin-up* and *pull-up* are interchangeable, technically a pull-up is a pronated grip and a chin-up is a supinated grip.)

Notice all of these examples are an open-kinetic-chain exercise coupled with a closed-kinetic-chain one. It comes down to this: A variety of exercises need to hit the muscle at a variety of angles.

PRIORITIZATION

A common joke in the fitness industry is Monday is National Chest Day. Bench presses are occupied like a war zone, but squat racks resemble a ghost town.

Why is this?

Priorities!

Chest is a "beach muscle" extremely important to the lay gym population. But legs? Not so much. As a bodybuilder, you must not fall into this trap. While some guys desire development of certain muscles over others, the complete bodybuilder wants a complete symmetrical package.

Prioritizing doesn't just mean working what is most important at the beginning of the week; it takes a bit of creativity and planning.

For example, chest is your best body part and legs are your weakest. What's the solution? Well, surely by now you have figured out it ain't hitting chest on Wednesday! You will be freshest on Wednesday, so train legs then. Learn to love them, or learn to love subpar results.

BREAKING OUT OF YOUR COMFORT ZONE

Many people will interpret this as "go hard or go home," and this is not the case. Some people only know one speed: full speed.

Sometimes doing a deload, working out with less intensity, will be needed. Don't skip the workout or go all out; do what you are supposed to do.

Even though you love to train hard and heavy, you may have always had an embarrassing weakness doing chin-ups. This does not mean do endless sets of lat pull-downs with cheating force to oblige your ego; go hit the chin-up bar!

The biggest problem is training with a lack of intensity. If you want to maximize muscular development, at some point you're going to have to grow a pair and attack the pig iron with ferocity.

BOSU BALL AND STABILITY BALL TRAINING

Performing exercises on stability balls and BOSU balls has increased in popularity over the past decade. Not only have these techniques been implemented by fitness folks and athletes, but they are now somewhat common in physique and strength athletes.

Do these techniques have a place in your program if you hope to pack on serious muscle?

Many strength coaches will say, "Absolutely!"

Studies have been performed on this subject, so let's take a look at what has been found.

High profile celebrity trainers and misguided strength coaches alike have perpetuated the belief that the best way to recruit the muscles that stabilize the core is to perform traditional strength-training exercises on unstable surfaces.

Recently, James Kohler of California State University Northridge (CSUN) led a study showing that training on stable surfaces overloaded and best-recruited core muscles.

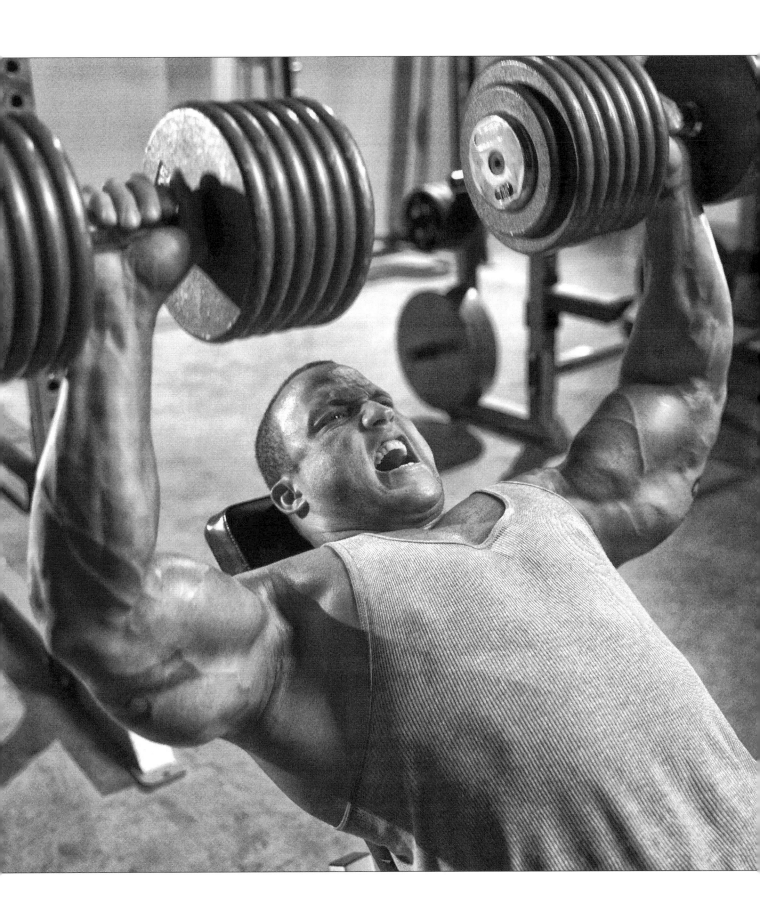

Both prime movers and stabilizers were assessed. Thirty resistance-trained subjects performed both barbell and dumbbell shoulder presses on stable and unstable surfaces for 3 sets of 3, with what equated to equal intensity.

The same protocol was used for the bench press. Core muscle activation was measured by using electromyography (measurements of the electrical activity of muscles). As the instability of the surface increased, the recruitment of core musculature decreased.

Scientific studies confirm that training on a stable surface is the most efficient way to load core muscles. Other studies echo this finding.

Athletes who are required to compete on unstable surfaces can look at occasionally training on them. However, they are misinformed if they believe they are overloading their core. Since your goal is size and strength, there is no reason to train on an unstable surface.

A FEW LAST WORDS

A number of strategies have been outlined to maximize the development of uncooperative parts; use them. Be sure to review Chapter 1 on bodybuilding methods.

If heavy bench presses aren't maximizing chest development, try a pre-exhaustion technique. Rest pauses, drop sets, or a reverse pyramid may be the answer. Review sections thoroughly; sometimes just eccentrically overloading might spark muscle growth beyond your wildest dreams. These techniques are outlined to help you! When traditional approaches aren't providing the bang for your buck, open up and try new things with the outlined strategies.

SOURCES

Bishop, P., M. E. Guillams, and J. R. McLester. "Comparison of 1 Day and 3 Days Per Week of Equal-Volume Resistance Training in Experienced Subjects." *Journal of Strength and Conditioning Research* 14, no. 3 (2000): 273–81.

Bryant, Josh, and Brian Dobson. *Metroflex Gym Powerbuilding Basics*. Arlington, TX: JoshStrength.com, 2011.

Gondin, J., M. Guette, Y. Ballay, and A. Martin. "Electromyostimulation Training Effects on Neural Drive and Muscle Architecture." *Medicine & Science in Sports & Exercise* 37, no. 8 (2005): 1291–99.

Gregory, Chris, and Scott Bickel. "Recruitment Patterns in Human Skeletal Muscle During Electrical Stimulation." *Journal of the American Physical Therapy Association* 85, no. 4 (2005): 358–64.

Hatfield, Frederick C. "Symmetry and Exercise Funk" (Home). *Dr. Squat* (n.d.). http://www.drsquat.com.

Poliquin, Charles. "Smart Training: Size vs. Strength Rep Ranges. *Iron Man Magazine* (n.d.). Free download. http://imbodybuilding.com/articles/size-vs-strength-rep-ranges/?p=2.

Siff, Mel C. *Supertraining*. 6th ed. Denver, CO: Supertraining Institute, 2003.

Waterbury, Chad. *Huge in a Hurry*. New York: Rodale, 2008.

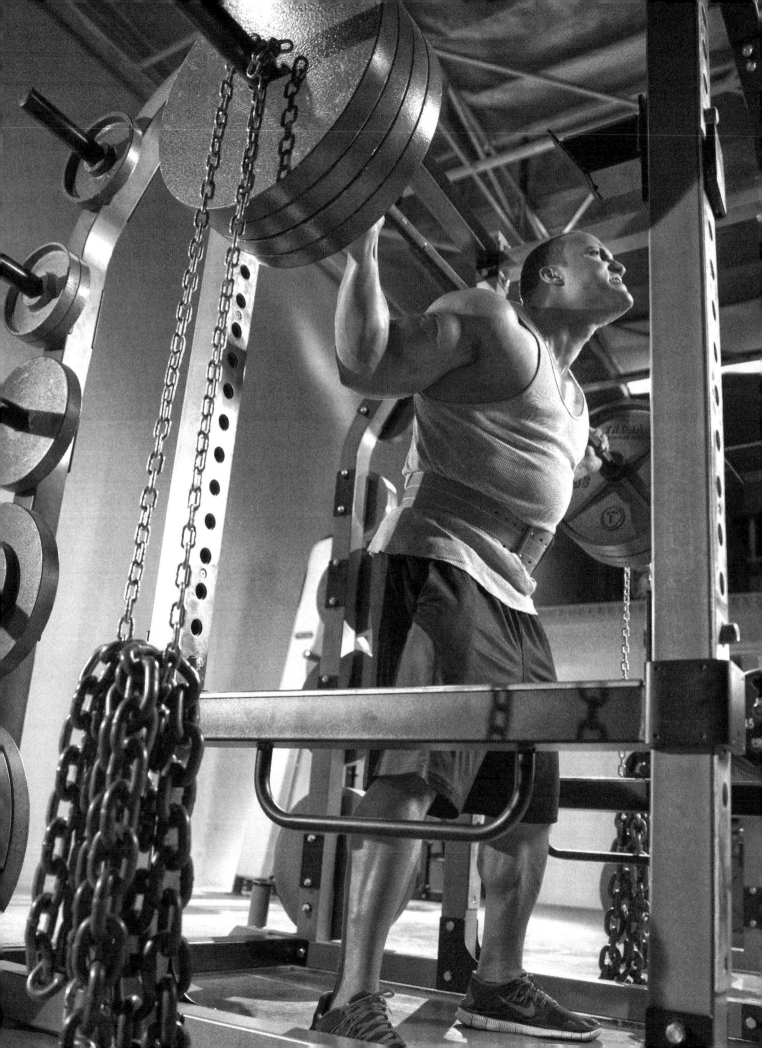

CHAPTER 6.

Bands and Chains Break into Bodybuilding

Bands and chains for bodybuilding?

You can't be serious, right?

Read on.

You just might be surprised how far back they go with the sport.

Back in the early 1900s, Eugene Sandow, the founding father of bodybuilding, was selling a home exercise device that used rubber resistance bands for strength training. Decades later, elastic bands could be purchased in the 1970s and were marketed as a cheap, safe, effective method for duplicating isokinetic resistance machines.

Yuri Verkhoshansky wrote about elastic bands in his 1977 book, *Fundamentals of Special Strength-Training in Sport,* a truly classic masterpiece from the fabled Soviet Bloc.

By the late 1980s and early 1990s, Powerlifting Guru Louie Simmons was writing about adding bands and chains to barbells. Unknown to many prior to Simmons, ISSA co-founder and world-renowned strength coach, Dr. Fred Hatfield, was using bands with elite athletes in the early 1980s.

Prior to this, Fred's business partner and ISSA president, Dr. Sal Arria, had marketed a band system in the 1970s. Some evidence from Weider's publications suggests Americans learned about bands from the Soviets in the 1970s.

BANDS FOR POWERLIFTING

Elite-level bodybuilders and powerlifters find stuff that works, then the ivory tower figures out why it works later. Such is the case with providing accommodating resistance with the use of adding bands and chains to barbells.

Elite-level powerlifters have used these tools to help push the limit of superhuman strength. While these accommodating resistance tools were around prior to 2000, since then they have become more popular in mainstream strength and conditioning circles. An increasing number of powerlifting world records, whether they be raw or equipped, have been broken post 2000.

In the 1990s, if a collegiate strength coach at a major Division-1 University had bands and chains in the school's facility, let alone fantasized about his athletes' using them, in a best-case scenario he would have been considered too powerlifting oriented, and in a worst-case scenario, he would have been ostracized by his peers.

Never mind that these devices can provide substantial overload to athletes, enhance rate of force development, allow athletes to work around injuries, deliberately attack sticking points, and effectively complement a human strength curve. We must let science be our guide, not peers who have probably never trained seriously and whose success is most likely dependent on a good recruiting class and knowing the right people. Thankfully, now a vast majority of universities and mainstream strength and conditioning facilities have bands and chains.

Similar opposition was experienced in the 1990s when strength coaches like Mark Phillipi implemented strongman events in the training of his athletes at the University of Nevada, Las Vegas. While strongman events go back as far as Milo of Crete in ancient times, this was viewed as some sort of new-age blasphemous epiphany. Now, every major college and even most high schools have tires to flip. The same can be said of those of us who, early on, opposed Olympic lifting for large football group settings because of a lack of technical proficiency. This belief in opposing Olympic lifts for football is increasingly mainstream now.

Bands and chains have started popping up in gyms around the globe, similar to the way Spandex did in the 1980s. The difference is, unlike Spandex, bands and chains can *actually help* your workout.

One study presented at the 2004 National Strength and Conditioning Association Convention demonstrated that athletes who did band-resisted bench presses had a significantly greater increase in their bench press max, as well as power produced, compared to athletes who trained only with straight bar weight.

Another breakthough study performed by the University of Wisconsin–La Crosse found that athletes had 25% more leg power than when compared to performing traditional free weight squats without the addition of accommodated resistance.

Hey, wait. This is all fine and dandy, but isn't this book about bodybuilding?

Yes, it is!

However, we must remember our limit strength is our base.

A study has been performed by Ithaca College (Ithaca, New York), where researchers directly confirmed the anabolic effects via the implementation of band training. The study demonstrated that athletes combining bands with bench presses and squats had strength gains that were more than double those of their counterparts who only used free weights without additional bands; the band group doubled the amount of muscle gained!

That directly applies to you as a bodybuilder.

USING BANDS AND CHAINS

Let's take the squat as an example.

As the lifter squats the weight down and then back up to an erect starting position, the resistance (from bands/chains) decreases on the way down and increases on the way up; by how much depends on the strength of the bands or the weight of the chains.

As you get toward the completion of the lift, more force will be required to complete the lift; in turn, more muscle fibers are required to complete the lift. So the benefits to the bodybuilder are apparent: As the range of motion lengthens, resistance becomes more powerful. In turn, you are forced to recruit more muscle fibers, which translates into more growth; and, of course, you become stronger.

Chains feel much more like a barbell using straight weight than bands do. Chains perform almost like the missing link between band-resisted movements and movements that use traditional iron.

Again using the squat as our example, chains are draped from the end of a barbell, so as you descend to the floor, the chain will subsequently unload link by link on the floor. This means as you descend into the bottom position, resistance is the least where you are the weakest,

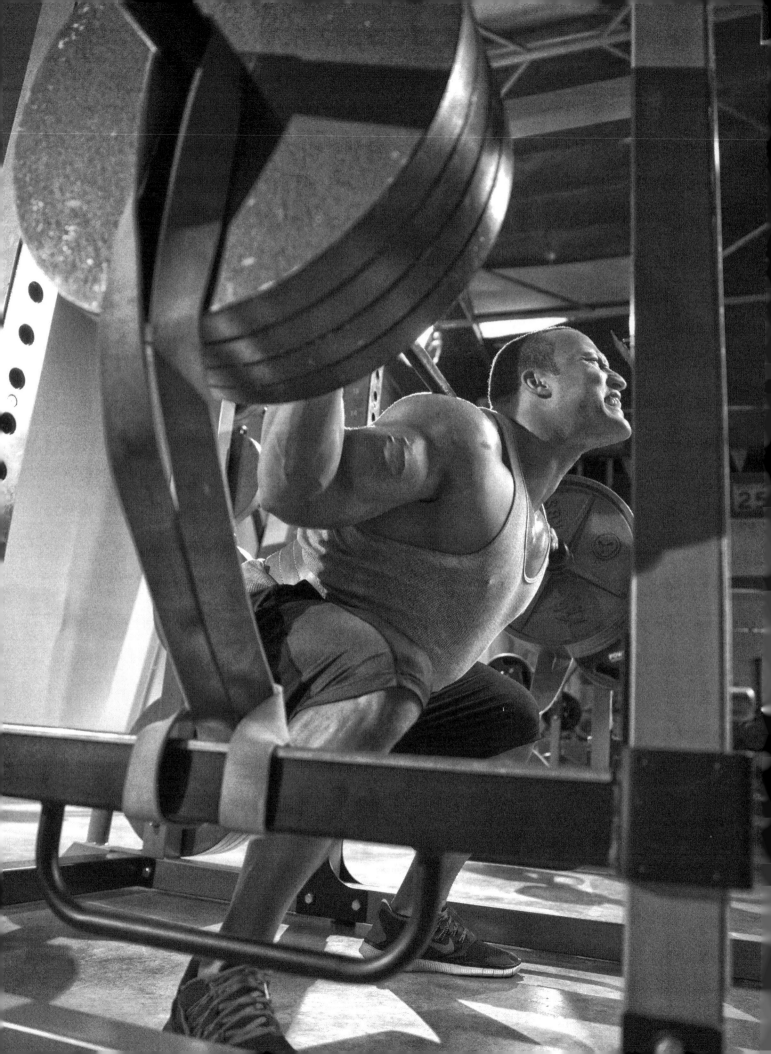

not to mention that you are more likely to achieve full depth because of the lightened load. As you lift the weight back up on the ascent, the resistance increases as each link is lifted off of the floor. You can quarter squat more than you can full squat, as your leverage improves in the quarter squat position; and during the completion you will be lifting more and more weight where you can handle it.

Bands work similarly to chains: As leverage improves, resistance increases. But in the squat, bands don't just hang off the bar onto the ground; they are actually attached to the floor, whether it is around a dumbbell, a specialized attachment, or even the bottom of a rack. As the two ends of the band get closer together on the descent of a squat, the resistance decreases; as you squat the weight back up and the bands pull farther apart, resistance increases. Bands do, however, cause an over-speed effect on the eccentric portion of the movement; so remember this: Performing greater than 8 reps or using them too frequently puts you at a greater risk of overtraining.

Here are some tips on setting up bands/chains for common movements:

Setting Up Bands

The way you set up bands depends on the equipment at your disposal and what exercise you are training.

If you are squatting in a power rack, you have a couple of options: Set the safety pins at a low position and loop the bands around them and attach them to the barbell; or loop the bands around the bottom of the safety rack. Some higher-end racks even have a special peg attachment for bands.

If you are in free-standing jacks and have to use dumbbells, make sure you place a barrier like plates around them so they do not roll when you walk the weight out. The bench press may also need to be performed in a power rack with the bands set up as suggested for the squat, or you can loop the bands around very heavy dumbbells. Regardless of what setup you use, make sure the bands are set evenly.

My favorite technique for bench press is to attach only one band to each end and slide it under the bench. For deadlifts, Jump Stretch actually makes a platform specifically for deadlifts; this is a great investment. Other options are to use one band and step on the band to make sure it stays in place; this is becoming more common.

Setting Up Reverse Bands

Bands need not be applied only to a barbell in a bottom-up fashion. They can also come from the top down; this method, if using the bands in a reverse fashion, is actually known as the *lightened method.*

Taking a look at the squat, attach the bands to the top of the squat rack instead of the bottom. The farther you squat down, the more the band helps you; so as you are in the deepest, most difficult position, the band will help you the most; and as you squat the weight back to the starting position, the band will help you less and less. This is the same accommodating resistance concept, just in reverse order.

Just think: If you have strong quads, odds are your quads are not getting a huge overload as you complete a squat; if your chest and anterior deltoids overpower your triceps, it will be very difficult to sufficiently overload your triceps with a compound movement like a close-grip bench press.

Whether it's chain resistance or reverse bands, you will now be able to effectively overload your triceps with a compound movement because of the additional resistance. As you lock the weight out, your triceps are the prime mover; at this point in the movement, they will be overloaded.

In a way, bands and chains can provide the benefit of a compound movement, but at the same time overload individual muscles in compliance with the principle of isolation. This is exciting, groundbreaking stuff for bodybuilders, so don't get left behind.

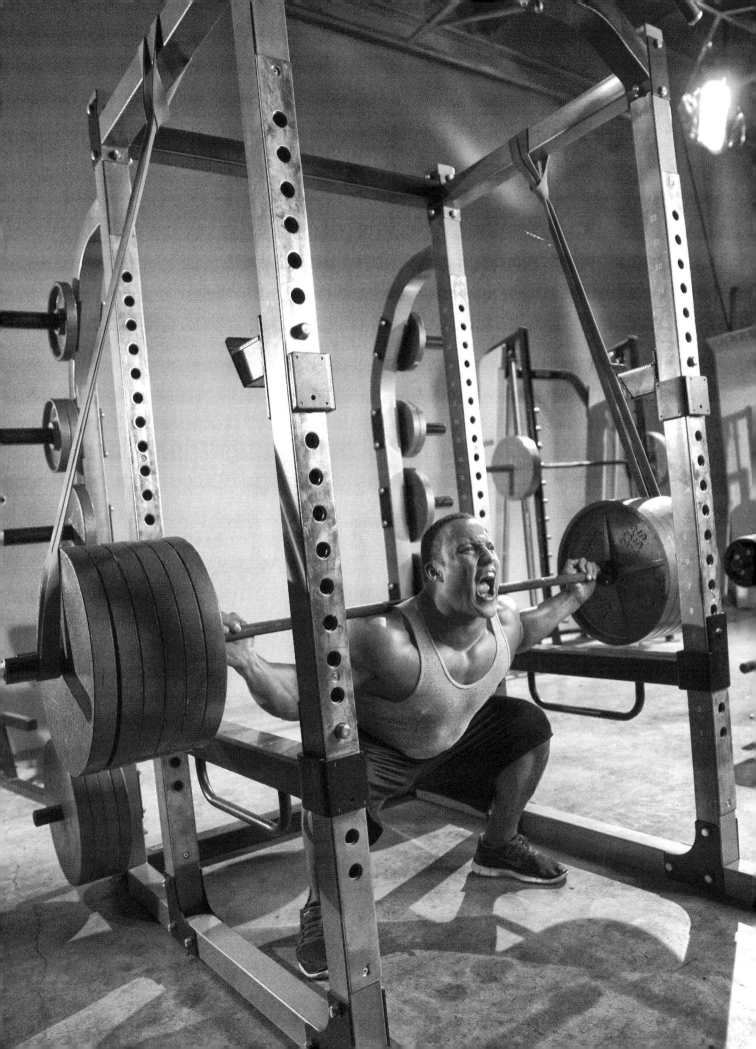

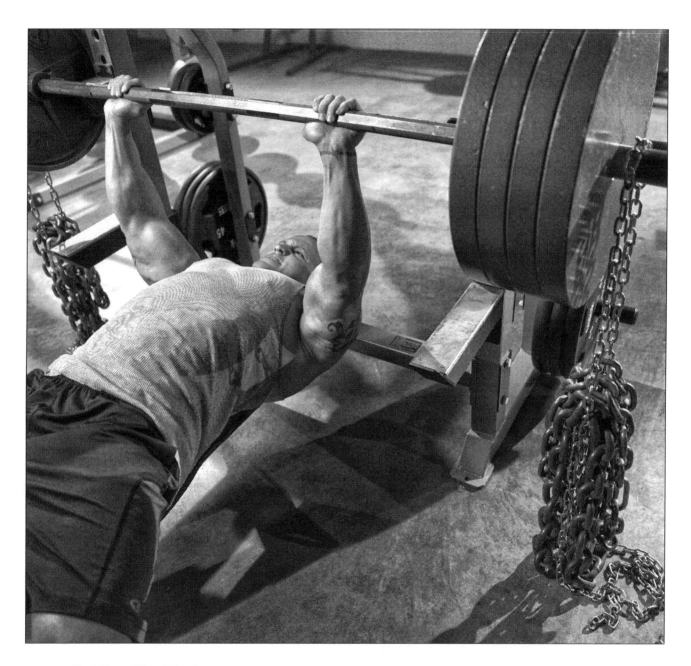

Setting Up Chains

Setting up chains is much easier than setting up bands. Double A Weightlifting Systems has made a device specifically for setting up chains. It's very helpful and has made my job training athletes much easier.

For the squat/bench, to attach the chains to the bar, most lifters use a smaller chain. The smaller chain allows you to form a loop and fasten the loop with a carabineer. You will attach the larger chain/chains to the loop. For the deadlift, if you do not have the Double A Weightlifting Systems device, just drape the chain over the barbell sleeve.

SOME KEY POINTS ABOUT BANDS AND CHAINS

- Bands cause an over-speed/more powerful eccentric part of the movement than chains do

- Chains feel much more like straight weight than bands

- It's easier to overtrain on bands than on chains

- It is easier to overtrain with bands and chains than with traditional resistance

- Avoid sets of more than 8 reps with bands

- Unlike chains, bands allow non-linear resistance (i.e., they can be attached to a pec dec or diagonal leg press and still work like they do with a linear barbell movement)

- Neither bands nor chains should be used more than 3 weeks in a row, because of potential overtraining

BANDS AND CHAINS IMPROVE STRENGTH CURVE

A human strength curve has seven distinct features that can be improved with the addition of bands and chains.

1. **Angle Q (starting strength).** The Angle Q involves starting strength (being able to turn on as many fibers as possible at once, instantaneously). Think throwing a punch as fast as possible or lifting a weight from a dead position in a rack, like a dead bench press. While acceleration can be "gradual," starting strength is not—it happens all at once. Compensatory Acceleration Training, plyometric training, or various Olympic lifts (assuming the athlete has proficient technique) could be used to enhance starting strength. So with bands and chains, if you do not start the weight with sufficient force, you will not be able to complete the repetition; every inch the bar moves, resistance increases, so poor starting strength is not an option with the addition of bands and chains.

2. **Sudbangles of A (acceleration).** Acceleration is best achieved by improving explosive strength (your ability to turn on as many muscle fibers as possible and leave them on). In the strength curve, the Angles of A should become greater and greater (positive acceleration). It comes down to one thing: To improve acceleration, you must compensatorily accelerate while you train! This means to lift the submaximal weight with maximal force. It should be noted that compensatory acceleration training (CAT) does have a big drawback: the negative acceleration phase, which is the deceleration of the bar over the final portion of the lift. Studies have shown that the bar can start to

decelerate up to 50% of the range of motion during CAT training. If you pull a deadlift as fast as possible, the final 50% may be decelerated because of your body's built-in safety mechanism. That's where bands and chains come into play. As an elastic band stretches off ground, resistance increases so you have to keep pulling with maximum force and acceleration. The same thing applies with chains: As each link comes off the bar, resistance increases. Bands and chains can essentially circumvent the negative acceleration phase of compensatory acceleration training. They also force you to use more muscle fibers; cruise control is not an option as leverage improves.

3. **Limit strength (your absolute limit of strength).** Limit strength is how much musculoskeletal force you can generate for one all-out effort. The only athlete who displays limit strength in competition is the powerlifter. As a bodybuilder, it is your base! *All* athletes do need a certain level of limit strength, and therefore it should be the first objective on your list in altering the strength curve. Bands and chains are very beneficial for enhancing limit strength, as countless studies now show. Think about it logically: Can you half squat or full squat more? Of course you can half squat more. A full squat will provide sufficient overload on the bottom portion of the lift, but certainly not on the top half. How can we overcome this? Simple: by adding bands or chains; as leverage improves, resistance increases, so more force (rather than a deceleration) is required to complete the lift. Furthermore, this continuous tension provided is similar to what a cable does, yet you still retain the benefit of the free weight movement, unlike the cable.

4. **Amortization (the brief period between the eccentric and concentric contraction).** The amortization phase is that brief moment between the eccentric and concentric contraction. When squatting, this is the brief period between descent and ascent. Bands particularly cause an over-speed effect on the eccentric phase of a movement: A fast movement produces a fast countermovement. Because of this, the efficiency of the amortization phase is enhanced.

5. **F-max (maximum amount of force produced).** Because of the negative acceleration phase with CAT training with straight barbell weight, ultimately the amount of force you produce in your strongest portion of the lift (think the top half of the squat after you come out of the hole) is compromised. This is your body's built-in safety mechanism. Bands and chains are a game changer; you have to continually produce more force to keep the weight moving concentrically because the bands/chains are continuing to increase in resistance.

6. **T-max (the time it takes to reach F-max).** As a barbell with a band or chain is lifted, additional resistance, as discussed, is rapidly applied. Because of additional resistance and the effect of the over-speed eccentric, the time allotted to reach maximum-force output is reduced. This is the relationship that Soviet sports scientists worshipped.

7. **F/T (the relationship between F-max and T-max, or "power").** Because more force can be produced with additional band and chain resistance, with a faster rate of forced development (RFD), bands greatly enhance power production; studies overwhelmingly confirm this.

Science, as well as obvious anecdotal evidence from the trenches, confirms the effectiveness of bands and chains for becoming more powerful. Let's look at how this directly benefits your muscle building quest by comparing a full-range-of-motion deadlift to a quarter-rack pull (a quarter top-end range-of-motion deadlift). You can obviously handle much more weight for a quarter rep than for a full rep. By adding bands or chains to the bar, as you lift the weight toward lockout, every inch of the way has additional resistance applied to the barbell. This means the rep will be challenging throughout the entire range of motion. Essentially, it is like a synergistic hybrid-blend exercise because you are getting the benefit of a full-range-of-motion exercise and essentially the benefits of an overload partial movement. Because of maximal overload throughout the entire movement, proper implementation will result in maximum muscle growth. Proper periodization is paramount to success because an exercise with additional band or chain resistance makes the exercise much higher intensity than the movement being performed in the traditional sense. Because of greater tension throughout the entirety of the movement, at no point can you put on cruise control.

Bands and chains can help injured lifters perform core movements through a full range of motion in some instances where they may not otherwise be able to perform.

Shoulder injuries are common among iron game veterans who have performed heavy pressing movements, year in, year out. Use the bench press as an example. Many of these lifters experience pain on the bottom portion of lift, so in the past they have generally had the option of dropping the movement altogether or performing partials.

Once again, bands and chains are a game changer because the weight will be much less at the bottom portion of the lift (where it needs to be) and resistance will increase as the weight approaches the top end of the lift. This will help produce sufficient overload, along with letting this lifter continue to train injury free. The same can be said of deadlifts. Many lifters with lower back problems are able to perform deadlifts because of the lighter load off the bottom.

BANDS AND CHAINS FOR MORE THAN CORE MOVEMENTS

If you haven't already, I highly recommend you read Steve Holman's *Train Eat, Grow: The Positions-of-Flexion-Muscle-Training Manual.* Holman does a great job of describing three different kinds of movements.

The first type of movement discussed (referred to as mid-range movements) is compound movements. These movements target a large number of muscles and force them to work together to lift the weight. Synergists assist in lifting the weight.

A practical example would be the bench press. The target muscle is the chest, but the deltoids and the triceps play significant assisting roles. Because of this, the heaviest weights can be used, thus providing a maximal overload. These exercises provide the best bang for your buck; when building your base and bulking up, it is paramount to concentrate a majority of your efforts here.

Examples of these types of movements are:

Quads: Front Squats
Back: Deadlift
Shoulders: Overhead Press
Chest: Bench Press
Triceps: JM Presses
Biceps: Barbell Curls
Hamstrings: Romanian Deadlifts

Anyone who has spent any time around a hardcore gym or serious training facility has seen people use bands and chains on core movements like squats, bench presses, and deadlifts.

As discussed earlier, these devices can be advantageous to you, the bodybuilder. Generally, for raw powerlifters, I recommend using 10%–25% additional band or chain resistance for core movements.

Many times you will hear about powerlifters literally using more accommodated resistance than weight on the bar. The issue here (and what you don't read in the fine print) is that these lifters literally double the amount of weight they can legitimately lift without supportive equipment.

The first man to "bench press" 1,000 pounds in competition with supportive gear could reportedly bench press 550 raw without his super suit. Another lifter dropped from an over 1,200-pound squat in gear to 600 pounds raw in competition.

As bodybuilders, we are trying to work the muscle, not manipulate equipment and leverage for a competitive situation or to satisfy the ego.

Generally, bodybuilders will do well within these recommendations for raw powerlifters. Of course, if you are going for a specific overload effect, you might go outside these guidelines; just keep in mind that, with an excessive amount of band tension and the over-speed effects it causes on the eccentric portion of the movement, you will be sore and will take longer to recover.

The same holds true with doing very high reps with band resistance. A general recommendation is to do fewer than 8 reps; if you exceed this number, you will have more success with chains.

STRETCH MOVEMENTS

These movements put a muscle at a position of maximal elongation. The idea is to activate the stretch reflex so you can recruit muscle fibers that may not have been directly hit with the compound movement.

Stretch position movements are theorized to produce a very favorable IGF-1 response, a very anabolic hormone. While hyperplasia has not been proven 100% in humans, many believe that stretch movements would have the best chance of inducing it.

Some examples are:

Biceps: Incline Dumbbell Curls (palms supinated the whole time)
Triceps: French Press
Hamstrings: Stiff Leg Deadlifts (also a compound movement)
Chest Dumbbell Flyes

CONTRACTED EXERCISES

I like to call these peak contraction exercises because constant tension is placed on the muscle throughout the movement.

A great example of this type of movement is the idea of a cable or accommodated resistance in general. Basically, as leverage improves, resistance increases; so the muscles have to contract maximally throughout the entire movement, not just in optimal leverage positions.

Usually, when bodybuilders talk about feeling reps, squeezing reps, and shaping reps, they are referring to peak contraction style movements. The whole idea is to feel the muscle, not ballistically perform the movement.

Here are some examples:

> Triceps: Triceps Push-downs
> Biceps: Cable Concentration Curls
> Chest: Cable Flyes
> Lats: Stiff-Arm Pull-downs

You have to hit muscles from different angles to maximize your physique. It will require compound movements, exercises performed in a stretched position, and, of course, peak contraction ones.

Exercises that have classically fallen into one of these categories with the addition of bands and chains can cross over and suddenly fit into two of these categories. This makes the sum greater than the individual parts, producing a wonderful synergy, and you will have one up on your competitors.

Here are some practical examples for the chest.

Dumbbell Band Resisted Flyes

You will put a resistance band around your back, holding it in your hands. You will also place a dumbbell in each hand while the resistance band is still across your hand. You still receive the maximal stretch the solid, dead pig iron provides, but as you squeeze the dumbbells together you now get a peak contraction-like effect. Dumbbells give a maximum stretch, solidly hitting the outer pecs. But as you squeeze them together, you basically go on cruise control, getting robbed of a true peak contraction. Bands change this—you now get that. Give this synergistic chest builder a try!

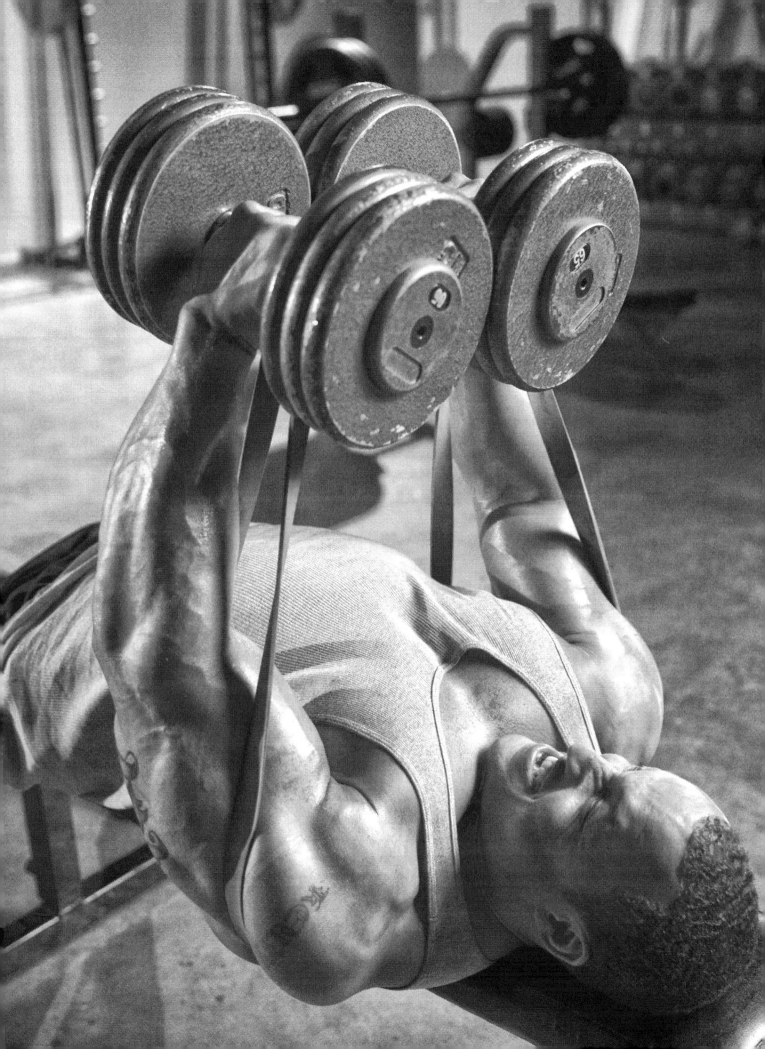

Chain Flyes

Flyes are undoubtedly a great chest exercise. However, they may fall on the risk side of the risk-to-benefit ratio for bodybuilders with shoulder problems because of the excessive strain in the stretch position.

Many bodybuilders in the situation will opt to train only with cables or mainly a pec deck. Chain flyes change that. Chain flyes are performed by attaching the same handles you use to perform cable crossovers to chains. You still get some of the stretch you feel with dumbbells that are lost with cables, but it is very moderate in comparison. As your arms abduct to the fully stretched position, the chains unload on the floor, removing much of the strain from the shoulders. As you adduct or squeeze your arms back together, the chains start to lift off the floor again, giving you the peak-contraction advantage of the cables.

A FEW LAST WORDS

There are plenty of other movements where bands and chains can be used, whether it is a band-resisted bar dip or doing drop-set chin-ups with multiple chains; as you fail, pull off chains and keep going. It might be chains on a barbell curl, bands on a leg press, or close grip bench press with chains. There are endless possibilities.

Remember, to be the best you are going to have to change with times, and the new frontier of bands and chains is here. Use them for great results.

SOURCES

Fleck, Steven J., and Kraemer, William J. *Designing Resistance Training Programs.* 3rd ed. Champaign, IL: Human Kinetics Publishers, 1997.

Hatfield, Frederick C. *Specialist in Sports Conditioning.* Santa Barbara: International Sports Sciences Association, 2001. (Unpublished ISSA edition.)

Zatsiorsky, Vladimir. *Science and Practice of Strength Training.* Champaign, IL: Human Kinetics Publishers, 1995.

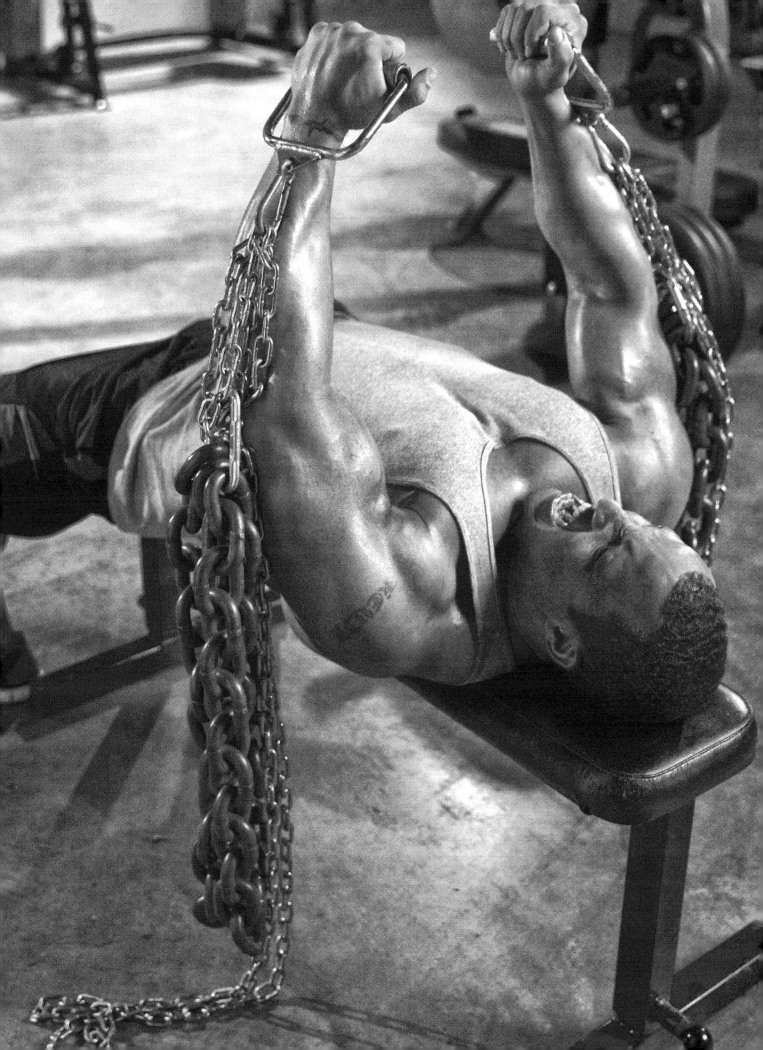

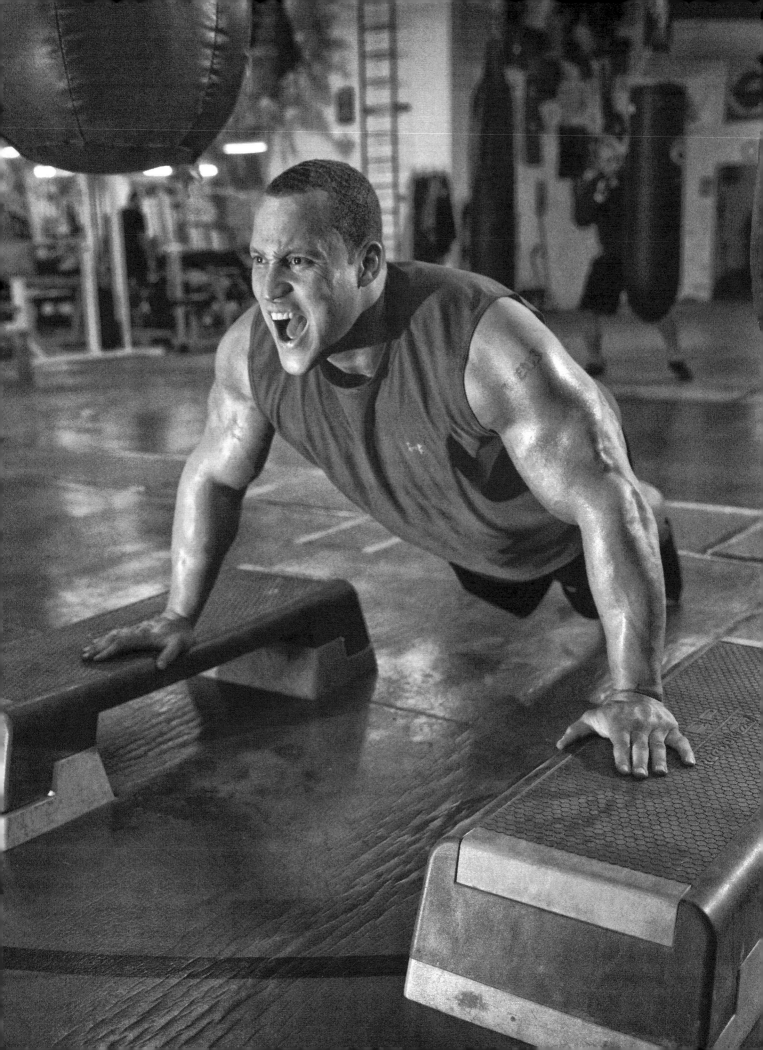

CHAPTER 7.

Aerobic Training

Aerobics are gospel to some in the fitness industry, yet to others aerobics is the complete antithesis of muscle building.

One camp tells us over and over about the proven benefits of aerobic training like strengthened heart, decreased body fat, lowered blood pressure, and lowered cholesterol, not to mention the claims that it synergistically helps prevent depression, disease, and even onset of osteoporosis, while increasing a sense of well-being.

The other camp believes that aerobic exercise decreases testosterone production, increases cortisol production, lowers immune system efficiency, decreases limit strength, and severely handicaps potential muscle gains from strength training.

With all this conflicting data, what is a bodybuilder to do?

The answer is certainly not to spend hours performing high-intensity aerobic exercises.

Studies have shown that intense aerobic exercise performed over long durations can greatly increase cortisol levels and oxidative stress; in other words, long-term aerobics performed at a high intensity will suppress your immune system and open up the catabolic door, counter to your muscle-building goals.

A 2004 study published in the *Canadian Journal of Applied Physiology* showed rats that swam intensely 3 hours a day, 5 days a week, for a period of 4 weeks, not only experienced decreased testosterone levels but, in fact, experienced a decrease in size of testes and other accessory sex organs. Next time someone wants you to run in the half marathon, your "no" answer can be backed by the science of shrinkage! I am, of course, joking; and this study does not give you license to avoid conditioning at all costs, but it would be unfair of me not to mention it.

Low testosterone levels can sabotage the potential gains in muscle mass. Besides decreased motivation and increased lethargy, hormones influence everything indirectly. With a less-than-adequate production of testosterone, your gains will be sub-optimal.

Studies have shown that aerobics in excess can potentially lower testosterone levels. One 2001 study published in the *Journal of Xi'an Institute of Physical Education* showed that moderate aerobic exercise did not have detrimental effects on testosterone levels.

Some studies show the superiority of aerobic training for fat loss over resistance training, others show a huge reduction in testosterone levels, and still others show virtually no effect.

The reason for conflicting information is study design.

Studies that show aerobic exercise as being superior to strength training for fat loss generally have subjects performing hours of intense cardiovascular exercise weekly, and the strength-training routine is rarely explained in detail.

Generally, the routine will be described as 3 sets of 15 reps, on whatever machine is popular at the time. Machines, while effective in some instances—for example, to overload a muscle through the principle of isolation—are generally inferior to barbells, dumbbells, and even bodyweight exercises. All stability is eliminated, and synergist muscles are robbed of the potential work performed.

Machines are generally performed in the most advantageous position: Leg presses are performed lying down, unlike the squat, which is performed standing. Except for isolation, machines are way easier! If we had to choose between machines and free weights, the choice would be simple: free weights; more work is performed.

This is study design flaw number one!

Secondly, aerobic protocols consist of specific parameters and variables (i.e., 45–60 minutes of swimming performed at 75% of heart rate max for 6 weeks straight, 5 times weekly). As your conditioning increases, 75% of your max heart rate will be adaptable; initially, you may have performed 30 laps at this intensity, but by the end of the study you may be completing 40+. As you adapt, the amount of volume you perform increases, even though relative intensity does not.

This variable adjustment is not made with resistance training. Besides, three sets of 15 reps with 50% of your one-repetition max on a machine are easy. Unless the subject is 100%

"green," no sort of overload will take place. In all seriousness, who in their right mind takes one-repetition maxes on a machine? Fifteen repetitions on the squat with 70% of your one repetition max will have your muscle fibers screaming.

There are many reasons why aerobic training protocols perform better on paper. Sometimes, it is outright bias!

If it came down to resistance training or aerobic exercise for improved health and body composition for a middle-aged client, resistance training reigns superior.

Obviously, this is a no-brainer for the bodybuilder.

After weight training, your metabolism is boosted for up to 36 hours, unlike with aerobics, so you will literally burn more calories while you sit and relax or even sleep. A few extra calories an hour for 36 hours, over the long haul, will add up.

Furthermore, each additional pound of muscle can burn up to 50 extra calories a day. Not to mention aerobic training benefits can be attained through intense PHA or circuit training. Strength-training benefits cannot be attained through aerobic training. It's not just calories burned during exercises, it's what happens after.

Outright bias sometimes plays a role in flawed study design.

Dr. Kenneth Cooper, who founded the Cooper Clinic in 1967, published the book *Aerobics*. Cooper and others like him pushed an aerobics-first agenda using selective science to help advance their dogma. Because of initial leaders like this in physical culture post World War II, Americans have always been spoon-fed the idea of aerobic superiority for health. Icons like John Grimek and Bill Pearl, who countered this notion, never received the mainstream acceptance of Cooper.

Obviously, with all these negatives associated with aerobic training, no sort of long, slow cardio has any place in the regimen of serious bodybuilders, right?

Not exactly.

Things are not black and white.

The studies that show the ill effects of muscle hypertrophy, anabolic hormonal deficiency, and decreases in strength have some commonalities. What it comes down to is that intense cardiovascular exercise for more than 30 minutes at above 75% max heart rate intensity, with a frequency of 3 times or greater a week, will be counterproductive to strength and muscle gains. An easy way to estimate max heart is 220 minus your age; so if you are 20 years old, $220 - 20 = 200$ max heart rate.

Long jogs are out as a way to optimally increase strength and muscle mass. Walking is great, but it does not constitute intense aerobics. And if your heart rate is over 150 simply when taking a leisurely walk, the programs and strategies outlined in the book may be way too intense for you, so please consult your physician before using these strategies.

Walking is a great leisure activity. Make it fun instead of slaving away on the treadmill. On days you are not training, go outside, get some fresh air, and even take the dog along. There is no need to spend hours on the treadmill to get lean. Interval training a few times a week, coupled with 20–30 minutes of walking 2–3 times a week, will keep you healthy, happy, lean, and mean. Shoot for keeping your heart rate in the 55%–70% range of your max heart rate.

Here are some benefits of aerobic activity, like moderate walking a few times a week:

- Increased general physical preparedness (GPP)
- Decreased delayed onset of muscle soreness (DOMS), thus enhancing recuperation
- Increased heart health
- Decreased stress
- Help in maintaining healthy joints/muscles
- Decreased body fat
- Increased energy levels

INTERVAL CONDITIONING

The conditioning fat loss wars people seem to fall into are two extremist camps. When it comes to conditioning for fat loss, there is the traditional long, slow cardio camp and, of course, the group that avoids the word "aerobic" like a deadly plague.

In 1994, at the Physical Activities Science Laboratory at Laval University in Canada, Angelo Tremblay and some of his colleagues tested the long-held belief among most exercise and medical professionals that long, slow cardio at a low intensity is superior for fat loss. In fact, they compared the impact of moderate/low intensity to high intensity interval training in hopes of finding what was superior for fat loss.

One group did 20 weeks of endurance training while the other group did 15 weeks of high-intensity interval training. The cost of total energy expenditure was much higher in the endurance-training group than in the interval group.

Additionally, Tremblay and his associates found that the endurance group burned nearly *twice* the amount of calories during training than did the interval group. Lo and behold, skin-fold measurements showed the interval training group lost more body fat than the endurance-training group.

This may not seem to make sense at first glance. However, the team found, "When the difference in the total energy cost of the program was taken into account... the subcutaneous fat loss was nine fold greater in the HIIT (interval training) program than in the ET (endurance training) program."

In layman's terms, interval training trumped long, slow cardio for fat loss!

The interval trainees got nine times the fat loss for every calorie burned during training.

The Laval University researchers found that metabolic adaptations that resulted from interval training may lead to enhanced lipid utilization post exercise, effectively accelerating fat loss.

Fat is the fuel for lower-intensity exercise, and carbohydrates are the fuel for higher-intensity intervals. While excess dietary fat can cause unwanted fat gain, so can excess in carbohydrates. This study confirms the need to look beyond the scope of what macronutrient is fueling the workout, or how many calories are burned during the workout. We must also look at what happens post-workout. Intervals stimulate your post-workout metabolism much more greatly than long, slow cardio. Additionally, studies have shown intense intervals have increased anabolic hormones post-workout.

This is why interval training has so many die-hard advocates and supporters. Science confirms that interval training is highly effective for fat loss. "Compare the physiques of top-level sprinters to top-level distance runners" is a simplistic, logical response many give when asked why they feel interval training is superior.

Izumi Tabata has conducted research for the National Institute of Fitness and Sports in Tokyo, Japan. In terms of aerobic benefits, Tabata demonstrated that a program of 20 seconds of all-out cycling followed by 10 seconds of low intensity cycling for 4 minutes was as beneficial as 45 minutes of long, slow cardio!

Tabata training is now a popular form of interval training that includes performing an activity all-out for 20 seconds, followed by a 10 second rest interval. Some popular methods of Tabata training include jumping rope, burpees, and kettlebell swings, along with many others. Numerous studies also confirm the effectiveness of interval training as an enhancement to aerobic capacity.

At this point, it probably sounds like a no-brainer; just do interval training all the time and get lean.

Not so fast.

Muscle grows from exercise via muscle damage, mechanical tension, and metabolic stress. Intervals generally work the same way, so they must be treated with respect.

The CNS is primarily affected by high-intensity work and takes at least 48 hours to recover, so interval training requires adequate recovery very similar to intense resistance training.

Interval training, in the true sense, is all-out.

The studies that confirm the effectiveness of interval training have subjects performing intervals with 100% intensity. From personal problems to intense training, all impose stress on you; when the right amount of stress is imposed from training, you adapt and improve. Remember, if you are training intensely multiple times per week and have a full-time job and a family, stressors are acting upon you in all directions. Without proper planning, training will no longer serve as a catalyst to meet your physical goals; it will break you down.

The more your training evolves, the more stress you impose on yourself. Studies have actually shown that the more weight someone can lift, the longer the recovery time needed.

If you can squat 200 pounds for a max, 75% of your max is 150 pounds; you may need only a couple of minutes to fully recover from a set of 10 reps. For a 700-pound squatter, 75% would be 525 pounds; over 5 minutes may be needed to fully recover.

While the relative percentage is the same, in reality squatting 525 pounds for reps will place a much greater strain on your CNS and musculoskeletal system than doing it with 150 pounds. The stronger you get, the less interval training you will be able to handle because of the heavy loads handled in training.

A beginning bodybuilder may be able to do 3 days a week of interval training, whereas a more advanced bodybuilder may be able to do only 1–2 days a week or none at all; high intensity, high volume strength training with short rest intervals is interval training in itself. Adaptations to your training are a consolidation of imposed stressors, which determine your muscle gains, fat loss, and strength levels.

Like intense resistance training, extreme stress is placed on the central nervous system and musculoskeletal system. Look at sprinters. They produce huge force while sprinting, and this places a large amount of stress on muscles, connective tissue, and the CNS.

Now imagine a 275-pound bodybuilder sprinting.

Be careful!

If you have health problems or have not been training on a regular basis, think twice about implementing intervals, and consult your physician before beginning interval training. The risk of overuse injuries will drastically increase if intervals are overdone. Rushing into these types of workouts before you have a sufficient base will great increase your chance of injury. Start slowly. Try just one or two high-intensity intervals at first. As conditioning improves, begin to challenge yourself.

Here are some interval training examples:

Barbell Complexes

You want to find out what you are made of? Try barbell complexes. Not only are these one of the greatest metabolic conditioners and fat loss modalities, they are also one of the best tests of pure guts. Time to "put up or shut up!"

If you are doing barbell complexes and find they are not challenging, you are not loading the bar with enough weight or not giving a sufficient effort. Barbell complexes potentially serve as a viable alternative to sprints for heavier athletes.

Barbell complexes are performed as quickly as possible, moving exercise to exercise with no break.

To construct a complex, you may do 5–8 squats, followed by 5–8 squats to presses, followed by 5–8 good mornings, followed by 5–8 power cleans, followed by 5–8 bent over rows, and finally finished off with 5–8 deadlifts.

The beauty of barbell complexes is they can be arranged somewhat specific to the muscle group being worked; if you train legs Monday and chest Tuesday, it would be counterproductive to do very intense intervals that emphasize legs and lower back; this will not allow the muscles to recover.

On a leg day, a barbell complex might look something like this: overhead squats, squats, reverse lunges, front squats, and Romanian deadlifts. On a back day, it might look something like this: good mornings, power cleans, hang cleans, deadlifts, and bent over row.

Sound tough? Your fortitude will be in for a test.

Some points to remember when performing complexes:

- Use compound exercises
- Perform exercises as fast as possible while maintaining proper technique
- Do not rest between exercises
- Try your best not to drop the bar
- Start with an empty bar and add weights in increments of 5 or 10 pounds
- Do 5–7 exercises per complex, each set consisting of 5–8 repetitions

- Rest 1 to 3 minutes between sets, do not exceed 4 sets, do not exceed 15 minutes' total duration

- Barbell complexes are intense interval workouts and are included in your total of interval workouts

Zen and the Art of Variable Manipulation

When progressing through barbell complexes, be intelligent in how you increase intensity! Just piling more pig iron on the bar every session will result in cessation of progress.

These are some variables you can manipulate to increase intensity:

- Rest periods—decreasing the rest periods increases intensity. If a 3-minute rest interval is becoming easy, try using the same weight but decreasing the rest interval between complexes; knock off 15–30 seconds between each session, eventually working down to a 1-minute rest interval. All of a sudden you are accomplishing 4 complexes in the same amount of time it used to take to do 2.

- Weight on the bar—increasing weight on the bar increases intensity. But remember, if you cannot complete more than one set, decrease the bar weight.

- Number of sets—increasing number of sets increases intensity. After you get up to 4 complexes, pile on more pig iron.

Barbell complexes can expedite fat loss but also expedite overtraining; I do not suggest you do them more than twice a week. These will test you mentally and physically. I have given you some practical examples, so try those. I have also laid out the variables taken into account when designing a complex. Play around and find out what works best for you.

Strongman Training

While top strongman competitors carry a much higher body fat percentage than top bodybuilders, many carry a much larger amount of lean body mass.

Strongman events are conducive for building muscle because they are very heavy, inducing extreme mechanical tension. Strongman events also cause enormous amounts of metabolic stress; generally, they take place for 30–60 seconds. Moreover, the movements are compound and cause extreme muscle damage. Svend Karlsen and Juoko Ahola look like lean, off-season bodybuilders, while Mariusz Pudzianowski basically looks like a competition bodybuilder year round, but bigger. Still need proof? Google images of Derek Poundstone or Bill Kazmaier, and you will have a whole new picture of what muscle hypertrophy looks like.

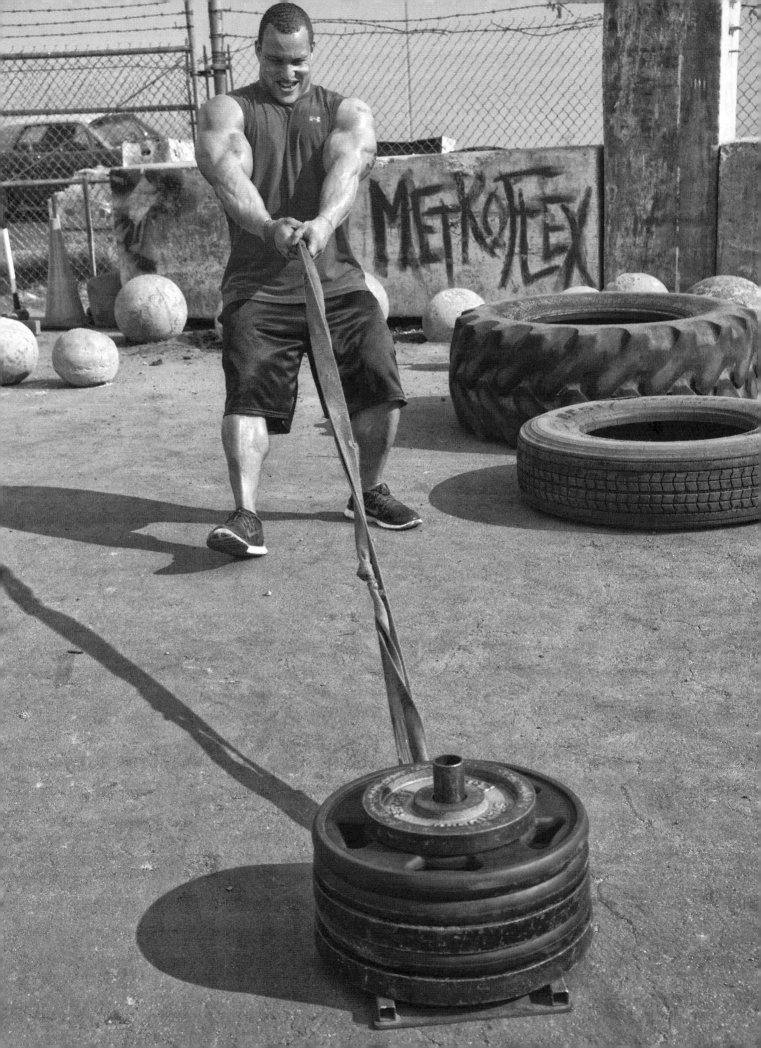

Strongman events can also be great for conditioning/fat loss as a finisher at the end of your workout and also aid in the muscle building process.

Here is an example of some strongman events that can be used as finishers in your training and what day they will correspond to:

Legs Day

Backward Sled Drags—facing the sled, lean back and pull with arms straight (never bend them). This has a huge emphasis on the quads. Perform 20–40 yards, 2–6 sets.

Forward Sled Drags—facing away from the weight, walk forward taking large steps, maintaining an upright posture. This has emphasis on glutes and hamstrings. Perform 20–40 yards, 2–6 sets.

Lateral Sled Drags—these can be performed with the sled attached to a weightlifting belt. Stand sideways to the sled and step laterally. This primarily targets the gluteus medius, but the gluteus minimus, tensor fascia latae (TFL), and sartorius play important assisting roles.

Other events like yoke and front yoke could be used. I included ones that most people will have access to.

Back Day

Farmers Walk—this will build the entire back, traps, and even forearms because of the grip. If you do not have access to farmers walk, implement by simply using dumbbells. Perform 2–4 sets for 20–50 yards. To make the exercise more difficult, add a turn.

Tire Flips—The best thing about tires is that they are free! Tires cost money for disposal, so anyone with used ones will be happy for you to take them off your hands. Tires work the entire body, particularly the posterior chain (back side of the body), and build explosive power. Do 5–8 flips for 2–4 sets. *Do not bend your arms* when lifting a tire off the ground; this exposes your biceps to an exacerbated chance of injury. Bicep tears are a common injury with tires, so proceed with caution.

Legs and back are the most common muscles used in strongman, but other techniques can be employed for other muscle groups. Other examples could be curl sled drags for biceps, crucifix hold for shoulders, and chest incline log press for chest.

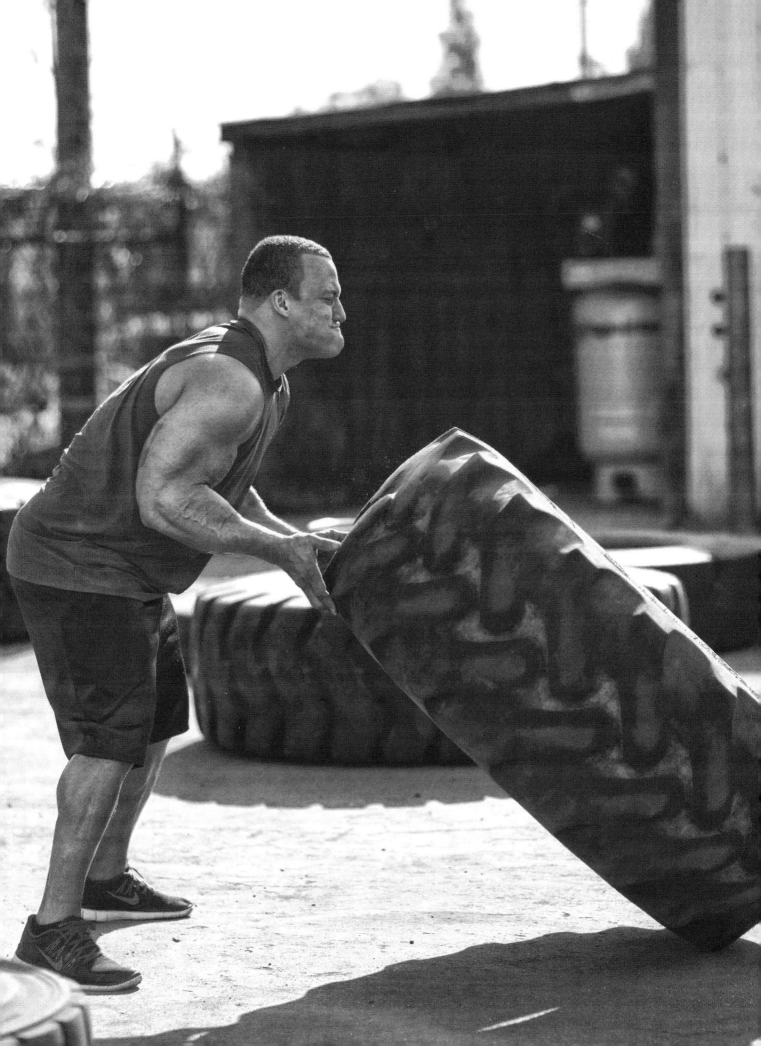

You are not trying to become a strongman, but some unorthodox training can produce some unorthodox results. Remember, the Wright Brothers were not aeronautical engineers, yet they were the first to fly. Sometimes superior results require outside-the-box techniques.

Kettlebell Interval Training

In the fitness industry, things run in extremes. Just take a look at flexibility; studies have shown static stretching pre-workout decreases force production, yet now some advocate if you ever stretch you will be weak and prone to injury.

On the other side are those who believe that yoga is more important to MMA fighters than sparring. Think of the other extremes: no carbs, low fat, BOSU balls, and the list goes on, my friends.

Kettlebells fall into this extremist camp.

Many times advocates will imply you can develop the endurance of a marathon runner, physique of a bodybuilder, strength of an elite powerlifter, flexibility of a yoga instructor, and speed of a world-class sprinter without pig iron or any other modalities.

This is false!

Kettlebells look sort of like a shot put or cannon ball with a handle welded to the top. For centuries, kettlebells have been used for strength training by top Russian athletes and for stress relief by those rotting in gulags.

If you are not sure what a kettlebell is, think of the old-time cartoons, like Bugs Bunny, where strongmen tossed around those odd shaped cannon balls with handles.

In the days of yesteryear, circus strongmen used these implements as part of their acts. Today, many folks are integrating kettlebell training into their strength and conditioning regimens.

Could they possibly benefit for fat loss?

Advocates of kettlebell training are quick to point out that kettlebells can simultaneously build core stability, coordination, endurance, strength, power, and flexibility.

Okay, but what about fat loss?

A recent study at the University of Wisconsin–LaCrosse demonstrated that intense kettlebell intervals burn calories at the same rate as a mile run at a 6-minute pace (that is, 1,200 calories an hour). Clearly, fat loss is a byproduct of intense kettlebell training.

Another study commonly cited to show the effectiveness of kettlebell training was conducted in 1983 by Aleksey Voropayev, famed Russian gymnast and researcher. This study showed that for a group of male soldiers, kettlebell training was more effective than traditional military training techniques.

In this study, one group followed a standard military regimen of chin-ups, 100-meter sprints, standing broad jumps, and distance runs. The other group used nothing but kettlebells and kettlebell training. Interestingly, at the end of the experiment, the kettlebell group scored higher on every exercise in which they were tested.

This study demonstrated that kettlebells not only enhanced the strength tests, as one would guess, but additionally increased endurance and power. This may explain why some believe that kettlebells are the magic bullet. Kettlebells are certainly not the magic bullet for bodybuilding, but they are fun and can help you burn body fat.

Three effective kettlebell exercises are clean and jerks, snatches, and swings. Here is a good circuit for conditioning and fat loss; complete the circuit without a break:

- 10 Kettlebell Swings
- 30 seconds of Jump Rope
- 5 Clean and Jerks (each side)
- 30 seconds of Jump Rope
- 5 Snatches (each side)
- 30 seconds of Jump Rope

Follow this circuit with a 1–4-minute break and repeat the circuit 3 times. Remember, these circuits are an intense form of interval training, if you give 100%. These count in your weekly total of interval workouts, so don't try and do a barbell complex twice a week, and then do this circuit 2–3 times. All intense training is a stressor; without recovery, you will be in a perpetual catabolic state.

Jumping Rope

The iconic image of the old pug getting ready for a prize fight by skipping rope is a beautiful image. Prize fighters have reaped the benefits of jumping rope for centuries. Jumping rope can burn up to 1,000 calories per hour, making it one of the most efficient fat-burning workouts available.

Unlike other forms of interval training that are much more stressful on the CNS, muscles and connective tissues are also spared significant stress while jumping rope.

Furthermore, jumping rope tones muscles throughout the entire body and develops lean muscles in all major muscle groups. Of course, jumping rope optimizes conditioning and maximizes athletic skills by combining agility, coordination, timing, and endurance. Most importantly for you, it can help burn body fat.

Jumping rope is very practical because, unlike advanced kettlebell exercises, the learning curve is easy. Jump-ropes are portable and inexpensive and can be purchased for less than $10. If you go on vacation, throw your jump-rope in your bag and you have no excuse to not do your conditioning work.

For your jump-rope program, start by jumping rope 30 seconds and resting 1 minute for 6 sets. Depending on ability, add 10 seconds per week or workout. Make it your goal to complete 6 sets of 3 minutes of jump rope, with a 30-second rest interval. When you are able to complete 6 sets of 3 minutes, body fat will have melted off and conditioning will be at a whole new level.

A FEW LAST WORDS

Old-time bodybuilding champions did much less cardio than many do today. There is no reason to spend hours a day doing long, slow cardio like some bodybuilders do.

The reason many of them are able to get away with this is because of drugs. These substances can literally change human physiology—both long and short term—and as many have discovered, not for the better. Countless studies show endurance athletes have much lower testosterone levels than their anaerobic counterparts, so if bodybuilding and packing on size and strength is your goal, endurance training should not be highest on your priority list.

Fat loss comes from strength training and dieting!

If you're depending on long, slow cardio or even interval training for fat loss, your body is telling you that your diet is not in check.

The age-old truth is still the same truth today: Strength training and diet are the keys to fat loss.

SOURCES

Bryant, Josh, and Brian Dobson. *Metroflex Gym Powerbuilding Basics*. Arlington, TX: JoshStrength.com, 2011.

"Fire Up Your Fat-Burning Furnace." (N.a.) *Joe Weider's Muscle & Fitness* 57, no. 1 (January 1996): 148. (Serial online.)

Kindermann, W., and A. Schnabel. "Catecholamines, Growth Hormone, Cortisol, Insulin, and Sex Hormones in Anaerobic and Aerobic Exercise." *European Journal of Applied Physiology and Occupational Physiology* 49, no. 3 (1982): 389–99.

Manna, I., K. Jana, and P. Samanta. "Intensive Swimming Exercise-Induced Oxidative Stress and Reproductive Dysfunction in Male Wistar Rats: Protective Role of Alpha-Tocopherol Succinate." *Canadian Journal of Applied Physiology* 29, no. 2 (2004), 172–85.

Thirumalai, T., and S. Viviyan Therasa, E. K. Elumalai, and E. David. "Intense and Exhaustive Exercise Induce Oxidative Stress in Skeletal Muscle." *Asian Pacific Journal of Tropical Disease* (April 2011): 63–66. http://apjtcm.com/zz/2011apr/16.pdf.

Tian Z. "Study on the Effect of Aerobic Exercise on Testosterone, Cortisol, High-Density Lipoprotein, Low-Density Lipoprotein, Angiotensin II and Myocardial Contractility in Rats." *Journal of Xi'an Institute of Physical Education* 18, no. 1 (2001): 28–31. Serial online.

Tremblay, Angelo. "Canadian Study." *Metabolism* 43 (1994): 814–18.

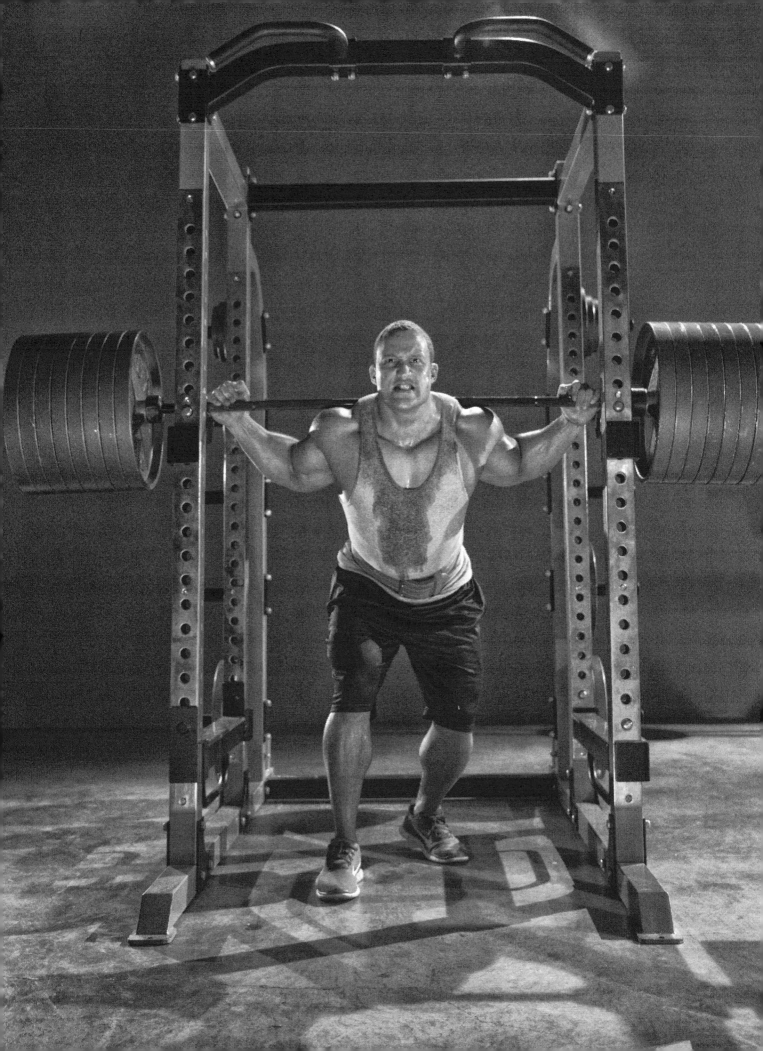

CHAPTER 8.

Injuries in
Bodybuilding

By Joe Giandonato, MS, CSCS

To the iron brethren, nothing is more demoralizing than falling victim to an injury. Those chasing milestone numbers in the gym might have their personal record journeys detoured or abruptly ended by an injury.

Competitive strength athletes, a group consisting of powerlifters, Olympic weightlifters, and strongman competitors, might be forced into an early retirement, or relegated to the purgatory of being the strongest person at their local commercial gym.

For bodybuilders, an injury might deliver a fatal blow to one's life on stage. Injuries might carry severe aesthetic implications that could prevent bodybuilders from ascending the competitive ranks.

Injuries, however, are largely preventable.

While the etiologies of common injuries will be discussed, the role of exercise, including the importance of adhering to proper form, incorporating corrective modalities such as self-myofascial release, and stretching, will also be discussed.

EXERCISE

Exercise is the catalyst of physiological and psychological change. Exercise in the form of strength training is capable of delivering immense gains in muscular strength and size as it triggers a cascade of neuroendocrine activity.

Strength training, like any other form of exercise, can be manipulated to achieve desired results. Bodybuilders enlist in the never-ending quest to maximize muscular hypertrophy.

Muscular hypertrophy is the expansion of a muscle's cross-sectional area, involving the concurrent increase in myofibrilar content; the accumulation of non-contractile matter, such as water, glycogen, and myoglobin, which are stored in the sarcoplasm of the muscle cell; and the densification of mitochondrial content.

Hypertrophy is achieved by exposing the muscle to stress, namely tension, via repeated external load. High-tension forces are experienced during eccentric muscle actions (i.e., descending into a squat or bringing the bar to your chest during a bench press). These eccentric muscle actions must be overcome with a concentric muscle action in order to complete the movement. These muscle actions are grouped together in blocks, which consist of sets and reps.

In order to yield continual progress, sets and reps, along with a plethora of soon-to-be-introduced overloading parameters, must be appropriately incorporated.

LOAD PROGRESSION

Load Progression entails the practice of simply adding weight to the bar. For example, say you performed 4 sets of 10 repetitions with 315 pounds on the barbell back squat during your last workout. For your upcoming workout, you would merely add weight to the bar, say 5 or 10 pounds, and perform the same number of sets and reps.

REPETITION PROGRESSION

The act of performing more repetitions per set with the same amount of weight previously used is another way you can challenge yourself and stimulate your muscles to respond. Instead of adding weight to the bar, you would again squat 315 pounds throughout all of your sets, but you would now add a repetition to each set, going from 10 repetitions per set to 11.

VOLUME PROGRESSION

If you do not want to increase the load or repetitions performed per set, you may tack on another set to your squat workout, going from 4 sets of 10 reps to 5 sets of 10 reps. More work is performed, therefore increasing the volume.

DENSITY PROGRESSION

Say you initially performed your squats interspersed with a rest period of 3 minutes, but were a bit short on time during your current workout. You could still use the same load you used in your previous workout but reduce the rest periods to elicit an improved training effect. Even seemingly nominal reductions in resting time will stimulate new growth. In fact, research indicates that shorter rest periods may maximize hypertrophy.

EXERCISE PROGRESSION

Advancing from one exercise to a different one that's more demanding is another way to challenge yourself and elicit new growth. Say you elected to perform front squats instead of back squats for your next workout but used the same load. Inevitably, you'd face a greater challenge using the same load for the front squats.

Additionally, intensification protocols such as supersets, drop sets, giant sets, and rest-pause sets, discussed earlier, could be implemented as method progression. Also, tempo progression, based on the Time Under Tension method, is yet another way you can challenge yourself.

Optimally, bodybuilders should permit ample time to accumulate new stress before intensifying. Novices should emphasize only one overloading parameter at a time. Concomitantly intensifying multiple overloading parameters or progressing too rapidly may result in injury.

Moreover, arbitrarily performing workouts throughout your training cycle, such as joining your buddies for an impromptu lift, typically disregarding progressive overload principles, may beget injury as well. Without a plan, you can plan on injury!

INJURIES

Simply stated, but just as easily ignored, is the fact that exercise breaks our bodies down. Rest and proper nutrition make our bodies and muscles stronger and bigger. If we fail to rest and refuel our bodies, we will make ourselves more vulnerable to injury.

Novice bodybuilders fall victim to a host of training mistakes. Most notably, novice bodybuilders mistakenly place a hefty premium on the loads they use for nearly every exercise. While continually progressing the load used on certain exercises is advisable, it frequently comes at the expense of good form among groups of novices.

As stated throughout the text, the quintessential pursuit of all bodybuilders is maximizing hypertrophy. Hypertrophy is achieved via mechanical tension, muscle damage, and metabolic stress, not by heaving barbells recklessly.

When form is compromised, ligamentous, cartilaginous, and osseous structures, which do not have contractile properties, are called into play to buffer the forces that muscles are designed to resist, which include tension, compression, extensibility, shear, and torsion. Injuries most indigenous to strength athletes affect bones, joints and their connective tissue, and muscles.

Bone Injuries

Bones provide the framework for our bodies. They cocoon organs and serve as the crux of our body's stability. Without bones we would die. Conditions that adversely affect bone health, such as osteoporosis, osteopenia, and chondromalacia, greatly impact quality of life. While exercise fortifies bone strength, exercise performed with poor form can slowly chip away at the bone's integrity.

Repeatedly performing heavily loaded squats, deadlifts, and overhead presses with less-than-stellar form might lead to the development of microfractures on the vertebral endplates of the spinal column.

Joint Injuries

Joints function as our body's movement centers. They are an intersection where collagen based structures, which include tendons, cartilage, and ligaments, all meet as they collectively stabilize the rounded head of the bone within the capsule of the joint.

Accrued stress from improperly performed and/or programmed exercise taxes these joint structures, while your collagen's water-containing extracellular matrix dries up, causing it to lose pliability as you age.

Articular cartilage, slivers of collagenous matter that encapsulates the ends of bones and permits seamless articulation, slowly begins to dry up as we age. Improperly performed exercise and poor program design can accelerate the degradation of collagen tissue.

Skeletal Muscle Injuries

Skeletal muscles serve as our body's first line of defense as they dissipate external forces imposed on the body. They surround and attach to bones via tendinous insertions, which they pull on to generate movement. When functioning properly, they keep our body's skeletal scaffolding upright and stable.

Additionally, muscles insulate our vital organs and assist with bodily functions such as respiration and digestion. Strong muscles may also compensate for weaker bones and joints. Since they are our body's first line of defense, they are more commonly injured than bones and joints.

Muscle injuries, which can be categorized as either acute or overuse injuries, are commonly sustained by active individuals and athletes.

Acute injuries can be further broken down into direct trauma and indirect trauma. Direct trauma is typified by a contusion that damages the muscle fibers and may lead to vasoconstriction or a hematoma. These injuries are commonly associated with contact sports. Indirect trauma disrupts the muscle fibers without contact. Indirect trauma results from excessive mechanical stress via eccentric overload.

Lifts performed with high loads, or those exceeding 70% of one's one-repetition maximum, have four phases. An *acceleration phase* is followed by a *deceleration phase*, also known as the "sticking point." A lifter who can successfully move through the sticking point will kick off another *acceleration phase* before hitting a final *deceleration phase* while completing the movement. If at any point the lifter cannot progress through one of the aforementioned phases, momentary muscular fatigue will be reached, which may precipitate mechanical stress that the muscle is not yet conditioned to handle.

Muscles are at the greatest risk of sustaining injury during an eccentric muscle action. That eccentric muscle action may occur prematurely, when the concentric muscle action is not great enough to resist gravitational and inertial forces.

Overuse injuries stem from repetitively performing a movement continuously and having an insufficient amount of rest between activities. Consequent adaptations are quite problematic. A muscle that is called on to work frequently may fatigue and call on neighboring muscles to pick up the slack and perform unintended roles.

In the general population, an example of such would be the sternocleidomastoid and the lateral flexors of the neck turning on and providing the neck stability, while the deep cervical flexors have either fatigued or aren't activated to keep the cervical spine stacked in its natural lordotic curve. Forward head posture results, and headaches soon follow.

Gym goers who fail to balance the force-couple relationship at the hip shared by the anterior core and posterior chain might end up relying on the muscles of the lower back for stability and movement.

AREAS OF CONCERN

Areas that are commonly riddled with overuse injuries among bodybuilders include the lower back, knees, elbows, and shoulders.

Lower Back

A tight lower back could inhibit neural drive to the glutes and hamstrings, which work in unison to extend and posteriorly rotate the hips. In the absence of hip extension, the body will try compensating with torso extension.

Ultimately an injury will occur if the bodybuilder is performing a deadlift variation with hundreds of pounds in his hands. The spine may contort and forcefully slip into extension as the bodybuilder completes his lift.

Lower back injuries that commonly afflict bodybuilders include spinal stenosis, which is a narrowing of the spinal canal, spondylolisthesis, which is characterized by slippage of the lumbar vertebral segments, and spondylosis, which is characterized by microfractures of the pars interarticularis, a section of the vertebra wedged between the articular processes of the facet joint.

Lastly, avulsion or herniation of the disc can occur, where the disc translates posteriorly, bearing down on the spinal nerves and creating unbearable pain. Typically, a lack of anterior core and posterior chain strength begets lower back injuries. If both of these areas are trained, the likelihood of suffering a lower back injury decreases.

Knees

The knees are two powerful, yet delicate hinge joints that are each overlapped by a dozen muscles, many of which share attachments with the hip. When the muscles that cross the knee or run alongside the femur, such as the adductors and IT band, become tight, knee alignment becomes altered.

Many old school bodybuilding programs heavily emphasize quadriceps training, practically ignoring the training of the posterior chain musculature, which includes the glutes and the hamstrings.

Insufficient hamstring extensibility and a lack of posterior chain strength won't permit a lifter to sit back into a squat properly and will impose shearing forces on the patella.

Compressive forces from tight muscles cause the patella to maltrack, forcing the foot and ankle to compensate. When the foot and ankle have to excessively pronate or supinate in response to what's going on above, movements that are influenced by quadriceps activity, such as jogging, walking, or gliding on an elliptical, are disrupted and may induce pain.

If the hip adductors (groin muscles) are too tight, and if the hip abductors and hip external rotators (lateral glute) are too weak, the ankle will collapse at the subtalar joint, causing pronation during static and dynamic activities. Tight hamstrings may enact more posterior force on the knee, forcing it to clamp down on the patella and the femur.

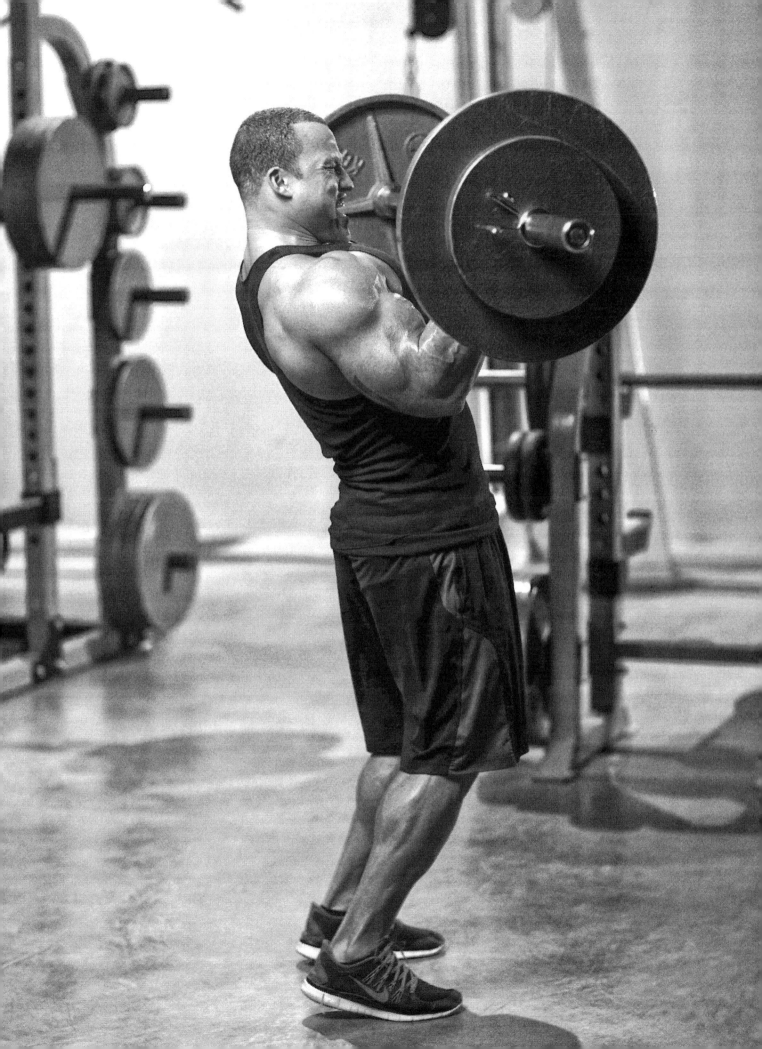

When muscles aren't firing properly or aren't working in unison to stabilize the knee, the body turns to the osteoligamentous structures for support. When an unstable knee is exposed to loaded dynamic exercises and high-impact activities, this spells a potential disaster.

All exercises performed from a standing position, such as squats, deadlifts, and presses, must be performed atop a stable base of support. The feet serve as the body's base of support.

Ideally, the feet should evenly distribute the person's bodyweight and external load throughout three points on the foot—the heel, the first metatarsal head, and the fifth metatarsal head.

Muscular imbalances further up the kinetic chain can interrupt this balanced foot position, making it difficult to get into position. If proper position cannot be achieved, the patella may mistrack and migrate laterally.

Ideally, the patella should track over the second and third metatarsal heads during all loaded activities, thus reducing the amount of stress imposed upon the knee.

Many bodybuilding programs tend to ignore the importance of posterior chain training and hamstring and adductor extensibility. Moreover, bodybuilding splits are designed to induce great amounts of mechanical stress to the muscle, from multiple angles, while not focusing on rather important aspects such as mobility, flexibility, and stability training.

Ideally, the time and effort spent developing the quadriceps should be equally matched with training the hamstrings and gluteals. If these groups are targeted, you can expect to use heavier poundages on squat and deadlift variations, as well as more mass on your wheels.

Elbows

The elbow is another powerful yet intricate hinge joint that often gets chewed up by the volume and variety of exercises that bodybuilders use in their training programs.

The elbow falls casualty to two common conditions, lateral and medial epicondylitis. Lateral epicondylitis occurs from repeated wrist supination and pronation with the elbows extended. Think performing pull-downs and rows with a supinated grip repeatedly. During the eccentric portion of the lift and through the return to the starting position, when the elbows fully extend, the muscles are still tensioned. Barbell presses, which lock the hands in a pronated position, stress the elbows at the end range of extension.

Medial epicondylitis stems from the overuse of the wrist flexors. Additionally, performing back squats with too narrow a hand placement on the bar, or routinely performing presses with a close grip, can exasperate the connective tissue of the elbows, contributing to inflammation and pain.

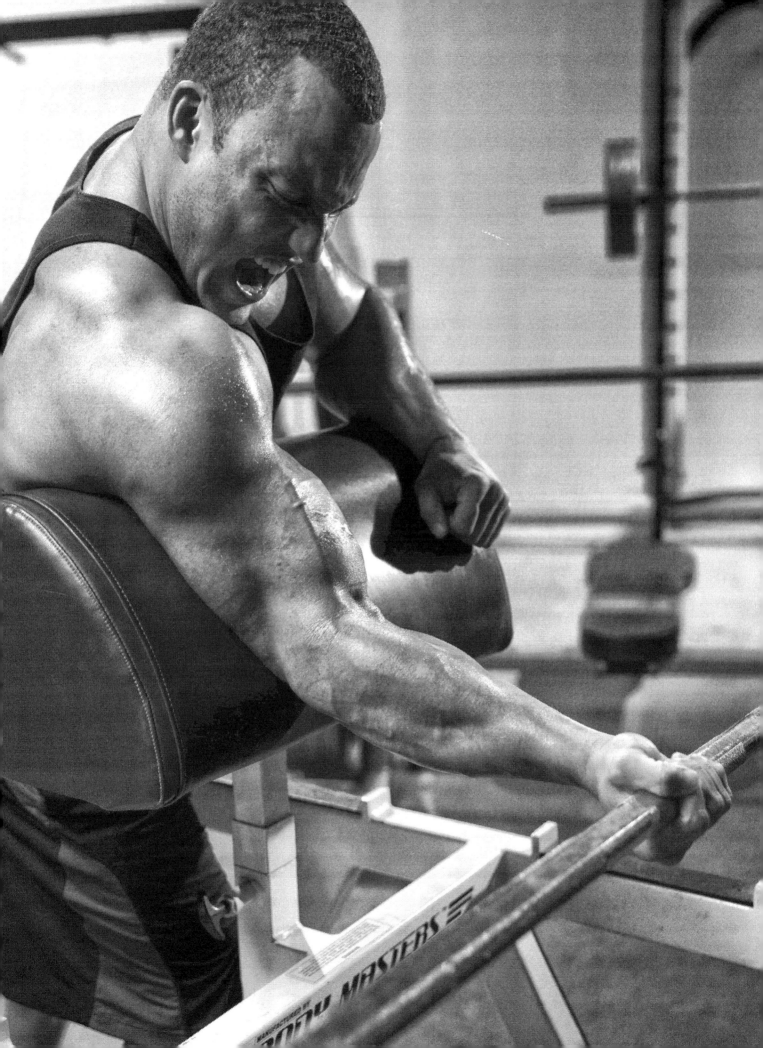

To alleviate elbow pain, bodybuilders should consider performing more rowing movements with rotating handles and dumbbells, pulling movements utilizing suspension systems, rings, and straps, and pressing movements with dumbbells and multi-handled bars.

While you might not be able to use the equivalent loads you'd be able to use on bilateral barbell movements, you'll spare the wrists by allowing them to move freely throughout the movement, which may cause the prime mover to contract even more greatly. Also, self-myofascial release can be incorporated as well as stretching the wrist flexors and extensors.

Shoulders

The shoulders actually consist of four separate joints: the scapulothoracic, glenohumeral, acromioclavicular, and sternoclavicular joints. Communally, these joints work to provide smooth articulation of the shoulder.

The main players, the scapulothoracic and acromioclavicular joints, will be discussed. Note that having mobility through the thoracic spine is also critical and, along with the synchronous proper functioning of the four shoulder joints, will keep the shoulders healthy.

Scapulothoracic Joint

Unlike the other three joints mentioned, the scapulothoracic joint has barely any ligamentous or capsular support. All its stability is derived from the optimal functioning of the 17 muscles that anchor themselves to it. The scapulothoracic joint is critical in keeping the shoulders healthy.

Experts suggest that the scapulae must be stable to permit optimal movement of the shoulders. When the dynamic or static stability of the scapula through its actions of retraction, depression, and upward and downward rotation cannot be achieved, the shoulders won't be able to properly rotate, which may lead to impingement over time.

Acromioclavicular Joint

The acromioclavicular joint, or rotator cuff, is regularly associated with impingement. An impinged shoulder will impact the load you can press horizontally and overhead and may be accompanied by pain. The joint, or cuff, is encircled by four muscles, which include the supraspinatus, infraspinatus, teres minor, and subscapularis.

Together these muscles compress the head of the humerus, or shoulder, into the cavity of the shoulder blade. These muscles counteract the pull of the pectoralis and latissimus groups, which are powerful internal rotators of the shoulder.

Bodybuilders many times disregard corrective exercise for the shoulders. Often they fight through the pain, risking considerable damage to their shoulders down the line. Bodybuilders and lifters in general could afford to insert more thoracic mobility drills (extension and rotation work) throughout their workouts and adopt a greater horizontal pull-to-press ratio.

The ratio should favor the horizontal pulling as it will strengthen the muscles that retract the shoulders, helping them gain the static and dynamic strength needed for pressing exercises. For every pressing exercise, one should perform two horizontal rowing exercises.

Once lifters become proficient at horizontal rowing, they may progress to face pulls, in which the shoulder is both externally rotated and abducted from the body, and lastly to vertical pulling. Also, substituting bench press variations (open chained) with push-up variations (closed chained), with or without added load, will force the rotator cuff to stabilize the shoulder, making the scapula retract while challenging the core musculature.

INJURY PREVENTION

Luckily, preventing injuries is quite simple. Though common sense practiced in the trenches of a gym is rarer than a parallel squat, it will help save you from the anguish of missed time in the gym. Following are 13 tips that will keep you from forking over copays and spending a couple of hours each week hanging out in dingy patient rooms with men and women in white coats.

Tip #1: Check your ego at the door. Certainly, pushing the envelope for strength gains will help you gain hypertrophy; however, using back-breaking weight week in and week out with horrid form will precipitate injuries.

Remember, if you're looking to optimize muscular hypertrophy, moderate to heavy loads (between 70% and 85% of your estimated or actual one-repetition maximum), performed within a range of 6–12 repetitions per set, is ideal.

Additionally, short rest periods, ranging from 1 to 2 minutes each, should be employed, as the short rest periods prompt a greater secretion of anabolic hormones, particularly growth hormone.

Tip #2: Pay close attention to your posture. Are you seated for the bulk of your workday, or are you standing? An optimal posture is one that's constantly moving. Get up from your desk, walk around, and stretch throughout the course of your work or school day.

Tip #3: Stretch! The S-word has evolved into a taboo among gym goers. However, stretching is necessary to restore muscles back to their natural resting lengths.

Regularly stretching can also help range of motion, alleviate post-workout soreness, reduce fatigue, and help the body relax. It is advisable to perform a thorough dynamic warm-up prior to your workout and conclude your workout with static stretching.

Additionally, you can perform some static stretches a couple of hours following your workout, or immediately before bed to help calm your body before sleep.

Tip #4: Perform self-massage. You know those weird things that resemble oversized pool noodles in the obscured corner of the stretching area of the gym? Well there's a reason that gym owners have started stocking their facilities with foam rollers.

Foam rollers, in conjunction with PVC piping, softballs, tennis balls, and lacrosse balls, are utilized to iron out nagging adhesions found in the multiple layers of the fascia, which sits beneath the skin and encapsulates skeletal muscle.

Improvements in soft tissue quality and musculotendinous extensibility, as well as gains in joint range of motion, are a number of benefits that self-myofascial release packs. Self-myofascial release also shifts cellular fluid balance, promotes blood flow, and helps reduce sympathetic tone, allowing the body's muscles to relax following exercise.

Tip #5: Hydrate. Hydration directly impacts soft tissue health. Muscles and their surrounding fasciae consist largely of water. The extracellular matrix, which contains collagen, elastin, and colloidal gels, needs to be hydrated in order to permit smooth movement. Water also significantly contributes to the elasticity of the fascia and the muscle it covers.

We know that dehydrated individuals are more apt to cramp, but they are also more prone to injury. Bodybuilders should aim for a gallon or more of fluid on training days, increasing fluid intake in warmer climates and/or if they're performing extensive cardiovascular exercise.

Tip #6: Learn proper biomechanics of exercise. Nuances include learning how to pack the shoulders during pressing movements, sitting back into a squat, and learning how to properly brace your core musculature during full-body compound movements.

Novices should strongly consider linking up with a qualified personal trainer or a bodybuilder who has years of experience in the trenches and actually knows how to perform various exercises correctly.

Tip #7: Don't get too caught up in the numbers you move. While gaining strength is important, bodybuilders should be dogmatic in their pursuit of gaining muscle mass, not surpassing their previous personal records each workout.

Muscles don't know how much load you're lifting; they only know tension.

Tip #8: Learn how to breathe properly. Often times breathing incorrectly begets injury. Ideally, you want to learn how to breathe through your belly and keep the muscles of the core tight, creating intra-abdominal pressure. This constant pressure provides the core musculature the rigidity it needs to keep your body stable throughout the course of the lift.

Remember to breathe during sets, inhaling during the eccentric and exhaling during the concentric, blowing through the second phase, or "sticking point" of the repetition.

Additionally, proper breathing during exercise and throughout the day will help control autonomic nervous system activity, will prevent the body from overalkalyzing, and will decrease acidity.

Tip #9: Don't shy away from bodyweight exercises. Bodyweight exercises will pack a tremendous value for the bodybuilder.

First, they help establish relative strength, which many novice bodybuilders and heavier bodybuilders lack.

Second, they require little to no equipment. Examples include push-up variations, sit-up variations, planking, lunging, and squatting variations. If you have a set of parallel bars and a chin-up bar available, or have access to a playground, you can add in pull-up and chinning variations as well as dips.

Bodyweight exercises can be incorporated in the dynamic warm-up or as finishers to conclude the workout. They also serve as a novel way to break up the inevitable monotony of working out at the gym.

Tip #10: Know when to deload. Your CNS, musculoskeletal system, joints, and connective tissue all need a rest. Often times, when strength and size is gained too rapidly, the musculotendinous junction, the force-generating component of functional movement where the muscle blends into the tendon, becomes inflamed as it struggles to support the muscles that have swelled in size.

Merely ramping up the repetitions per set and scaling back the intensity on movements for a few months out of the year will help you establish tensile strength of connective tissues. Substituting loaded exercises for bodyweight exercises will also help the cause.

Tip #11: Prioritize and periodize. Ask yourself what you, the bodybuilder, need to work on. Do you suffer from any muscular imbalances? Are there some aesthetic flaws you'd like to address?

Honestly assess yourself and devise a plan to help you get to where you need to be. The plan will come in the form of a periodized program.

If strength and hypertrophy are desired, remember there are no shortcuts. However, there are two surefire means of accomplishing those goals: systematic progressive overload and consistency.

Tip #12: Get more athletic. While professional bodybuilders are heaping mountains of chiseled muscle, it's doubtful that many of them could engage in a game of pickup basketball or flag football. Although bodybuilders want to gain as much muscle as possible, gaining a bit of athleticism won't necessarily hurt.

Consider embedding elementary agility drills and low level plyometric exercises within your dynamic warm-up. Jumps and short sprints will help excite the CNS, fostering a brief training effect that will permit you to lift heavier during your workout.

Tip #13: Warm up extensively. A pre-workout warm up should be thorough and should encompass directed mobility and flexibility work, as well as movement patterning and arousal activities.

Foam-roll and stretch what's tight, perform some bodyweight movements, pattern the movements you'll load heavier later in your workout, crank up the music, and get going. While the music is pumping, perform all of your warm-up sets in the fashion you'd perform your work sets.

Treat the light weights heavy and imagine that the heavier weights are light. Execution should look identical on each lift. The stronger you are, the more time you'll need to devote to your warm up.

Additionally, do not perform warm up sets with high reps. The goal of the warm up is to get the body acclimated to the heavier loads and more intense work that takes place later in the workout.

A FEW LAST WORDS

Bodybuilders must be cognizant that their quest to add muscle doesn't end at a destination; it's a continuous journey, and a surefire way to ensure longevity is to take care of the body you have.

If you adhere to the aforementioned tips, you'll safeguard yourself against the injuries, both acute and chronic, that bodybuilders face throughout their careers.

ABOUT THE AUTHOR

Joe Giandonato, MS, CSCS, is the Head Strength and Conditioning Coach at Germantown Academy in Fort Washington, Pennsylvania, where he develops and oversees the programming for 88 sports teams. In the off season, Giandonato also works with a number of the school's alumni who are competing collegiately and professionally. Previously, Giandonato served as an Intern Assistant Strength and Conditioning Coach at Saint Joseph's University and worked as a health coach, where he implemented wellness programming, at the Children's Hospital of Philadelphia and the University of Pennsylvania. Giandonato has authored over 100 articles that have appeared on a number of popular fitness websites, and he has served as an adjunct instructor at a number of Philadelphia-area colleges. He aspires to ascend to the collegiate or professional ranks as a head strength coach one day.

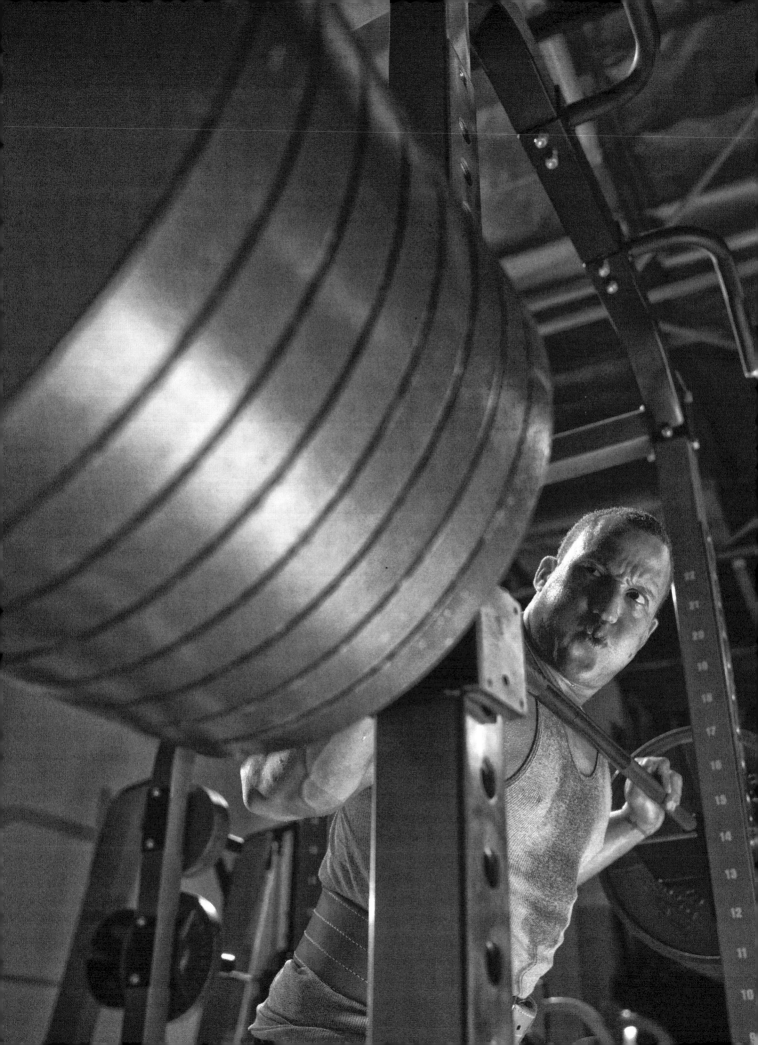

CHAPTER 9.

Bodybuilding Sports Psychology

Your hard work and commitment have given you a body with a new level of muscularity, proportion, and definition. Yet, in the process, you have completely abandoned any social life you once had. Incredible dedication indeed, but it comes with a price.

BODYBUILDING DIFFICULTY

After a great football practice, the team can go out and celebrate by grabbing pizza. Celebratory meals are not an option for you as a bodybuilder, though, as minimizing body fat is your objective. A missed tackle by a defensive lineman can be picked up by a linebacker. Team sports, to certain degree, allow for a mistake to be corrected by a teammate. This is teamwork in action.

If you cheat on your diet, you and only you will pay the price. The upside is you are truly the master of your destiny.

Bodybuilding is a lifestyle that takes a huge mental commitment. No matter how great your genetics may be, they will matter little if your mental game isn't top-notch. When you're bringing your A-game mentally, the physical will follow.

Let's talk about how you can do that.

CONDITIONING YOUR MIND FOR SUCCESS

The mind and body are a team. If you want to build your ultimate physique, you can never forget that. If you consistently visualize success, you will consistently succeed. To become a winner, you should practice the skill of "thinking like a winner."

Associating Sacrifice with Success

According to self-help guru Tony Robbins, pain and pleasure are the guides you use to make decisions. When you have been dieting for months and training hard, what do you think about? Moving towards pleasure or away from pain?

Some view this process as complete self-deprivation and torture to the point of obsession. This is all they think about, all they talk about. Every time they espouse these negative thoughts and words out loud, they become like a prayer or powerful chant. By hailing themselves as some sort of martyr, their chance of success decreases.

Diet is associated with pain and suffering, which is why this country has a skyrocketing obesity rate. Even for those who survive the "suffering" of diet, usually the weight is gained back rapidly.

Why?

Someone can only endure self-torture for so long. In *the paradigm of pain and pleasure,* as I call it, diet and training cannot be viewed within the spectrum of pain. Unless you are some sort of masochist, this is a quick path to not reaching your goals.

What about bodybuilders who are routinely successful?

Generally, they envision the great benefits derived via training and diet by painting a mental picture of themselves walking up to get the first place trophy at a contest. For a non-competing college student, the mental picture might be having the best body at spring break in Panama City; and for a fat guy, he may just see himself talking to pretty girls with confidence.

All these scenarios operate within the pleasure paradigm. These examples focus on the positive results achieved through hard work instead of the discomfort of hard training and extreme dieting.

What do you focus on?

Hard training and dieting are physically demanding and mentally exhausting; the right mindset increases your chances of success and, more importantly, helps you enjoy and appreciate the process.

Failure does not exist. There are only results.

When Thomas Edison was asked if he was frustrated after trying to construct a light bulb 9,999 times without achieving his desired result, his response was, "I have learned 9,999 ways not to make a light bulb" and further added, "Every wrong attempt discarded is another step forward!"

In the past, if your training goals have not panned out with the desired results, you can view this as a blessing. You now know what not to do.

Here are six strategies I believe can be beneficial to achieving your goals.

Step 1: Define your goal clearly and write it down. This means being specific about what you want. Gaining size is not a goal, but adding half an inch to your arms is. Increasing your squat by 50 pounds in 12 weeks has a higher outcome of success than "getting your legs stronger." Goals need to be clear, concise, and measurable.

Step 2: Devise a series of short-term goals, which will ultimately lead to realizing your main goal. It's easier to attain a short-term goal that's within reach than to try and make great leaps and bounds of progress all at once. When you try too much at once and fail, you tend to get discouraged. Instead, set a number of short-term goals that you can accomplish, and then knock them off one at a time. Focus with tunnel vision on the task at hand, one goal at time, knock one off, then move to the next. Each one of your short-term goals should lead you to completion of your major goal. And, as you complete each short-term goal, you motivate yourself to continue training.

Success breeds success!

A 1998 study published in the *Physiology & Behavior Journal* had participants give a saliva sample before and after their favorite team played. The average testosterone level significantly increased in the fans of winning teams but decreased in the fans of losing teams.

Imagine what happens to *you* personally when you succeed. Stress/losing produces cortisol, and success/winning increases testosterone production; so not only is the right mindset important, but by repeatedly experiencing success, a more anabolic environment is created.

Step 3: Create strategies for your success. This is your game plan. On the same sheet where you wrote your long-term goal and listed the short-term goals that will get you there, you should break down your daily activities into the best means to get you where you're going. This means the routines, exercises, sets, reps, intensity, rest periods, diet, and so on. Keep a training journal. Follow your own plan to success. Prepare a daily schedule that takes you in the direction you want to go. Keep your goal sheet current and review it day by day.

Step 4: Visualize yourself succeeding. No one would attempt to build a house without a set of blueprints. Likewise, you must plan your success strategy, and actually "see" yourself, in your mind's eye, accomplishing your goals. Your inner feelings, your thoughts, your daydreams, must all be filled with images of your ultimate success. Twice a day—once after training and once before bedtime—read your goal sheet out loud. Then, close your eyes and with crystal clarity, see yourself performing perfectly, exactly as you want to. See yourself actually accomplishing your goals, not just wistfully thinking about accomplishing them.

Step 5: Align your mind, body, and spirit with achievement. By affirming your commitment to your stated goals, and actually visualizing and verbalizing your commitment, you will find that your mind, body, and emotional self all become one. The power of this union will send an emotional supercharge to your body by actually stimulating secretion of your body's "emotion producing" biochemicals. The alignment is accomplished by actually verbalizing your commitment while visualizing it. Repeat your commitment statement before, during, and after your success visualization every day.

Step 6: Give yourself a reward for your accomplishments. After you've achieved a sub-goal or goal, give yourself a reward or treat of some sort. Buy yourself new clothes or a needed item, or even a luxury one. Reaffirm the good feelings in your mind and dwell upon your achievement and your success. Congratulate yourself and savor the feelings of pride and confidence in having taken direct action to make yourself better and stronger.

The key to mental conditioning is to make your new thoughts and new approach a habit. Thoughts become words, words become actions, and actions become your destiny. The more regular your new habit becomes, the more quickly old and destructive habits fade away. The only way to continue making progress is to regularly reinforce your new, goal-directed training. Remember the old cliché, "Once is an accident; twice is a pattern."

It usually takes about three weeks to implement this revised way of thinking. During that time, you're likely to feel tempted to return to old patterns and habits.

Don't do it!

The more you resist old habits, the stronger you'll become, until you develop an iron will to succeed and you no longer even think about returning to those old habits.

Remember to create a goal, visualize it as real, and work regularly to attain it. You will get there!

12 Motivational Strategies for Workout and Bodybuilding Success

1. Set short-term goals in writing. In a famous survey of Harvard Graduate students upon graduation, only 3% had written goals and plans; 97% had not. Ten years later, the 3% with written goals made 10 times as much money as the other 97% put together.

2. Short-term goals should lead you to a long-term goal. Allow for occasional setbacks along the way, but regard them as learning experiences, thereby turning those setbacks into something positive.

3. Set a training schedule and stick to it.

4. Make pain and fatigue work for you. You see them as signs that your all-out effort is helping you attain your goals; again, remember the pain-pleasure paradigm.

5. Challenge yourself in your training.

6. Devise your own, personal definition of success. It's what you say it is, not what someone else says.

7. Believe in yourself and foster positive aggression in your training.

8. Keep track of training personal records (PRs). You will feel good when you break them.

9. Listen to a mentor's advice and apply it to your workouts.

10. Take pictures. They can be worth a thousand words.

11. Build strong self-confidence.

12. Take action!

MENTAL CONDITIONING PROGRAM

Mind power and successful mental conditioning come only with a sustained and sincere effort. You can't make a wish and hope that it comes true and then forget about working on it.

The mind reacts much the same way the body does. If you train and condition it regularly, it will respond with a performance that you can always count on and be proud of.

Some of the key ingredients to an effective mind conditioning program are motivation, incentive, visualization, and, most important of all, belief.

A 2009 study published in *The Perceptual Motor Skills Journal* showed that when athletes believe in their competition training plans, they are more likely to be victorious in their given sport.

The power of belief may even be related to fatigue.

A 2009 study published in *The European Journal of Applied Physiology* entitled "The Limit to Exercise Tolerance in Humans: Mind over Muscle" challenged the notion that fatigue causes exhaustion and showed that exhaustion might be caused by perceived rate of effort.

What does this mean to you?

It means *you've got to believe.*

You've got to believe in yourself, in your talents and capabilities, in your goals and all you hope to achieve, and in your methods for achieving them.

The beginning of understanding what your mind holds in store for you is a simple realization. You must realize that within you is all the power you need to succeed both in training and dieting, which will ultimately lead to success in competition. Within you is all the potential for success. Within you is the brain power of a superman or superwoman.

Once you make this realization—that your mind holds a vast wealth of knowledge, information, control, power, ability, and potential—you can start to tap into that power. You can delve into your own secret depths and find out what you're really made of.

The Incentive Factor

Motivation begins and ends with incentive. You have to know what you want and why you want it. In conditioning, this means you must desire a specific improvement. Better symmetry, reduced body fat, or sheer muscle mass are various incentives, and they are part of larger incentives such as being liked and admired, being a winner or achiever, enjoying success, shaping a personal identity, gaining peer acceptance, and so on.

The Emotional State of the Bodybuilder

Your mind and your emotions are tightly tied together. It's up to you, as the athlete, to find a balance between them and exert some degree of control over them.

Your emotional state plays a large role in your overall bodybuilding success or lack of success. The way you feel inside has repercussions for your behavior and performance on the outside.

Many different factors go into the makeup of a solid emotional base. Some of these are personal life, sexual life, family life, job, daily schedule, diet, financial matters, health concerns, and, most importantly, self-esteem.

Your own self-esteem contributes greatly to your success level in bodybuilding and in life!

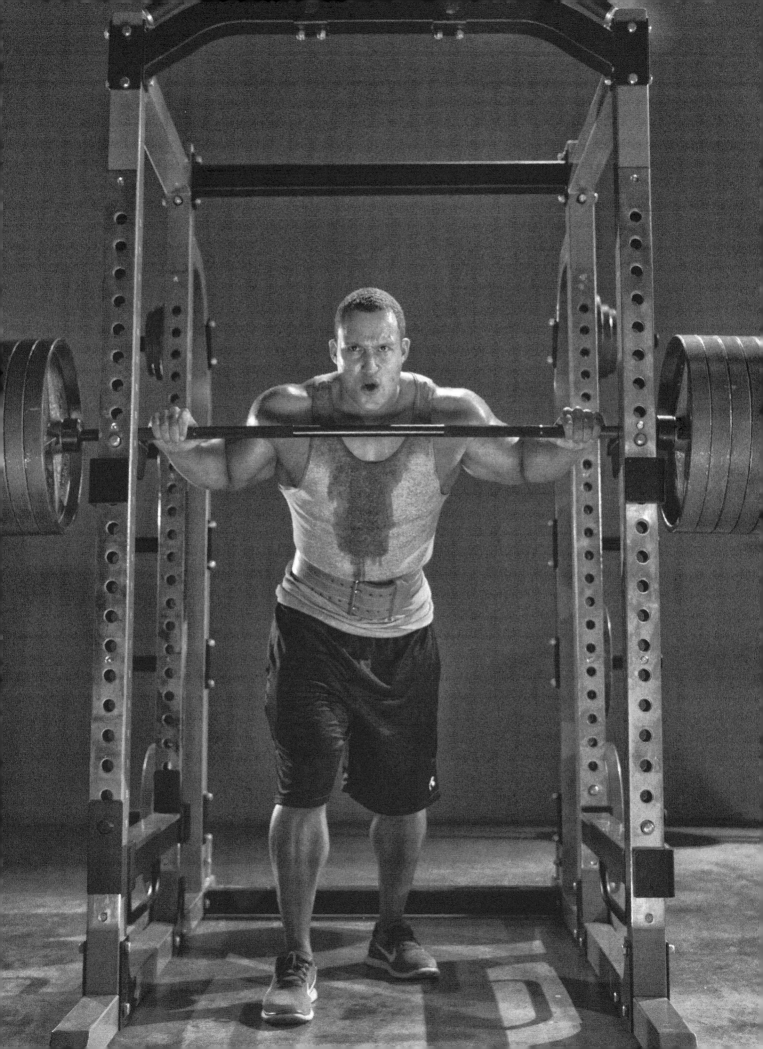

Concentration

Success in bodybuilding can almost be likened to the practice of Zen masters. The concentration is so complete that there is no consciousness of concentration. Frank Zane has talked extensively about this. Branch Warren's career has been said to be over numerous times, yet he keeps coming back better and better. This is purpose-driven focus and concentration.

You have no doubt been in a situation where your attention was so rapt and absorbed in one thought that you completely blocked out all others. This was probably due to your high concentration level on some thought of great importance to you.

For anyone who wants serious results, the gym is not a social club.

Enjoy seeing your friends, but always remember that you go to the gym to train.

In other sports, generally, the best performances are nearly always those that are executed just below total consciousness. This is how training needs to be focused and has to be purpose driven.

Approach training this way retreating to your own mind, a magical place where there is no pain, no discomfort, and where only positive forces loom.

In the antiquated world of the Samurai, this was called "mindfulness." When you are in a state of mindfulness, you are aware of all that surrounds you, but all that is around you does not deter the focus that is within you.

This kind of focus builds confidence.

The more you focus on what you're working to achieve, the less distractions will enter your awareness. This lifts you out of the state of mind that can't "see" success. Once you begin to "see" success, you consider yourself potentially better than the competition.

Little by little, you concentrate more and more, until you're unaware of anything in your way. You see your way clearly to victory and success.

This is total concentration.

It is this kind of total concentration that comes to those who develop total self-confidence. You must have high self-esteem and high motivation, and be consistent in your training and sports conditioning program.

You must develop your mind conditioning to the point that total concentration is merely a learned response, one you no longer consciously think about.

In other sports, if you don't do your best, you share the blame with the team; in bodybuilding, everything is on you. If you enter a contest in sub-par condition, you alone will suffer the consequences and humiliation.

THE PERILS OF OVERLOOKING MENTAL PREPARATION

I can't over-emphasize the degree to which mental preparation is often overlooked by iron disciples around the globe!

Your conscious mind deals with things at face value such as reasoning, logic, communications, and things of that nature. Most people believe they operate only in this part of their mind. This part of your mind, however, is only a very small percentage of your total mental capacity.

The subconscious mind directly influences your concept of self. The power to achieve and do great things is in your subconscious mind. The simple truth is you must believe in order to achieve.

In the 1950s, clinical and experimental psychologists proved that the human nervous system is unable to differentiate between a real experience and a vividly imagined detailed experience. This does not mean that you can repeat 10 times a day, "I will be a Mr. Olympia," and it will happen. That would be a passive experience.

For the nervous system to believe it is doing what you are imagining, you must create a vivid mental movie, complete with the feelings, the sights, the sounds, and the smells that would accompany the experience in real life. You need active experiences to positively affect your subconscious mind.

The discovery of self not only can help your training but, more importantly, can even aid you when you pose on stage in front of a crowd.

T. F. James was quoted more than 50 years ago in *Cosmopolitan* magazine as saying, "Understanding the psychology of the self can mean the difference between success and failure, love and hate, bitterness and happiness."

Our triumphs, our failures, and other people's reactions to these triumphs and failures form our concept of self. In other words, our experiences shape our self-image. It isn't so much the actual experiences but the way we perceive these events.

The good news is that the human nervous system can't tell the difference between real and imagined experiences, so start seeing yourself and everything you do as a success!

The limits you place on yourself literally become a self-fulfilling prophecy. If you prophesize championships, they are much more likely to come to pass.

Bad genetics?

Generally, those who don't experience success believe they are a product of bad genetics. Clearly your genetic blueprint can enhance your chances of success. The flip side is, though, very few have even scratched the surface of maximizing their genetics.

To experience positive change, a metamorphosis at our core's being must take place. Once we establish a healthy self-image, it is easier to accomplish things within the realm of this new self-image.

Prescott Lesky, who is considered one of the founding fathers of self-image psychology, conceived personality as a system of ideas that seem to maintain consistency with one another.

Thoughts and goals that are inconsistent with this system of ideas are not acted upon, while ideas aligned with this system are acted upon. Lesky emphasized that at the nucleus of this system of ideas is an individual's concept of self.

The creative mechanism within every individual is impersonal. It can work automatically to achieve success or failure. Yet, this depends on the goals you set for yourself. Present it with positive goals and the "success mechanism" will set in. Present it with negative goals and the "failure mechanism" will set in. Our goals are mental images developed in the conscious mind. Self-fulfilling prophecies, whether positive or negative, are real!

The great Scottish philosopher, Dugold Stewart, once said, "The faculty of imagination is the great spring of human activity and the source for human improvement."

That old Scotsman was on to something.

A study in 2009, published in *The Journal of Exercise Psychology and Human Perception Performance*, echoed Stewart's words. The study was called "Evidence for Motor Stimulation in Imagined Locomotion." It showed that people who imagined movements prior to performing them performed these movements better.

Think about this.

For you to optimize results, optimal exercise technique is a necessity.

Mental imagery, if one wishes to be the best, should become a regular component of training. Know what your current goal is and know, without a doubt, that you will accomplish it. After that, look to the future. Find a new target and focus in with laser-like precision.

According to the late Dr. Maxwell Maltz, author of the famed book, *Psycho Cybernetics*, man is a teleological, goal-oriented being. We are engineered to always be seeking and achieving goals.

This means you must set specific goals for yourself as a competitor and in training. Training goals need to be specific, measurable, and realistic.

Goals need to be established for the microcycle, mesocycle, and macro training cycles. Each unique phase has a unique goal that helps you to achieve the ultimate goal of reigning victorious on or off stage.

Do you know where you want to be a year from now? "To do my best" is not a proper goal. It is very convoluted and open to interpretation. In general, people with no goals feel their life isn't worthwhile. The truth is, they have no worthwhile goals.

Man is hardwired to achieve goals and conquer obstacles. Losers whine about their best. They make excuses about their jobs, money, or training partners, while the winners are victorious and keep doing their thing.

Brain activity precedes movement, and it is vital that correct movements are visualized long before those movements are performed.

Weight training exercises are movements; they are your sport! Visualization techniques were used by top Russian and Eastern Bloc coaches for decades before the rest of the world accepted them.

They work!

THE MENTAL IMAGERY PROGRAM

Each day, set aside 20 minutes for mental imagery training. Find a dark, comfortable place to lie down and relax your muscles. This should be a place where all the anxieties and troubles of everyday life can be forgotten.

Start developing a "movie" in your head; a movie where you are the star. Successful visualizations benefit from as many details as possible. This can be of you training at the gym or posing on stage, hitting every pose with perfect precision. If it is training at the gym, envision details of the gym, the look, sounds, and smells—make it real!

This experience should be like a vivid dream, the kind where you wake up and feel it has actually happened. You want your central nervous system to have a real experience. After experiencing this vivid dream, the real life experience may seem like déjà vu. You have already experienced this. Your subconscious mind says so, and that is where the power of achievement lies.

Visualization will not be accomplished through strain or effort. It is instead achieved through relaxation.

Try to systematically relax your muscles, one muscle group at a time. Then start to develop the movie in your head. Play back in your mind your past successes like a successful competition or any event that was positive.

Reflecting on past victories and successes is helpful in defining a positive self-image. The key is to help these positive experiences build a base for your psyche. Realize with proper focus that the future will be better, and begin to view that with nostalgia.

Louie Pasteur once said, "Chance favors the prepared mind." Moreover, Napoleon Bonaparte role played, and so did General George Patton. Both these men were prepared for almost any situation that could arise, because they had mentally prepared for them.

If you have the freedom, it can be helpful to decorate your workout facility. Posters of past greats can serve as a great motivational tool. You should have heroes you admire and who will motivate you to become better.

Today's training methods are far more advanced in many ways than those of yesteryear, so you can conceivably surpass these past greats.

Just remember, those titans of the past were way ahead of their time for their era. Be thankful that they paved the way for you, and never lose respect for these iron game heroes.

You now know how to create a positive self-image, but what about negative people and the negative energy they bring?

The key is to distance yourself from these negative energies as much as you can.

If you can't, simply pay them no mind.

Do not hate these people. Hate and contempt breed resentment; and resentment, in and of itself, is a negative energy. Remember, the opposite of hate is not love, but apathy. Let go of those who try to influence you negatively; wish them the best as they travel on their life journey and you on yours.

Let your energy flow in a positive direction, not in the direction of someone you don't like. Save all the energy for yourself and the ones you love and the ones who support you.

A FEW LAST WORDS

Many years ago, the YMCA was onto something powerful when it proclaimed "sound mind, body and spirit." All three must be exercised in concert to produce synergistic results.

Truly, you are what you believe!

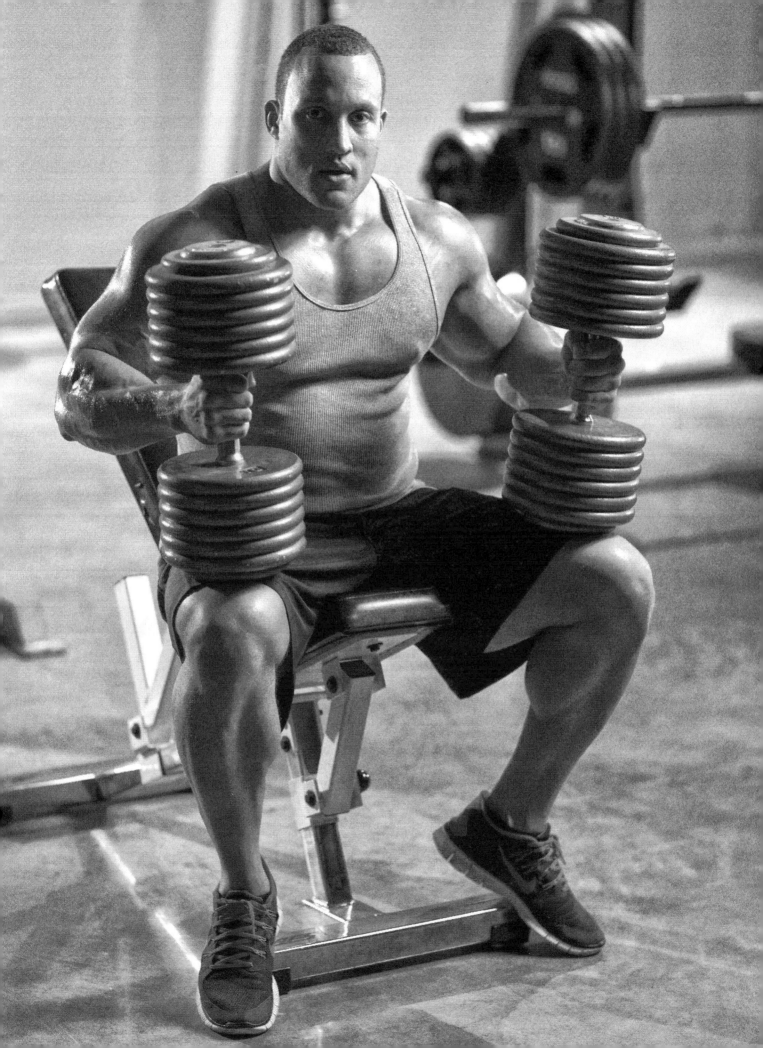

SOURCES

Anbar, R. D., and J. H. Linden. "Understanding Dissociation and Insight in the Treatment of Shortness of Breath with Hypnosis: A Case Study." *American Journal of Clinical Hypnosis* 52, no. 4 (2010): 263–73.

Arruza, J. A., S. Telletxea, L. G. De Montes, S. Arribas, G. Balagué, J. A. Cecchini, and R. J. Brustad. "Understanding the Relationship Between Perceived Development of the Competition Plan and Sport Performance: Mediating Effects of Self-Efficacy and State Depression." *Perceptual and Motor Skills* 109, no. 1 (2009): 304–14.

Attrill, M. J., K. A. Gresty, R. A. Hill, and R. A. Barton. "Red Shirt Colour Is Associated with Long-Term Team Success in English Football." *Journal of Sports Sciences* 26, no. 6 (2008): 577–82.

Bernhardt, Paul C., James M. Dabbs, Jr., Julie A. Fielden, and Candice D. Lutter. "Testosterone Changes During Vicarious Experiences of Winning and Losing Among Fans at Sporting Events." *Physiology & Behavior* 65, no. 1 (1998): 59–62.

Hardy, James, Craig R. Hall, and Lew Hardy. "Quantifying Athlete Self-Talk." *Journal of Sports Sciences* 23, no. 9 (2005): 905–17.

Hatfield, Frederick. *Specialist in Sports Conditioning*. Santa Barbara: International Sports Sciences Association, 2001. (Unpublished ISSA manuscript.)

Hays, K., O. Thomas, I. Maynard, and M. Bawden. "The Role of Confidence in World-Class Sport Performance." *Journal of Sports Sciences* 27, no. 11 (2009): 1185–99.

Karageorghis, C. L., D. A. Mouzourides, D. Priest, T. A. Sasso, D. J. Morrish, and C. L. Walley. "Psychophysical and Ergogenic Effects of Synchronous Music During Treadmill Walking." *Journal of Sport & Exercise Psychology* 31, no. 1 (2009): 18–36.

Kunz, B. R., S. H. Creem-Regehr, and W. B. Thompson. "Evidence for Motor Simulation in Imagined Locomotion." *Journal of Experimental Psychology: Human Perception and Performance* 35, no. 5 (2009): 1458–71.

Maltz, Maxwell. *Psycho-Cybernetics*. New York: Pocket Books, 1960.

Marcora, S. M., and W. Staiano. "The Limit to Exercise Tolerance in Humans: Mind Over Muscle?" *European Journal of Applied Physiology* 109, no. 4 (2010): 763–70.

Mullen, R., and L. Hardy. "Conscious Processing and the Process Goal Paradox." *Journal of Sport and Exercise Psychology* 32, no. 3 (2010): 275–97.

Parmigiani, S., H. Dadomo, A. Bartolomucci, P. F. Brain, A. Carbucicchio, C. Costantino, P. F. Ferrari, P. Palanza, and R. Volpi. "Personality Traits and Endocrine Response as Possible Asymmetry Factors of Agonistic Outcome in Karate Athletes." *Aggressive Behaviour* 35, no. 4 (2009): 324–33.

Schücker, L., N. Hagemann, B. Straub, and K. Volker. "The Effect of Attentional Focus on Running Economy." *Journal of Sports Sciences* 27, no. 12 (2009): 1242–48.

Verkhoshansky, Yuri, and Mel C. Siff. *Supertraining,* 6th ed. Denver, CO: Supertraining Institute, 2009.

Stoeber, J., M. A. Uphill, and S. Hotham. "Predicting Race Performance in Triathlon: The Role of Perfectionism, Achievement Goals, and Personal Goal Setting." *Journal of Sport & Exercise Psychology* 31, no. 2 (2009): 211–45.

Warnick, J. E., and K. Warnick. "Specification of Variables Predictive of Victories in the Sport of Boxing: II. Further Characterization of Previous Success." *Perceptual and Motor Skills* 108, no. 1 (2009): 137–8.

Weiss, S. M., A. S. Reber, and D. R. Owen. "The Locus of Focus: The Effect of Switching from a Preferred to a Non-Preferred Focus of Attention." *Journal of Sports Sciences* 26, no. 10 (2008): 1049–57.

Williams, S. E., J. Cumming, and M. G. Edwards. "The Use of Imagery to Manipulate Challenge and Threat Appraisal States in Athletes." *Journal of Sport & Exercise Psychology* 32, no. 3 (2011): 339–58.

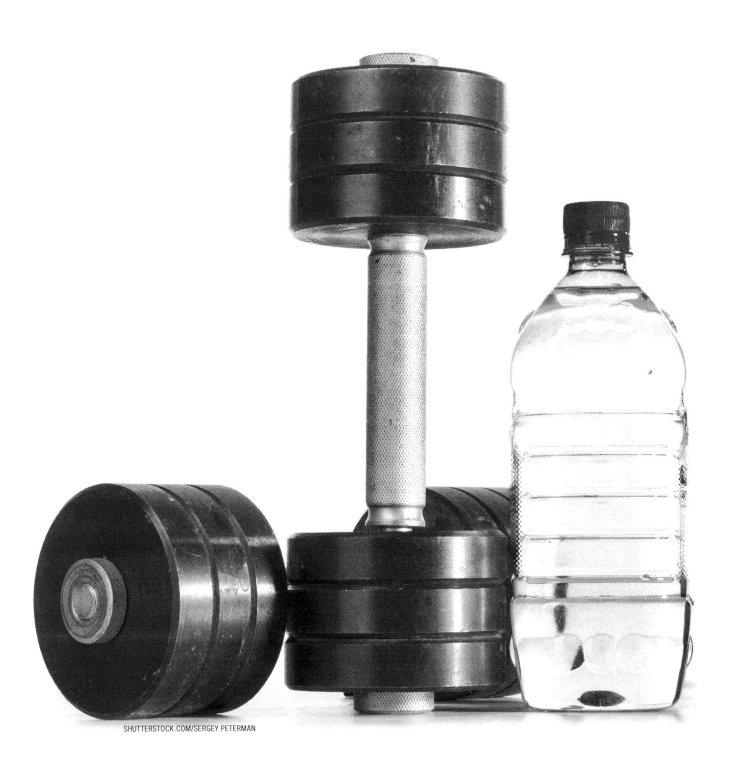

CHAPTER 10.

Nutrition

Intense bodybuilding workouts that routinely spend time in an anaerobic hell via advanced bodybuilding techniques and lifting heavy weights with high volume can't be fueled by Mickey D's!

Nutrition is important in any sport, and every sport has champions who defy the odds and break every dietary guideline.

With one exception.

Bodybuilding.

You cannot expect to be a champion unless you eat like one.

HYDRATION

You will never perform your best unless you are properly hydrated. It is nearly impossible to set an exact general fluid requirement, however.

The rate of water loss is affected by weather, diet, exercise, obesity, drugs, and a host of other factors. Dehydration will drastically affect mental and physical function and performance. In some cases, when water loss is as little as 1%, physical performance can be significantly compromised.

The following guidelines are for healthy, active individuals, and they are estimated based upon daily energy expenditure, provided by the International Sports Sciences Association.

Table 10.1. Minimum Daily Water Intake

DAILY ENERGY EXPENDITURE	MINIMUM DAILY WATER INTAKE
2,000 Calories	64 to 80 oz
3,000 Calories	102 to 118 oz
4,000 Calories	138 to 154 oz
5,000 Calories	170 to 186 oz
6,000 Calories	204 to 220 oz

As temperature and humidity surpass 70 degrees, fluid loss is increased. Special attention must be paid to hydration status. Many hardcore gyms have no air conditioning. For instance, the new Mecca of Bodybuilding, Metroflex Gym in Arlington, Texas, is proud of the fact of not having air conditioning; when heat index is factored in, this is one of the hottest areas in the world.

WHAT TO EAT

For bodybuilding, the classical recommendations are a diet composed of 50%–60% carbohydrates, 25%–30% protein, and 15%–30% fat.

Some nutritional guidelines literally advocate zero carbohydrates, some take a more cyclical approach, and others a more traditional approach.

With zero carbs, no matter how mentally tough you are, you will not be able to train as hard as you could with adequate carbohydrates. Fat has about 9 calories per gram, while protein and carbohydrates have only about 4 calories per gram.

Following a traditional approach, if you needed 3,000 calories to continue slow muscle growth during the off season, for example, you'd be getting 450 calories from fat (15% of your daily calories), 750 calories from protein (25%), and the remaining 1,800 calories from carbohydrates (60%). Of course, these calories are divided by the number of times you eat each day (5–6 times).

NUTRITIONAL GUIDELINES

Even if you do not compete, here are some considerations to help with dietary choices to help you look and feel your best.

- Eat high-quality complex carbohydrates several times throughout the day. This is sort of an insurance policy to make sure you are getting all the energy your body requires. Try to get some high-quality complex carbohydrates every 2–3 hours.

- Consume high-quality protein every 2–3 hours. You are putting lots of stress on your muscles, and they need to repair and grow stronger. High-quality protein does just that.

- Fats are an essential part of your diet. However, carbohydrates are your body's preferred energy source, and fat alone is not a sufficient energy source for high-intensity weight training.

- Eat 5–6 meals a day.

- Eat vegetables.

Review the pre-, intra-, and post-workout nutritional strategies included in the recovery section. They are crucial for recovery.

In bodybuilding, for years some have believed that nutrition is responsible for as much as 80%–90% of bodybuilding success.

Think about it.

If that was true, all bodybuilders would need to do is spend 80%–90% of their time on nutrition and just 10%–20% of their time on the unimportant things like going to gym, doing the right exercises in the right way at the right time with the right intensity, blah, blah, blah… and they'd be champions.

Yes, nutrition is very important, but so is training; it's at least half the equation.

You can't just simply eat your way to a great physique!

The key is to follow sound nutritional strategies and do your best to avoid having to bulk up too fast with a "dirty bulk" or having to cut weight rapidly.

It is sad, but true, that some recreational gym lifters ignorantly dismiss the importance of nutrition. No matter what workout routine they follow, they will never look or feel their best without a sound nutritional strategy.

While 3 meals a day is certainly a better plan than what is followed by many sedentary folks, that strategy will not fuel a hard-training bodybuilder.

Remember, your goal is not to sustain life, but to maximize muscle mass and minimize body fat. By eating 1–3 meals a day you can stay alive, but your physique and strength will suffer.

You need to eat 5–6 meals daily, or every 2–3 hours. This allows your body the necessary amount of time to utilize, digest, and oxidize the nutrients in the meal.

Additionally, spreading out your calories steadily throughout the day, over 5–6 meals, will decrease the chances that excess calories will be converted to fat and your body will cannibalize your muscles for the nutrients it lacks.

More frequent meals will cause your metabolism to speed up and minimize body fat, while helping maximize muscle and strength gains.

Carbohydrates

Carbohydrates are not just the body's preferred source of energy, but they are the most easily digestible macronutrient. A carbohydrate is composed of hydrogen and oxygen. There are two kinds of carbohydrates: the simple ones (sugars) and the complex ones, which include starches and fibers.

Ever hear of the glycemic index (GI)? The glycemic index is the blood glucose response for 2 hours after food is eaten, compared to a 2-hour response of the equivalent amount of glucose eaten. It is important to eat primarily low-glycemic carbohydrates. The lower the GI, the less rapid the glucose response. By eating foods with a lower GI, your body will maintain more stable blood glucose levels. High-glycemic carbohydrates that are easily converted to adipose tissue should be avoided.

Hey, wait a second. What about during and immediately post workout?

Good thinking. This is an exception to the rule.

Potatoes, brown rice, oatmeal, cream of rice, Ezekiel bread, yams, and quinoa are quality carbohydrates recommended for the bodybuilder. A majority of your carbohydrates should come from complex sources. Your mother always used to tell you to eat your vegetables; she was right!

Vegetables are fibrous carbohydrates that help aid in digestion of food and the defecation process and additionally serve as an abundant source of nutrients. Carbohydrates, under normal circumstances, should make up 30%–50% of your diet; but carb cycles and contest prep would not be classified as "normal" circumstances.

The 1980s and '90s were nutritionally dominated by the low fat zealots, but in the last decade, the low carbohydrate zealots have made their presence known.

All sorts of exotic low/no-carb weight loss fad diets have been advocated. Before you jump on the anti-carbohydrate bandwagon, remember: Carbohydrates are your body's first choice of fuel for physical activity. Additionally, carbohydrates fuel the brain and central nervous system.

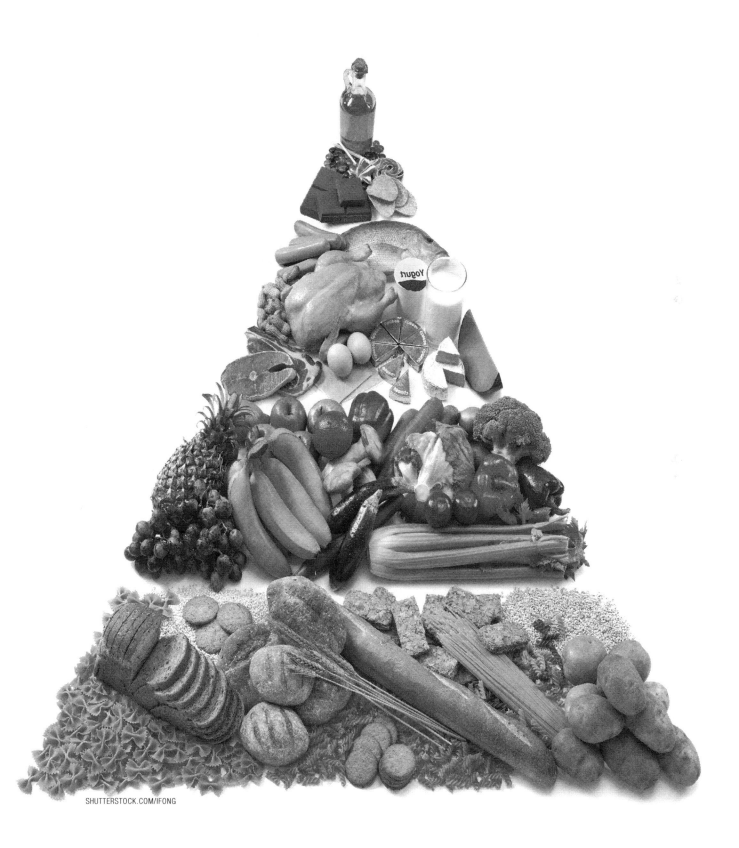

Fiber

Most people, regardless of goals, do not eat enough fiber. Fiber is found in various plants, fruits, leaves, grains, nuts, seeds and legumes. Fruits and vegetables are your best choices for sources of fiber. There are many functional benefits from eating a high fiber diet, and numerous studies confirm that high fiber diets reduce the rate of cardiovascular disease, colon cancer, and diabetes.

Fiber is not an energy source; in fact, the human gut cannot digest it. However, it has protective qualities. It helps promote efficient intestinal function such as regulation and absorption of sugars into the bloodstream. Also, fiber helps soften the stool and promotes normal defecation patterns. Many health agencies recommend 20–30 grams of fiber a day. This may be sufficient for a person with a low calorie diet, but for someone attempting to add muscle bulk on a high calorie diet, 50 to 80 grams of fiber maybe needed.

Quality Protein Sources

The following foods are quality protein choices for the bodybuilder's diet: eggs, chicken breast, turkey breast, fish, and lean read meats. If finances permit, I would highly suggest buying organic poultry, grass-fed meat, and cage-free eggs. Fish should be wild caught, not farm raised.

Quality protein supplements are convenient, work well, and often are more economically feasible than buying the aforementioned protein sources. Whey protein powder, casein protein powder, and egg protein powder are conveniently available. Generally, multi-blends are preferable.

Avoid soy protein powder because, aside from not being a complete animal-based source of protein, numerous studies have shown that it lowers testosterone levels. Not what any self-respecting musclehead wants!

Some key points to remember about protein:

- Protein is essential for growth and recovery.
- Branch-chained amino acids are required to keep muscle breakdown to a minimum.
- High quality protein should be consumed, such as grass-fed beef, fish, lean poultry, and cage-free natural eggs with 350 mg of omega-3 fats minimally per egg. Unless you are on highly restricted calories, eat the yolk.
- Protein should be consumed with every meal.
- High quality protein supplements can be used, but remember the real thing is always better than a synthetic product. The keyword is supplement, not

substitute. Consider natural foods as a supplementation option whenever they are available.

- Not all protein is created equal! Protein in whole dairy products and fatty meats is very difficult to digest, if your body even digests it at all. Stick to lean, natural sources of protein.

Fats

Keep your consumption of fats between 15% and 30% of your daily diet. Avoid fried foods, fast food, processed lunch meats, extremely fatty meats/poultry, margarine, shortening, and many salad dressings, even in the off season.

Your fats should be from unsaturated sources like olive oil, flax oil, salmon, and grass-fed organic meats. If you are unsure of the fat content, read the nutritional label on the food. It should say the number of fat grams and the number of calories from fat per serving. If this information is not included, remember that a gram of fat has 9 calories. So, if there are 30 grams of fat, just multiply 9 x 30 and you will realize there are 270 calories of fat.

If your goal is to consume 20% of your calories from fat and you are eating 5,000 calories daily, you would need 1,000 calories from fat. This would be approximately 111 grams of fat, so 111 gm x 9 calories = 999 calories.

If your goal is 20% protein, that would be 250 grams of protein, so 250 gm x 4 calories = 1,000 calories. Therefore, even though you are consuming more than twice as many grams of protein than fat, you are consuming the same amount of calories from each.

A protein gram has 4 calories, while a fat gram has 9 calories. While this may seem elementary to someone with a nutritional background, this is a common mistake that even experienced personal trainers make. Attention to detail is very important here.

"Choosing the right types of dietary fats to consume is one of the most important factors in reducing the risk of developing heart disease," said Alice Lichenstein, DSC, a renowned researcher from Tufts University in Boston.

For a long time, especially in the 1980s and '90s, low fat diets were the fad. This did not yield better physiques or better health.

Actually, the opposite happened as the obesity level skyrocketed.

The rate of obesity in America has doubled in the last 20 years. In the 1960s, fat made up around 45% of the average American's diets—and less than 15% of the U.S. population was obese.

Average Americans now get less than one-third of all of their calories from fat, and approximately 34% of Americans are obese. Therefore, there is more to the obesity epidemic than an increase in dietary fats. Fat has gotten a bad rap because of its caloric density. One gram of fat yields 9 calories, compared to just 4 in carbohydrates.

In regard to obesity, this simple solution should be remembered: if you take in more calories than you burn, you will gain weight. Every 3,500 calories in surplus of your daily maintenance level will cause you to gain 1 pound. It is a lot easier to get into a caloric surplus with fats than the other macronutrients, but as a bodybuilder you must be diligent and disciplined with your diet.

You must have fat in your diet; your body uses fatty acids to do things such as building cell membranes and performing key functions in the brain, eyes, and lungs.

Some other functions of fats include functioning as a fuel source during exercise, providing insulation, aiding in absorbing fat-soluble vitamins, supplying essential fatty acids, providing protective padding for body structures, and protecting your nerves.

Additionally, it is essential in keeping your lungs and eyes working properly, and fats also help your immune system and metabolism function properly.

Not all fats are created equal.

I would recommend avoiding trans fatty acids at all costs. Monounsaturated fats (found in olive oil, nuts, and avocados) have definite health benefits.

Numerous studies have attempted to show a link between heart disease and saturated fat intake; the majority of these studies have failed to show any sort of correlation whatsoever. The studies that have shown such a correlation usually have some flaw in them. An example of flawed studies would be ones that lump together artificial trans fat consumption with saturated fat consumption, which the body absorbs completely differently. I would not recommend consuming excessive amounts of saturated fats; but to be fair and impartial, the jury is still out on saturated fat.

NUTRITIONAL GUIDELINES FOR MAXIMIZING YOUR PHYSIQUE AND PERFORMANCE

Remember, dieting is not just 12–16 weeks before a contest or your high school reunion. It's a long-term commitment to make a part of your lifestyle.

Your eating habits will either support or sabotage your training efforts. Science can show you how; your job is to take advantage of this knowledge and reach the next step of your maximum hypertrophy and minimal body fat.

Always Eat at Least Five Meals a Day

Two or three meals just aren't enough. If your body is not getting the calories it needs through your meals, where will energy come from?

Muscle tissue!

That's right—the same muscle tissue you spent weeks and months sweating for in the gym. The body is a conservative machine, and it won't grow unless (a) you give it a reason to (through weight training) and (b) you provide plenty of calories so that the body is convinced it can afford to add more lean mass.

Caloric Distribution

Calories must be ingested according to your upcoming activity level. Therefore, prior to every meal, ask yourself, "What am I going to be doing for the next 3 hours?"

If you plan to sit at a desk at work, eat less. However, if you plan to train, eat more. By carefully manipulating your caloric intake in this way, meal after meal, day after day, week after week, month after month, pretty soon you'll look in the mirror and see something you've been waiting to see for a long, long, time: a well-defined, muscular physique.

Guidelines For Bulking

"If you cannot see abs or veins on your arms and legs you are getting too fat!" Branch Warren once exclaimed in a conversation with me.

Rules like "Never exceed 15 pounds over your competition bodyweight" generally are rendered useless. The look and size of a bodybuilder can be an illusion, and Branch's words of wisdom ring true. Adding muscle mass is important, but never at the expense of getting fat.

Dieting is tough enough, and excess body fat will require an aggressive crash-course strategy to be competition ready, most likely dieting away the extra muscle or being in a prolonged state of caloric deficit. Neither of these scenarios is conducive to maximizing muscularity.

Here is a sensible guideline for bulking:

- Add 2 calories per pound of bodyweight to your daily caloric intake.
- The added calories should be from all macronutrients; a minimum of 1 gram of protein per pound of bodyweight should be consumed.
- Spread these added calories equally among 5 meals per day.
- For example, people weighing 150 pounds should add 300 calories per day to their diet over five meals, which equals about a 60-calorie increase per meal.

- The additional 300 calories will, with intense weight training, result in a gain of approximately 1–2 pounds of added muscle per month.

- Reduce your caloric intake 2 days per week by 2 calories per pound of bodyweight. (To ensure that excess fat is being removed, this should be on non-training days.)

- Right after a show or after a long diet is the best time to bulk because your body will act like a sponge, absorbing nutrients with maximum efficiency. This natural rebound effect, coupled with heavy training, will synergistically promote anabolism.

Fat Loss Guidelines

One pound of fat contains 3,500 calories. The logical assumption would be to reduce your caloric intake by 500 calories daily. 7 x 500 = 3,500 calories, so you will lose a pound of fat per week and will be lean and mean in no time, right?

Whoa… hold your horses.

Your body tends to use "excessive" muscle tissue for energy before fat. As you drop weight and lose muscle, your caloric needs will drop. This is why *calories must be cut very slowly*!

Follow these guidelines:

- Subtract 2 calories per pound of bodyweight from your daily caloric intake.

- The reduced calories should come mostly from carbohydrate and fat calories, and not protein. Eat minimally 1 gram of protein per pound of bodyweight.

- This caloric reduction should be applied to all of your meals; do not reduce the frequency of meals.

- For example, assuming a bodyweight of 150 pounds and you're eating five meals per day (highly recommended), you should reduce each meal by 60 calories (total of 300 calories' reduction over a full day).

- By reducing your daily caloric intake by 300 calories, you can expect to lose about 2.5 pounds of fat per month, assuming you're weight training for muscle-mass preservation or increase.

- Increase your caloric intake 2 days per week by 2 calories per pound of bodyweight to ensure that you're getting enough calories to put on lean muscle and that upward BMR adjustments are being made. This is the concept of the Zigzag diet explained in the next subsection. Even carb cycling, Body Opus, etc. follow this premise; although carbs are the macronutrient cycled, caloric intake is not linear.

Zigzag Caloric Approach

Trying to gain muscle and lose fat at the same time is difficult. The Zigzag diet, the brainchild of Fred Hatfield, was designed for this purpose. This strategy is designed to yield results over time.

Here's how it works: Let's say you presently weigh 240 pounds and your body fat is 20% and your goal is to weigh 240 with 10% body fat. Very simply, you up your caloric intake for 4–5 days, then cut back for a day or two. In this way, you gain (approximately) a pound of muscle and a pound of fat, and then lose the fat, retaining the muscle.

Let's look at when it's time to bulk.

The question remains: How do you do this without adding fat?

Here's how.

Simply reverse the Zigzag procedure just discussed. Reduce your caloric intake for four to five days, and then bring it back up to normal levels for a day or two. Provided that you have been eating at least 5 times daily, fat storage enzymes will be at very low levels.

Therefore, when you resume normal caloric intake for one to two days, the idea is your body will be unable to store the excess calories as fat. Continued over months and years, these procedures will result in added lean mass, without excess body fat.

Do not try to bulk too fast!

Plan ahead—don't wait until 3 weeks out to lose 15 pounds of fat. Be smart and remember: Rome was not built in a day.

Supplementation

In today's world, it is simply impossible for athletes to eat properly all the time, even under the best of circumstances. That's why many athletes supplement.

Which supplements do you need?

Although this depends on a variety of factors, a good multivitamin is a good place to start. Amino acid tablets are a very good source of basic protein in super-digestible form, and they can work wonders for your recovery rates.

And while we're on the subject of protein, it might pay to investigate the plethora of weight-gain shakes currently available. For athletes trying to add muscle mass, they can be invaluable.

A final note: Use caution when investigating the wide array of exotic-sounding miracle supplements with supposed steroid-like effects. They usually have no proven benefit for hard-training athletes and can sometimes have harsher side effects. The pharmaceutical industry is regulated, and the dietary supplement industry is not.

A FEW LAST WORDS

Here are some final guidelines:

1. **Never experiment with new or unusual (for you) foods as a show approaches.** If you do, you may discover a food that doesn't agree with you at the worst possible time. Instead, stick with familiar foods that work well for you. As stated earlier, low-glycemic carbs are best, exceptions being intra workout and immediately post workout.

2. **Don't try to fix things in the short term.** If you have excessive body fat, you will not magically become lean by popping a diuretic. It's what you eat over the long term that really counts.

3. **Take pride in developing a personal discipline when it comes to nutrition.** Many, many recreational bodybuilders are highly disciplined when it comes to training, but poorly disciplined in terms of nutrition. One facet of this discipline involves meal planning. Little is written about the fact that to eat properly, you must plan your meals in advance. Many athletes use excuses like "At work I just don't have access to good food," or "I'm always so busy." The list goes on and on. All of these problems can be solved through planning. Bring a cooler to work, or buy a small refrigerator. Cook up some chicken breasts and eat them throughout the day. Use meal replacement shakes—an easy, low-preparation way to eat well at work. Or, use workout bars as an occasional meal when time gets tight. The options are many, if you take the time to plan.

4. **If you have not already done so, buy a measuring cup and a scale.** You will need to measure carbohydrate grams, protein grams, and fat grams. This is very tedious and time consuming. You will need to use http://www.calorieking.com to find the values for each food. If you are getting ready for a contest, you need to weigh your food!

Remember, one of the biggest factors to this whole equation is genetic potential. It is hard to make a pit bull out of a poodle. No matter what cards you have been dealt genetically, if you put forth your best effort and follow the presented guidelines, you can still reach your potential.

Heredity may have dealt the cards, but nutrition and training will play the hand! Like the saying goes, "Hard work beats talent when talent doesn't work hard."

SOURCES

Bryant, Josh. "The Effect of Whey and Soy Protein Supplementation on Lean Body Mass (LBM) of Resistance Trained Young Men." JoshStrength.com (22 July 2010). http://articles.elitefts.com/nutrition/the-effect-of-whey-and-soy-protein-supplementation-on-lean-body-mass-lbm-of-resistance-trained-young-men/

Coburn, Jared W., and Moh H. Malek (Eds.). *Essentials of Strength Training and Conditioning,* 2nd ed. Champaign, IL: National Strength and Conditioning Association, 2000.

Gatorade.com. "Estimating Your Calorie Needs." http://drsquat.com/content/knowledge-base/estimating-your-calorie-needs.

Grandjean, A., K. Reimers, and M. Buyckx. "Hydration: Issues for the 21st Century." *Nutrition Reviews* 6, no. 8 (2003): 261–71.

Hatfield, Frederick C., and Daniel Gastelu. *Specialist in Performance Nutrition.* Santa Barbara: International Sports Sciences Association, 2000. (Book out of print.)

Kern, Mark. "Branched Chain Amino Acids (BCAA)." Pages 20–21 in *CRC Desk Reference on Sports Nutrition.* Boca Raton, FL: CRC Press, Taylor & Francis Group, 2005.

Kraemer, W. J., N. A. Ratamess, J. S. Volek, K. Häkkinen, M. R. Rubin, D. N. French, A. L. Gómez, M. R. McGuigan, T. P. Scheett, R. U. Newton, B. A. Spiering, M. Izquierdo, and F. S. Dioquardi. "The Effects of Amino Acid Supplementation on Hormonal Responses to Resistance Training Overreaching." *Metabolism* 55, no. 3 (2006): 282–91.

Maughan, R., P. Watson, G. Evans, N. Broad, and S. Shirreffs. "Water Balance and Salt Losses in Competitive Football." *International Journal of Sport Nutrition and Exercise Metabolism* 17 (2007): 583–94.

Newell, Kyle. "How to Use the Body Opus Diet!" *Bodybuilding.com* (19 April 2010). http://www.bodybuilding.com/fun/how-to-use-body-opus-diet.htm.

Passe, D., M. Horn, R. Murray, and J. Stofan. "Palatability and Voluntary Intake." *International Journal of Sport Nutrition and Exercise Metabolism* 14 (2004): 266–78.

Spano, M. "Functional Fooods, Beverages, and Ingredients in Athletics." *Strength and Conditioning Journal* 32, no. 1 (2010): 87–93.

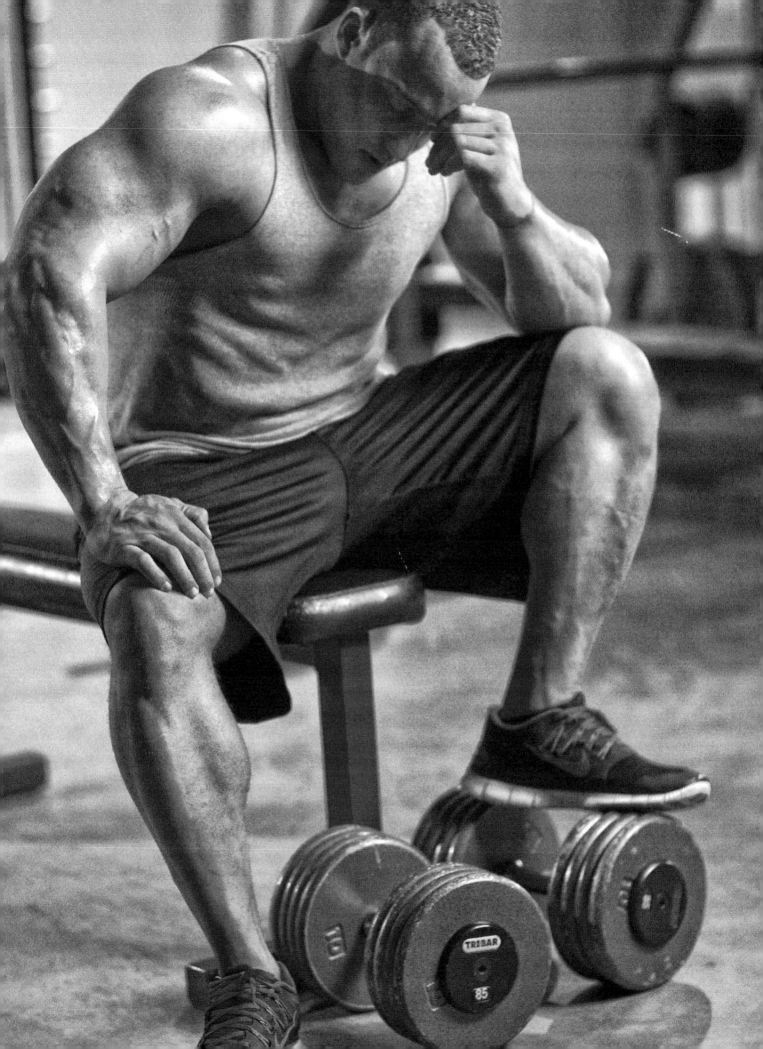

CHAPTER 11.

Recovery

All athletes, particularly bodybuilders, benefit from a properly planned recovery period. Far too many of them are not recovering properly, leaving them with less-than-optimal gains in size and strength.

A few questions heard time and time again are: "When is muscle developed?" "Do we get stronger during heavy deadlifts?" And "Do muscles get bigger with endless heavy bench presses?"

Without proper recovery, the answer to all three is *no!*

Recovery is when our muscles grow and become stronger. The muscle actually begins breaking down during training and is in a catabolic state. Once recovery begins, the body flips the switch, so to speak, and muscle is then in the preferred anabolic state.

Intense weight training forces the muscle fiber to adapt to the intense strain placed on it, break down, and prepare for muscle hypertrophy once recovery begins and the anabolic window is opened.

To take a holistic approach to maximize muscular development, use multiple exercises, tempos, rep schemes, and intensity levels. Because bodybuilders stress many muscle fibers at different levels of intensity, optimizing recovery is like gospel. The object is not to adapt to training, like so many other sports; it's to prevent this from happening so you can keep breaking down muscle fibers and keep making them grow.

UNDERSTANDING THE PRINCIPLE
OF INDIVIDUAL DIFFERENCES

It is not surprising that recovery rates will vary among bodybuilders. Bill Pearl and Arnold Schwarzenegger often prescribed hitting muscle groups every other day. Ronnie Coleman trained muscle groups twice a week. Branch Warren trains muscle groups only once a week.

Why are there so many different recovery periods for athletes in the same sport?

Recovery is mostly determined by the athlete's genetic blueprint. Ectomorphs typically are hard gainers, mesomorphs gain the easiest, and endomorphs typically gain fat more rapidly than muscle.

A number of other factors can determine adequate recovery periods. One factor is intensity. Doing 25 sets per body part, taking a majority of sets to momentary muscular failure, is harder to recover from than doing 10 sets in a workout with reps to spare at the end of each.

STRESSORS

Overtraining is not just training too intensely too often; it is an accumulation of all of life's events. Every day in our lives we are bombarded with a variety of stressors. Frequently, these stressors are of low enough "intensity" or subtle enough that they don't affect us.

What's worse, of those stressors that do have a more immediate negative effect, their intensity is often compounded by the mere presence of the many other stressors.

For example, any number of environmental stressors can have physical or physiological consequences. And one's psychological state is inextricably intertwined with one's own biochemistry.

Consider some of the more common stressors listed below that can directly influence overreaching and overtraining.

Environmental stressors stemming from:

- Excessive heat or cold
- Excessively high or low humidity
- Excessive altitude (above or below sea level)
- Challenging terrain
- Ultraviolet irradiation
- Environmental pollution
- Poorly designed clothing

- Poorly designed equipment
- Airborne pollen and other allergens
- Poor training facilities

Psychological/sociological stressors stemming from:

- Job problems
- Depression
- Mental illness
- Neurological disorders
- Pain
- Aging
- Anger
- Fear or anxiety
- Problems with academic studies
- Shaky financial status
- Family problems
- Sex problems
- Personality conflicts
- Schedule conflicts
- Boredom
- Lack of encouragement
- Psyching up too frequently
- Pressure to perform
- Lack of adequate coaching

Physiological/biochemical stressors stemming from:

- Environmental stress
- Psychological stress
- Anatomical/structural stress
- Aging
- Disease
- Myriad genetic factors
- Sleep disorders

- Poor nutritional status
- The use, misuse, or abuse of prescription or recreational drugs
- The use, misuse, or abuse of herbs (phytochemicals) and nutritional supplements

Anatomical/structural stressors stemming from:

- Surgically altered tissue structure
- Injury-induced alterations in tissue structure
- Environmental stress
- Physical defects
- Poor genetics
- Aging
- Overuse stress
- Poor exercise technique
- Ill-conceived training program
- Exertional stress (especially eccentric muscle actions)
- Too much training volume
- Too much training intensity
- Too much training duration
- Too much training frequency

As a rule of thumb, you want to eliminate (or, if you can't eliminate it, minimize the ill effects of) all stressors except the last five. These, you want, but *only* if you can *control* them.

A lot of mechanisms are believed to be responsible for fatigue (long term as well as short term). By cursorily reviewing the mechanisms of short-term fatigue, we can gain a more complete perspective of the dynamics of long-term fatigue—burnout.

You will see that short-term fatigue can involve any or all of the various mechanisms involved in movement, from the thought process to the final contraction of the muscle.

Back in 1978, exercise scientists in England divided short-term fatigue into two groups: central fatigue and peripheral fatigue. The causes of central fatigue include diminished motivation, impaired transmission of nerve impulses down the spinal cord, and impaired recruitment of motor neurons.

In a 2007 article in *Experimental Physiology*, Ross et al. explained that central fatigue in the brain still activates the muscles, but the muscles are a "potent competitor."

The causes of peripheral fatigue, on the other hand, involve impaired function of the peripheral nerves serving the individual muscles, impaired transmission of electrical impulse at the neuromuscular junction, and impaired processes of stimulation within the muscle cell (including metabolite changes resulting in depletion of ATP and thereby the function of the contractile machinery of the cell).

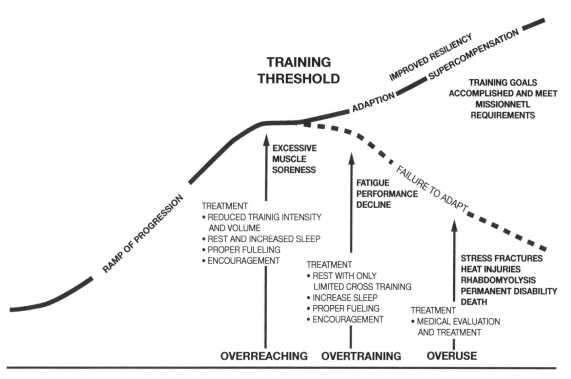

OVERTRAINING SYNDROME

"CHALLENGE IS TO PROVIDE A RATIONAL TRAINING PROGRESSION THAT ELICITS THE DESIRED TRAINING EFFECT"

(USARMYPT.COM)

Figure 11.1 Burnout and overtraining.

Folks, listen up!

There are two ways to cope with cumulative microtrauma.

You can avoid it, or you can treat it.

You avoid it *not* by avoiding lifting or by avoiding a small amount of (normal) cellular destruction, but instead by not letting microtrauma accumulate.

You do this the same way you treat cumulative microtrauma:

- Sensible, scientific weight training and light resistance systems of training, which employ a carefully devised "periodicity" or "cycle" method
- Sensible, scientific application of the many therapeutic modalities at your disposal that will be described throughout this chapter
- Sensible, scientific nutritional practice (especially maintaining an adequate amino acid pool to effect protein turnover, adequate energy foods to replace those depleted during intense training, and a minimum of 5 meals daily)
- Sensible, scientific nutritional supplementation (especially the branched chain aminos, adequate protein, vitamin and mineral intake, and other state-of-the-art supplements designed to aid tissue recovery and healing)
- Using good technique in your lifting and skills (especially avoiding excessive eccentric contractions ["negatives"] and uncontrolled ballistic movements)
- Getting plenty of rest both between workouts and at night (trying to get at least 9 hours of sleep per night, plus at least 1–2 short 20-minute "cat naps" during the day)
- Taking advantage of various psychological techniques that promote restoration (especially meditation, visualization training, hypnotherapy, or self-hypnosis techniques)

So, it all boils down to a simple plan.

The plan is to do things the best way science can provide. The above list ought to at least get you thinking along some reasonable pathway in that regard.

CALORIC INTAKE

Adequate caloric intake with the right nutrients gets the recovery ball rolling. If you are not eating enough to give your body the energy and protein it needs to rebuild the muscle, it won't grow or become stronger. Inadequate caloric intake will result in overtraining and, even worse, increasing the chance of injury. Not only is it important to know what to eat and how much of it, but *when* you eat plays a huge role in *how* you respond to exercise.

I highly recommend the book *Nutrient Timing* by Drs. Robert Portman and John Ivy. Nutrition guru Dr. John Berardi has done an excellent job publishing a number of articles on this subject; check out his website, www.precisionnutrition.com.

Contemporary science generally focuses on calories in versus calories out, and if you lift weights and eat enough calories and protein, muscle hypertrophy will take place. This is great for the average couch potato hoping to buff up a little for the high school reunion; it is not so simple for you, the muscle-building elitist. Consume the wrong nutrients at the wrong time, and you can potentially incapacitate your hard work in the gym. Simple carbs before bed is not the path to a championship physique, but consumed post workout they can expedite recovery and open the floodgates to anabolism.

Intra-Workout Nutrients

The authors of *Nutrient Timing* break the day down into three phases: energy phase, anabolic phase, and growth phase. The *energy phase* is when you need fuel during a workout. Your body's acute hormonal response to weight training is increased GH, IGF-1, and testosterone secretion, but not all anabolic hormones are abundantly increased; insulin concentrations are reduced, and increased skeletal blood flow takes place.

During exercise, the following acute catabolic effects take place: increased cortisol levels, decreased net protein balance, depleted glycogen, depleted insulin, and increased metabolic rate.

The idea is to counteract these effects but maximize the anabolic ones. This can be aided by consuming a sports drink that contains branch chain amino acids (BCAAs), like Gatorade, during your workout. Gatorade will help replenish glycogen stores. BCAAs have also been shown to reduce fatigue in hard-training anaerobic athletes—that is, you, the bodybuilder. It has also been noted that leucine may be the most critical BCAA because of its anti-catabolic properties and vital role in protein synthesis.

World-renowned William J. Kraemer led a study showing that, in a state of overreaching for two weeks, strength performances were not compromised for a control group supplementing with BCAAs, whereas strength performances were significantly compromised for the group taking a placebo.

Purposeful overreaching is a component of many periodized bodybuilding training plans. Supplementation with BCAAs has huge implications for performance, which indirectly aids in the acquisition of hypertrophy.

Countless other studies confirm the effectiveness of BCAAs. During the energy phase, Dr. John Berardi recommends consuming 0.8 grams of simple carbs per kilo of bodyweight and 0.4 grams of a fast-acting protein, like whey, per kilo of bodyweight.

Following Berardi's recommendations, a 100 kg bodybuilder (220 pounds) would consume 80 grams of carbs and 40 grams of protein during his workout.

Post-Workout Nutrients

The *anabolic phase* lasts up to 90 minutes post workout. This is when your muscle cells are ready to grow; if your muscles are fed with the right nutrients post workout, abundant muscle growth will take place; if they are not, catabolism will be magnified and prolonged, and that's not a good thing!

Insulin sensitivity and glucose tolerance peaks post workout, so up to 2 grams of carbohydrate per kilo of bodyweight and 0.5 grams of protein per kilo of body weight can be consumed.

This means for a 220 pound (100 kg) bodybuilder, this would be 100 x 2 = 200 grams of carbohydrates, and 100 x 0.5 = 50 grams of protein. During workout and post workout, this would equal 280 grams of carbs and 90 grams of protein.

This would look like 280 + 90 = 370, and 370 x 4 = 1,480 calories; this is a lot of calories and carbohydrates, so when employing this strategy, carbohydrates will need to be reduced throughout the day. This is on the extreme high end; but obviously, when cutting, it is important to pay attention to calories in versus calories out.

What About the Rest of the Day?

A couple of hours after the completion of training, while the anabolic window is not wide open, carbohydrates do not need to be consumed to excess because of the intra-workout and post-workout consumption of fast-acting carbs; a majority of glycogen stores are restored. Throughout the rest of the day, a 1:1 protein-to-carbohydrate ratio can be consumed, along with complex carbs with a lower glycemic index (GI) rating.

PERFORMANCE-ENHANCING DRUGS (PEDS)

Another factor to consider is the use of PEDs.

Testosterone, an androgenic hormone produced by the body, is paramount in creating an anabolic environment for muscle. If athletes choose to introduce PEDs to their training regimen, the workload on the muscle can be increased as the recovery period is accelerated. It is important to remember, regardless of muscle-building drugs cycled into your regimen, that PEDs accelerate muscle recovery; they do not enhance the recovery of your central nervous system.

Vladimir Zatsiorsky, in his book *Science and Practice of Strength Training,* espouses that when training a core movement at above 90% of one's maximum with the maximal effort (ME) method more than three weeks in a row, progress will cease and start to actually go backward.

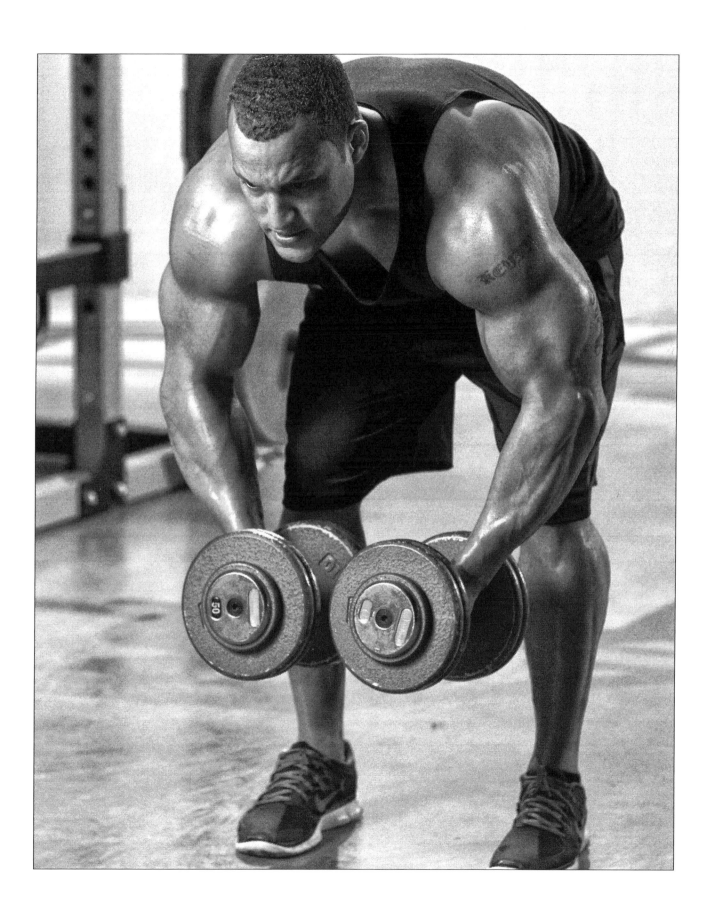

This is why after three weeks with 90% plus, it would be important to switch core movements or take a week of less intensity, less than 70%. This happens because of central fatigue and inability to perform because of factors of the central nervous system. Peripheral fatigue/muscular-related fatigue can be somewhat counteracted with PEDs, whereas central fatigue cannot.

You can increase volume with submaximal weights on non-neuromuscular taxing exercises while on steroids; but training deadlifts to failure with 90% or greater of your one-repetition max, week in, week out, steroids or not? Good luck recovering from that.

Regardless of drug status, carefully monitor volume at 90% of core lift maxes. Because steroids *may* enhance neuromuscular factors, this is one more reason to be aware of central fatigue if you are using.

DELOADS FOR BODYBUILDING

Powerlifters typically train movements with little purposeful isolation of muscle groups. The individual lifts typically involve multiple muscle groups. Typically, the core exercises are only done once a week, sometimes twice. Some popular Eastern Bloc programs, however, suggest performing each lift multiple times per week, but very submaximal weights are used and assistance movements are very limited.

Many powerlifters utilize a "deload week." I have trained many world-record-setting powerlifters and have implemented some form of deloading with all of them. The deload is an excellent tool to rest connective tissue and muscles but, most importantly, to rest the central nervous system (CNS).

A simple guideline to follow for deloading is less than 70% intensity (lighter weights used) and less than 70% volume (sets and reps). It is not uncommon for powerlifters to take anywhere from 7 to 14 days off prior to a meet so that they are fully recovered prior to a maximum-effort lift.

It is also not uncommon for powerlifters, following the meet, to take the week off from training to rest the CNS after a maximum effort. After all, many Russian researchers have concluded maximal competition lifts can take weeks to recover from because of the tremendous stress on the CNS.

As a bodybuilder, you must train core movements as well as isolated muscle groups. Bodybuilders can typically follow a deload recovery protocol similar to that of powerlifters.

Deloads for powerlifters provide a chance to perform lifts in compensatory accelerated style with submaximal weights, along with the opportunity to refine technique.

Bodybuilders, of course, need great technique, but the object is much more sophisticated than simply moving the weight from point A to point B; the object is muscle hypertrophy of the specific muscle groups you are using. If your anterior delts are very powerful, they may overpower your pecs on the bench press. This may call for a pre-exhaustion protocol, or even eliminating the movement from your arsenal.

It is important to pay attention to kinesthesia, Weider's Instinctive Principle, and, of course, physical changes that are taking place. I highly suggest opening a Photobucket account (they are free) so you and your coach or training partners can make honest assessments of your aesthetic progress.

Deload workouts give bodybuilders a chance to perfect movements because intensity is not a concern. These workouts are not blow-off workouts, they are technique workouts. Follow periods of high intensity with periods of low intensity using the provided guidelines, and you will look, perform, and feel better.

Some folks may feel deloads are not for them. Should the skinny guy just trying to add a little muscle deload? Of course! As stated earlier, without adequate recovery, the muscle cannot grow or become stronger. Recovery opens the anabolic window.

How about the guy who is leaning out? Is recovery important to him?

Yes!

If this guy is dieting, his body is automatically in a catabolic state. That means that fat is reducing, as well as muscle. The idea is to save as much muscle as possible, so adequate recovery is a must.

There have been famous bodybuilders who do not deload; and prison yards are full of inmates who pack on slabs of muscle mass by hitting the pig iron hard, day in, day out.

"The Austrian Oak," Arnold Schwarzenegger, has talked about times when he walked into the gym and felt like he shouldn't train, so he walked out.

Most of the guys on the prison yard train off of an intuitive feel, meaning when they feel beat up mentally and physically, they take a couple of days off or go lighter and do fewer sets/reps (volume).

This is basically Weider's Instinctive Training Principle in action.

With deloads, there will be fewer "off days"; periods of reduced intensity will be systematically cycled in your training, so you won't have to abruptly stop training when your body feels broken down.

ACTIVE RECOVERY

Active recovery is spawned from the notion that you recover more efficiently when you are active. Numerous studies have demonstrated that elevated muscle blood flow through low-intensity exercise is highly beneficial; it helps minimize the delayed onset of muscle soreness (DOMS), and it enhances muscle healing.

Powerlifters are light years ahead of bodybuilders when it comes to active recovery. Sled dragging with light weight, performed the day following a heavy squat, is a popular strategy for active recovery. Some powerlifters will drag a sled with extremely light weight for 10–20 minutes straight; others will do sled-drag trips of 20–60 yards with light weight and short rest intervals. Even a low intensity 15–20 minute walk can serve as a resourceful active recovery modality.

Active recovery after a heavy chest workout could vary from extremely light dumbbell bench presses to increase blood flow to a dynamic stretch or even foam rolling.

Light activity can enhance recovery; the key is not to add an additional stressor. The day after bench pressing 400 pounds for reps, doing dumbbell bench presses with 15 pounds can aid in recovery, whereas doing 1,000 push-ups will not. Common sense must be applied to active recovery.

WEIDER SYSTEM

The Weider system was developed to guide you in developing your own personal system based on your own unique recuperative ability, experience, goals, strengths, weaknesses, and "guts" to go the distance. Initially, many in the lab chose to scoff at the Weider Principles, yet science has confirmed many of them.

The Weider System guidelines come in the form of a series of training methods collected (and in many instances named) by Joe Weider personally over many years, which became widely known as the Weider Principles.

In fact, of the Weider Principles that were developed by Joe personally, one in particular had a major impact on the world of bodybuilding. That was the concept of splitting your workouts to train specific body parts. The Split System, Double Split System, and Triple Split System, as they became known, are Joe's unique contribution to bodybuilding science.

Joe was a true pioneer, the founder of modern bodybuilding, and he has done more for the sport than anyone.

We cannot forget Joe Weider!

The Weider Principles encompass three broad categories:

- Principles to help you plan your training cycle
- Principles to help you arrange your exercises in each workout
- Principles to help you perform each exercise

This is periodization in action.

It is easy to discern whether this orderly collection of training methods, both in the aggregate and individually, adheres to the seven Granddaddy laws.

The simple truth is that individually, they do not. But when you look at them in the aggregate, and the guidelines as to when and how to apply them, then they most certainly do.

Here's why:

The simple fact that you are training at all assumes you know (a) you're going to grow (Overcompensation Principle), (b) you're going to train regularly (Use/Disuse Principle), and (c) weight training is the most efficient method of doing (a) and (b), as opposed to, say, riding a bicycle (Specificity Principle).

Both the type and amount of adaptive stress that each of the Weider Principles delivers to the organism can be manipulated efficiently and effectively (SAID and Overload Principles, respectively).

Each method listed in the Weider System has its strengths and weaknesses in regard to the specific muscle components it targets (SAID Principle), so you must use your instinct and experience in discerning when to apply each, or whether to apply it at all (Individual Differences Principle); and the list of methods is totally flexible.

Within the instructions for each are listed guidelines to aid you in discerning whether to use it and how often to employ it in your day-to-day training microcycles (GAS and Individual Differences Principles).

RECOVERY: THE PLANNING FACTOR

The three categories of principles discussed in the Weider System are listed n the next subsections with a brief explanation of each. One of the principles appears in all three categories. That's the Instinctive Training Principle.

When planning and carrying out a training program, use your own training experience and knowledge of how your body responds to exercise stress. This must take place on a cycle-to-cycle, day-to-day, and quite literally minute-to-minute basis!

This does not mean not having a plan; it means being able to adapt your plan. This is why it is important to keep a training journal; the more detailed the journal, the more effectively you will be able to prescribe training variables.

Principles for Planning Your Training Cycle:

- *Cycle Training Principle* (breaking your training year into cycles for strength, mass, or contest preparation, you help avoid injury and keep your body responsive to adaptation)

- *Split System Training Principle* (breaking your workout week into upper versus lower body training, for example, will result in more intense training sessions)

- *Double or Triple Split Training Principle* (breaking your workout down into two or three shorter, more intense training sessions per day)

- *Muscle Confusion Training Principle* (muscles accommodate to a specific type of stress ["habituate" or "plateau"] when you continually apply the same stress to your muscles over time, so you must constantly vary exercises, sets, reps, and weight to avoid accommodation)

- *Progressive Overload Training Principle* (the basis of increasing any parameter of fitness is to make your muscles work harder than they are accustomed to)

- *Holistic Training Principle* (different cellular organelles respond differently to different forms of stress, so using a variety of rep/set schemes, intensity, and frequency will maximize muscle mass)

- *Eclectic Training Principle* (combining mass, strength or isolation-refinement training techniques into your program, as your instincts dictate, often helps you achieve greater progress)

- *Instinctive Training Principle* (eventually, all bodybuilders instinctively attain the ability to construct diets, routines, cycles, intensity levels, reps, and sets that work best for them. Of course, they should still seek outside counsel. The more you advance, the more important it is to receive input and implement it in the training cycle. To make instinctive training work, you have to be objective)

Principles to Help You Arrange Your Workout:

- *Set System Training Principle* (performing one set per body part was the old way; the Set System calls for multiple sets for each exercise in order to apply maximum adaptive stress)

- *Superset Training Principle* (alternating opposing muscle group exercises with little rest between sets)

- *Compound Sets Training Principle* (alternating two exercises for one body part with little rest between sets)

- *Tri-Sets Training Principle* (doing three exercises for one muscle group with little rest between sets)

- *Giant Sets Training Principle* (doing 4–6 exercises for one muscle group with little rest between sets)

- *Staggered Sets Training Principle* (injecting 10 sets of boring forearm, abdominal or calf work in between sets for, say, chest or legs)

- *Rest-Pause Training Principle* (using 85%–90% of your max, do 2–3 reps and put the weight down, then do 2–3 more, rest, 2–3 more, and rest for a total of 3–4 rest-pauses; the short rest-pauses allow enough time for ATP to be resynthesized and permit further reps with the heavy weight)

- *Muscle Priority Training Principle* (work your weaker body parts first in any given workout; alternatively, work the larger muscle groups first, while you're fresh and energy levels are still high)

- *Pre-Exhaustion Training Principle* (e.g., superset flyes, a chest isolation exercise with bench presses, and a compound exercise involving triceps and chest, in order to maximize chest development by pre-exhausting the triceps)

- *Pyramiding Training Principle* (start a body part session with higher rep/ low weight and gradually add weight (and commensurably reduce the reps), ending with a weight you can do for 5 reps or so)

- *Descending Sets Training Principle* (lighter weights from set to set as fatigue sets in; called stripping)

- *Instinctive Training Principle* (Eventually, all bodybuilders instinctively attain the ability to construct diets, routines, cycles, intensity levels, reps, and sets that work best for them)

Principles to Help You Perform Each Exercise:

- *Isolation Training Principle* (all muscles act as stabilizers, synergists, antagonist, or protagonist. By making any given muscle the prime mover in any given exercise, you've isolated it as much as possible, and therefore the stress applied to it)

- *Quality Training Principle* (gradually reducing the rest between sets while still maintaining or increasing the number of reps performed)

- *Cheating Training Principle* (swing weight past the sticking point at the end of a set in order to add stress)

- *Continuous Tension Training Principle* (maintain slow, continuous tension on muscles to maximize red-fiber involvement)

- *Forced Reps Training Principle* (partner-assisted reps at the end of a set)

- *Flushing Training Principle* (doing 3–4 exercises for a body part before moving to another body part)

- *Burns Training Principle* (2–3-inch, quick movements at the end of a set)

- *Partial Reps Training Principle* (because of leverage changes throughout any given exercise, it's sometimes helpful to do partial movements with varying weight in order to derive maximum overload stress for that body part)

- *Retro-Gravity Training Principle* (negatives or eccentrics as they're called, make it possible to get more muscle cells to respond because you can lower about 30%–40% more weight than you can successfully lift concentrically; this is important for increased IGF-1 production and satellite cell proliferation)

- *Peak Contraction Training Principle* (holding the weight through maximum contraction for a few seconds at the completion of a movement)

- *Superspeed Training Principle* (compensatory acceleration of movements to stimulate hard-to-reach fast-twitch fibers)

- *Iso-Tension Training Principle* (method of practicing posing, tensing each muscle maximally for 6–10 seconds for up to a total of 30–44 flexes in a variety of posing positions)

As you learn about the science of training and the art of programming, you can synergistically blend these principles into a holistic program.

Please review the periodization section near the end of Chapter 1. In discussions with Dr. Fred Hatfield on recovery, he repeatedly emphasized that periodization and planning are the most important factors in adequate recovery.

I agree with Dr. Squat!

BODYBUILDING DELOAD TAKE-HOME POINTS

- Volume (sets x reps x weight): Perform 60%–70% of total workload
- Perform reps in a peak contraction style
- Work on perfecting movement technique
- Deload every 3–6 weeks (this is a guideline, not the rule)

Here is a practical example of a chest workout for a bodybuilding deload. Workout A is the last intense chest workout; workout B is the deload version.

Workout A (Intense Workout)

1. Band Resisted Incline Dumbbell Incline Presses—4 sets x 8 reps (band resistance 25% of total dumbbell weight)

2. Weighted Dips (Forward Lean)—12, 12, 8, Rest Pause (3 total sets @ 80% of one-rep max)

3. Negative Overload Smith Machine Bench Presses (5-second negative); once this pace can no longer be achieved, do as many reps as possible without negative overload weight x 3 sets

4. Chain Flyes—12 reps/Dumbbell Pull Over—20 reps (3 super sets)

   Time Under Tension Incline Cable Flyes (40 seconds) x 3 sets

Workout B (Deload Workout)

1. Incline Dumbbell Incline Presses—3 sets x 8 reps (same weight as last week, minus bands)

2. Dips (Forward Lean)—Bodyweight x 8 x 3 (really work on feeling the movement)

3. Smith Machine Bench Presses (5-second negative) x 6 x 2 sets (use 70% of last week's weight)

4. Chain Flyes—12 reps/Dumbbell Pull Over—20 reps (2 super sets—use 70% of last week's weight)

5. Incline Cable Flyes x 10 x 2 sets (use 70% of last week's weight)

"Okay, I get it: Recovery is important! So what different factors of recovery are important, and how should I implement them in my program?"

Glad you asked.

NUTRITION AND CALORIC INTAKE

To recap: adequate caloric intake is vital to the body during recovery so that anabolism can occur. Protein is vital to protein synthesis, the precursor to anabolism. As high as 2 grams per pound of bodyweight can be needed. Carbohydrates and fats are necessary for the energy reservoirs for hardcore workouts.

There is such a thing as too much protein, and it can even hurt your muscle-building goals. Once your needs for muscle repair have been met, your body will actually break down and use protein for energy. Remember, carbohydrates are the body's preferred energy source. Consuming huge amounts of proteins is also very expensive. If something could potentially hurt your muscle-building goals, why risk it? And why waste the money? Some alarmists like to preach that if you go beyond a certain amount of protein, your kidneys could potentially fail very rapidly. Science does not support these claims for healthy people. Generally, you're not going to have to exceed 1.5 grams per pound of bodyweight. Just like training, more is not necessarily better when it comes to protein.

A rule of thumb for bulking is a minimum of 16–20 calories per pound of bodyweight (many times more will be needed). So, if you weigh 200 pounds (200 x 16 = 3,200, and 200 x 20 = 4,000), that means you will need 3,200–4,000 calories to bulk. This can vary depending on activity level, work, training and intensity and, of course, individual genetic blueprint.

Legal Supplements

I would recommend the following supplements: BCAAs, creatine, and glutamine; all of these supplements have been shown to work in numerous peer-reviewed studies.

And that's important because any Tom, Dick, or Harry on the street can sell you the hype, but it means nothing *unless* it is scientifically proven to work in *people* and not just mice or other lab animals.

I also like a high-quality, multi-blend protein powder.

Many pre-workout supplements exist; however, numerous studies confirm the effectiveness of caffeine on maximum strength as well as muscle endurance.

With pre-workout supplementation like high dosages of caffeine, your body will adapt quickly, so initially you can just keep increasing the dose (which is not good), but eventually this will no longer work.

Cycle on and off pre-workout supplements. Deload weeks are a great chance to cycle off stimulants and pre-workout formulas.

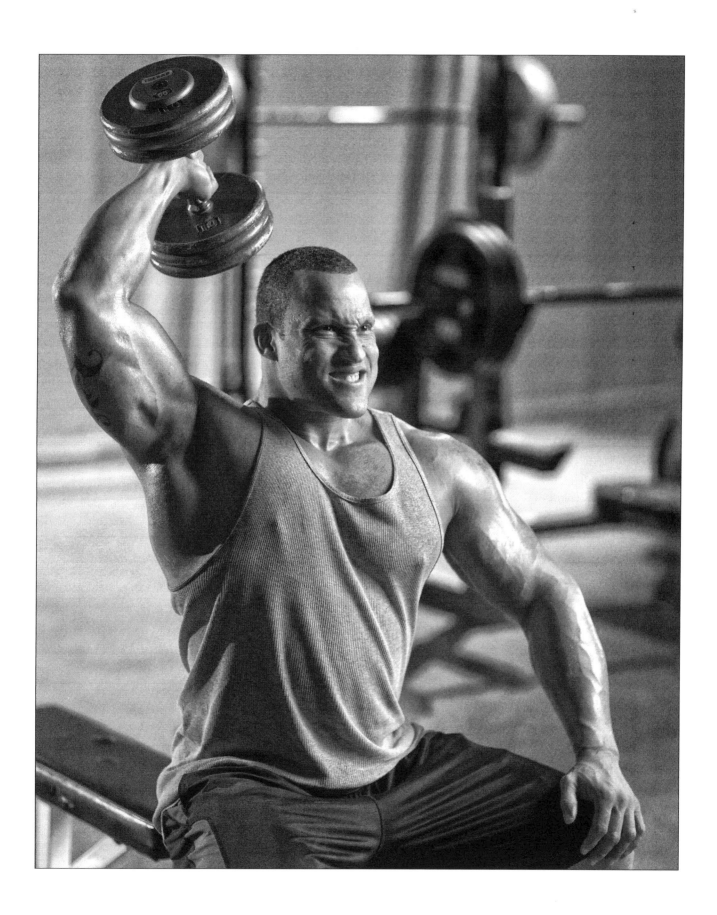

Illegal Supplements

I highly discourage the use of these compounds.

However, it would be unfair and naïve not to mention these anabolic agents.

Androgenic anabolic steroids (AAS) have been around forever. AAS are believed to improve recovery time, thus allowing the athlete to train longer and harder, and with greater intensity. Remember to consider possible adverse effects to your health as well as the legal consequences.

SLEEPING

Sleep is imperative to recovery. The body emits most of its natural growth hormone—as much as 70%—during REM (Rapid Eye Movement). Sleep has a profound effect on muscle growth and physical well-being.

I recently read an article that stated the body needs at least 7 hours of sleep in a 24-hour daily cycle. This article was aimed at "the average person." Bodybuilders certainly do not fit that category. At least 8 hours of solid, uninterrupted sleep is needed.

It is also recommended to nap as often as possible.

A recent study performed by the University of Chicago Medical School and published in the *Annals of Internal Medicine* reiterated this. The study consisted of two control groups, both on calorie-restricted, weight-loss diets. One group was sleep deprived, while the other had a full night's sleep every night. Both groups lost the same amount of weight in this study, but, the sleep deprived group had 25% less fat loss. Think about the potential benefits you are robbing yourself of while dieting, if you are not sleeping enough.

It is important for bodybuilders to understand how sleep cycles work, so the maximum anabolic effects of rest can take place. During sleep, the brain functions in cycles, with each one lasting approximately an hour and a half.

There are two separate types of sleep; REM and non-REM. A sleep cycle commences with four stages of non-REM sleep; then this will change to REM sleep. Generally, five of these cycles are experienced per night.

During REM, as well as stage three and four sleep, your body and brain are completely at rest and memory consolidation takes place. This literally gives your brain a chance to rest and recharge.

From a weightlifting standpoint, you will feel mentally alert and neuromuscular maximum efficiency will take place. Nearly 50% of sleep is REM for newborns; as we age, this number reduces. This is why it is important to get your rest: As we age, our sleep becomes less efficient.

The Importance of Nutrient Timing and Sleep

The first meal of the day is called breakfast, and if you break down this word, you'll see it means to break your fast; when you are sleeping you are obviously not eating.

While you are in this necessary fast, things turn catabolic because amino acids are converting to glucose. Regardless of the recommendations Granny made about not eating before bedtime, the longer you don't eat prior to falling asleep, the deeper you fall into a catabolic state; when you're properly fed, however, the opposite is true.

This can be prevented by consuming a casein protein shake before bed or eating it from a natural source like cottage cheese. Casein is a very slow-digesting protein, so it releases throughout the night, counter to what a fast-acting protein like whey would do.

Recent research from the Weider Group confirms this by showing that bodybuilders who drank a casein shake before bed gained significantly more muscle than bodybuilders who drank casein only in the middle of the day. This research can be practically applied to you by consuming 25–50 grams of casein protein prior to bedtime.

Tips to Optimize Sleep

Often it is hard to get a good night's sleep. Even when we do fall asleep, the quality of sleep may be insufficient.

The following tips can assist you in getting that good night's sleep:

1. **Pray before bed.** It is much easier to fall asleep and rest being at peace with your Creator.

2. **Avoid a pattern of sleeping 12 hours one night, then 6 the next.** This is not the same as sleeping 9 hours a night. A true sleep bank does not exist. Oversleeping and under-sleeping throw off your routine.

3. **Exercise.** Avoid intense, late-night sessions. If these were done early in the day, they would aid in a good night's sleep, but if they're done at night, the opposite is true.

4. **Avoid alcohol, caffeine, and other stimulants before bed.** Caffeine increases alertness, as do other stimulants. Alcohol, on the other hand, will actually help you fall asleep, but it will greatly disrupt REM sleep; after a night of heavy drinking you fall asleep early, but you are not really resting.

5. **Avoid sleeping pills.** These will create a dependency and should be a last resort.

6. **Get checked out for sleep apnea.** Many large, muscular men have sleep apnea that can easily be treated with a CPAP device that not only will improve sleep quality and performance but can lower blood pressure and greatly improve overall health.

7. **Optimize your sleeping environment.** Keep your room cool and dark. Sometimes even playing soft, classical music can help you doze off into a restful bliss.

8. **Relax at night and avoid extreme highs and lows.** Neither promotes relaxation. If every time a certain person calls you it always results in an extreme emotional reaction, then, when you see that person calling, do not pick up the phone.

FURTHER EXPEDITING RECOVERY

Sometimes a good night's sleep and a proper diet still aren't getting the job done. When you train hard, sometimes the body still has not healed completely during the recommended recovery period.

So what can we do to expedite the healing process?

Chiropractic Care

Over the years, chiropractic care has gotten a bad rap by some because of a few bad apples, but the fact remains that many top bodybuilders and strength athletes use chiropractic care regularly, as they should.

I have seen Ronnie Coleman, on numerous occasions, getting an adjustment at the chiropractor before or after I get mine. Good chiropractic care is one of the most valuable ergogenic aids for the athlete.

Chiropractic is a natural (that is, not employing drugs or surgery) healing system that treats the whole person rather than just the particular symptoms of a disorder.

By restoring proper alignment to the spinal column and the joints, the doctor of chiropractic can help the athlete operate at optimum biomechanical efficiency. The implications for the bodybuilder are of epic proportion.

The bottom line is, if you are not properly functioning biomechanically, you will not be able to lift the weights necessary long enough to stay injury free. Chiropractic care can help the bodybuilder strengthen muscles, improve coordination and balance, extend range of motion, restore proper biomechanical function, achieve greater mental focus, and have more energy.

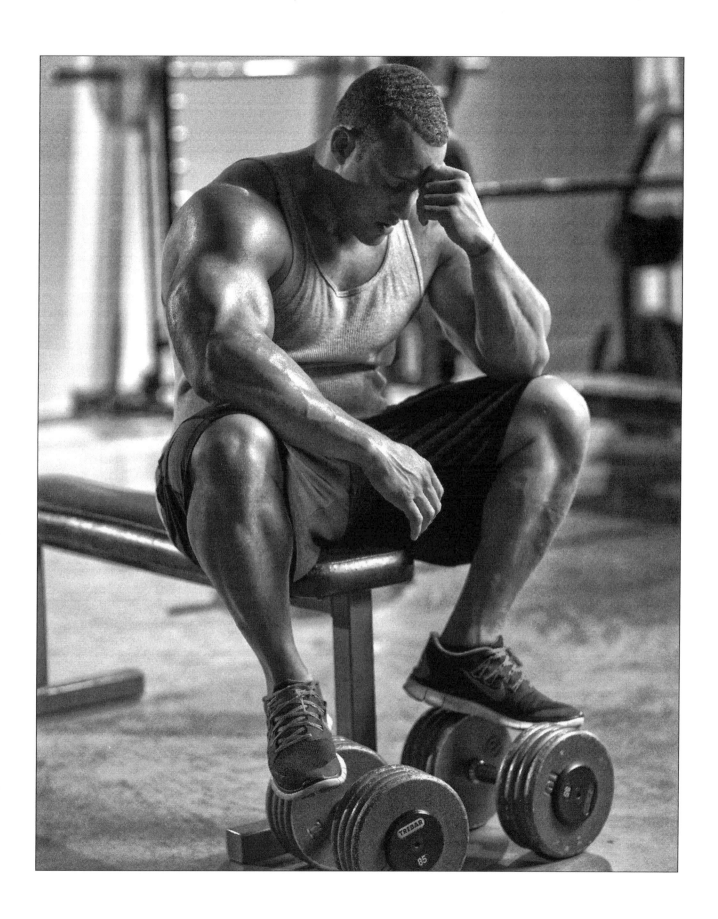

Competitive bodybuilders and recreational weight training enthusiasts alike are advised to seek out (by asking fellow athletes) a competent sports chiropractor; one who emphasizes the biomechanical aspect of treatment and injury prevention.

Massage

I train clients at Metroflex Gym, the home to IFBB Pros Ronnie Coleman, Johnnie Jackson, Branch Warren, Cory Mathews, and Stephen Fraizer, along with top strength athletes like nationally ranked bodybuilder/strongest raw bench presser in the world, Al Davis, and a host of other top bodybuilders and powerlifters.

We have an excellent masseur named Chris "Sarge" Stratton who stays quite busy due to the beatings our athletes endure. I am not talking about Swedish Massage or an Oriental Massage with a happy ending.

I'm talking about deep tissue massage.

All of the aforementioned athletes have used Chris on a regular basis for massage therapy. Many of these athletes are 40+ years old and train harder than men half their age and still are making improvements.

I believe this is due in large part to massage.

So wait a second: Massage is for more than relaxation?

Yes!

World famous sprinting coach, the late Charlie Francis, believed you could get up to 40% more maximal effort training with the proper implementation of massage therapy.

When Charlie stood at the throne of Canada's world-class sprint program by his own accord, the marathon runners had a higher injury rate than that of the sprinters.

This is huge!

Francis believed this was primarily because of the massage therapy and chiropractic care he implemented in his athletes' training.

How massage works. Massage works by applying mechanical pressure to the soft tissue; in turn, this can increase joint range of motion, improve muscle stiffness, and reduce delayed onset of muscle soreness (DOMS).

This is not just gym lore; science is beginning to confirm the effectiveness of massage.

In one contemporary study, researchers at McMaster University showed the profound effect deep tissue massage had on the cells' "powerhouse," the mitochondria. Post-workout, deep tissue massage caused muscle to enlarge and grow new mitochondria; and as you recall, mitochondria serve to convert nutrients into useful energy.

The subjects in this study were men who rode a stationary bike to exhaustion. Post workout, the men received a deep-tissue massage on one of their legs for 10 minutes. Pre- and post-training session muscle biopsies were taken from one quadriceps muscle, and then from both muscles right after a 10-minute massage of one leg, and then again 2.5 hours later.

The results were that the deep-tissue massage increased the number of mitochondria, as well as the muscles' size, significantly more than exercise alone. This means an increase in the efficiency with which muscles can utilize oxygen.

During a massage, blood flow can improve and increase the temperature of the muscle. Additionally, a massage by a licensed, skilled practitioner sparks a heart rate reduction and decreases blood pressure; this is monumental in the recovery battle and can be extra helpful to the bodybuilder abusing PEDs that have caused a spike in blood pressure.

Furthermore, massage can potentially reduce cortisol levels. Since the name of the game is minimizing body fat and maximizing muscle mass, I will redundantly pontificate the importance for the bodybuilder, particularly the natural one, to *use massage*.

Mental relaxation is a byproduct of a good massage; just like your muscles, your brain needs a rest.

Another 2012 study published in the *Alternative Medicine Alert Journal* confirmed the McMaster study findings on the effects of massage on mitochondria.

The study also found massage therapy modulates pro-inflammatory cytokines, which causes a similar effect to NSAIDs, but without the negative side effects. The study went on to show another large benefit for the bodybuilder, by demonstrating that massage enhances protein synthesis in exercised muscle tissue.

Selecting a masseuse (masseur). A good massage therapist needs to have knowledge of anatomy, physiology, and pathology, both theoretical and applied. Make sure your massage therapist has a current license. Experience is important with any profession, but hands-on experience is how one gets better. Find a masseuse who works with athletes, not someone whose sole responsibility is to help rich people relax at a health spa.

Foam Rolling

Massage therapy can be expensive. Self-Myofascial Release (SMR), better known as foam rolling, is much cheaper than massage therapy. A foam roller is a one-time investment that costs under $10. Similar to deep tissue massage, it works by releasing trigger points because of the principle of autogenic inhibition.

Practitioners of SMR believe that the foam roller is one of the most effective tools for releasing tension in muscles and effectively improving your overall range-of-motion.

Popular strength coach, Mike Boyle, has referred to foam rolling as a poor man's massage. Advocates of the foam roller believe it is nearly as effective as a massage.

The foam roller is believed to have the benefits of correcting muscle imbalances, reducing stress, reducing pain, increasing joint range-of-motion, relieving muscle soreness and stress, improving the extensibility of the musculotendinous junction, increasing neuromuscular efficiency, and maintaining normal muscle length.

Foam rolling technique. Foam rolling is simply performed by taking the foam roller and slowly rolling it across the muscle from which you want to release adhesions and knots. The foam roller is wedged between the floor and your bodyweight at the specific area you are focusing on.

You want to roll at a slow, controlled paced and stop on the most tender spots, directly focusing on the localized area where pain is most persistent. Once pain ceases, then move onto rolling out another area. Increasing the intensity of foam rolling is simple: Just put a larger percentage of your body on the roller. To decrease the intensity, do the opposite.

Expert trainer Mike Robertson recommends rolling from the proximal to the distal attachment of a muscle. When rolling the thighs, roll from the top to the bottom, focusing on one specific area; do not do the whole targeted area at once. Robertson believes this sequence is important because, as you gain proximity to the distal muscle-tendon junction, there is greatly increasing tension.

In summary, you work the top half of the muscle first; then, after it has loosened up, roll the bottom half. This will decrease the tension that is ensuing at the bottom of the muscle.

Foam Rolling Guidelines:

- Breath slowly and controlled; this will relieve tension.

- Perform foam rolling exercises post workout and off training days. Some in the field advocate this as a warm-up. However, not enough studies have been performed on SMR effects on force production and potential injury prevention when foam rolling is used as a warm-up.

- Spend approximately 1–2 minutes per foam-rolling technique per spot.

- Spend 30–45 seconds on a painful/tender area.

- To get the most out of foam rolling, do it daily.

Few peer-reviewed studies have been conducted on the effectiveness of SMR. A number of trainers and physical therapists in the field swear by the effectiveness of foam rolling techniques. This is why they are included in this text. Some advocate these for both warm-up and cool down.

If integrating SMR into your holistic program, remember this: The Golgi Tendon Organs (GTOs) are proprioceptors that are sensitive to tension and rate of tension change.

Stimulation of GTOs will inhibit muscle spindle activity and decrease tension in the muscle; this is called *autogenic inhibition.* That is because the contracting prime mover muscle is inhibited by its own receptors.

In layman's terms, like static stretching, SMR activates the GTOs and potentially limits the ability to produce maximum force and maximum power.

Although many swear by this method as an effective warm-up, no direct studies currently exist on force production effects from using foam rolling prior to training.

The following is an example of an SMR cool-down program after an intense workout.

SMR (Foam Rolling)

Roll tender spots for 30–45 seconds, 1 set each spot:

Hamstrings and calves
Gluteus medius
IT band/Tensor fascia latae
Quadriceps/Hip flexors
Adductor
Low-back/Erector spinae
Rhomboids
Latissimus dorsi

Contrast Baths

Contrast bath therapy, also known as *hot/cold immersion therapy,* is a therapeutic modality where a portion of your body, or your entire body, is immersed in cold water followed by warm water; this is done for several alternating cycles.

This is the theoretical basis of how a contrast bath works: It increases local blood circulation by vasodilatation caused by the warm water, followed by vasoconstriction caused by the water. Cold water causes lymph vessels to contract, and they relax when exposed to warm cold water. Because of the alternating temperatures, the lymph vessels help remove stagnant fluid; in turn, a favorable effect on inflammation helps expedite the recovery process of broken-down tissues.

A 2007 study published in *The Journal of Science and Medicine in Sport* showed contrast water immersion to be a valid method of hastening plasma lactate decrease during recovery after intense anaerobic exercise for both males and females. In 2012, another study confirmed the effectiveness of contrast baths.

In-the-trenches coaches and athletes from a variety of sports implement contrast baths and believe they are very effective to enhance recovery from intense training.

For contrast baths, the legendary, late Charlie Francis, who was considered revolutionary in many of the recovery methods he helped popularize in the west that he learned from his colleagues from the former Soviet Bloc, recommended 3 minutes as hot as an athlete could stand, immediately followed by 1 minute as cold as the athlete could stand; then repeat for two cycles, but always finish with cold. He recommended performing this activity up to twice daily. Treatment times were not set in stone; they varied depending on bath temperatures and how much of the body was submerged, and the availability of baths.

A sauna might be swapped for a hot shower that would then be paired with a cold whirlpool. This technique can certainly be alternated as an effective therapeutic means to help speed up recovery.

The idea is to alternate this recovery technique with other ones, and vary the time spent at each temperature; like training techniques, the same recovery methods done over and over without variation will eventually lose their effectiveness in enhancing recovery and will become more of a ritual.

Epsom Salt Baths

This regenerative modality is sort of self-explanatory by the name; the idea is to take a hot bath for 10–20 minutes, but the kicker is that you add 200–400 grams of Epsom.

Proponents believe this will reduce inflammation and it is very relaxing for your muscles. For chemically enhanced bodybuilders, or those who naturally retain water, this will help prevent extreme water retention and increase blood magnesium levels.

Charlie Francis used this technique with his sprinters when they were residually sore. He warned against using standard table salt because this would cause stimulation. not relaxation; and for recovery, that is not a good thing!

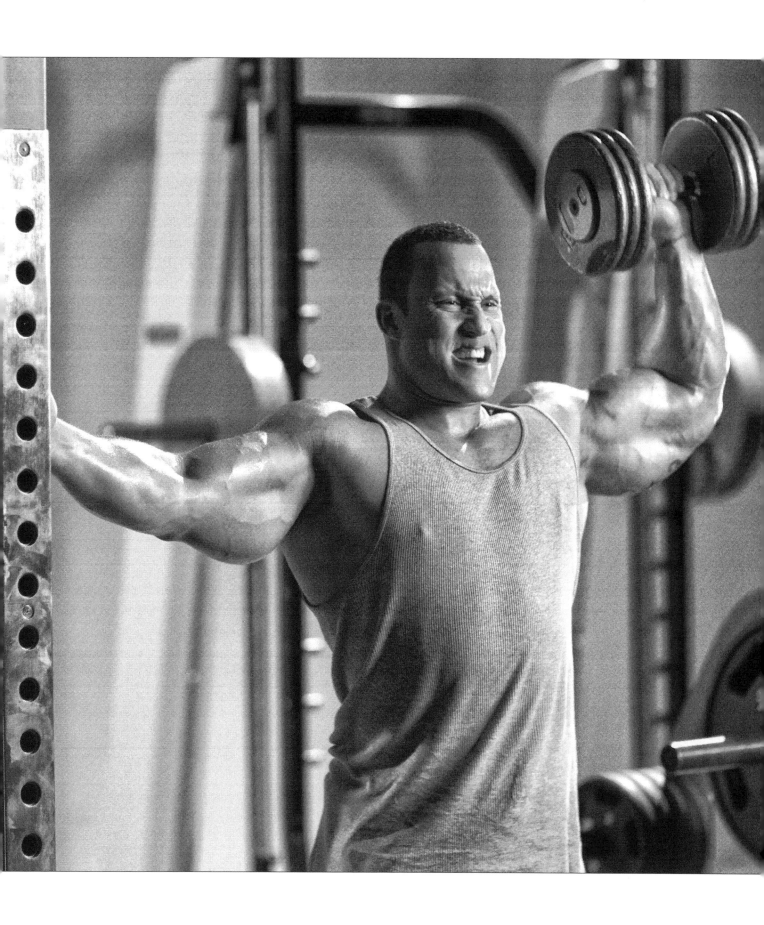

Electromyostimulation (EMS)

Performed with a low-geared pulse toward restoration, this can be an effective means to decrease recovery time. The discharge frequency on an EMS unit can range from 1Hz to 9Hz for restorative purposes and should be used for approximately 20 minutes.

The Compex Unit seems to be favored by strength athletes and has a setting to enhance power, strength, and resistance; and for this purpose, it has an actual active recovery setting.

The Russians have effectively used EMS for well over half a century. EMS has been used to enhance strength, as numerous studies have shown. This works because the stimulation is low intensity and pulses the muscles very gently, which massages the muscles.

According to both Siff and Verkhoshansky, EMS used in this way will help expedite the removal of waste products caused by intense training. Because of increased localized blood supply, nutrients to the muscles will be increased; this restorative method should be done the day after intense training on the area where you trained the day prior.

Cryotherapy (Ice Massage)

The term *cryotherapy* comes from the Greek and is translated as *cryo* meaning *cold*, and *therapy* meaning *cure*.

Cryotherapy has been around for over 300 years. In most gyms, athletes will simply refer to this method as ice massage. Ice massages are believed to decrease inflammation, pain, and cellular metabolism but increase cellular survival and cause vasoconstriction.

T-Nation contributor and well respected trainer/author, Christian Thibaudeau, gives these recommendations for the practical application of an ice massage: Commence by lightly massaging in a circular motion with the ice to the muscle; as you continue, gradually increase the area you are massaging, continuing in a circular motion; this is done for about 10 minutes.

Cryokinetics for Low Back and Leg Recuperation

Cryokinetics is therapy combining ice and movement to loosen muscles and stimulate the removal of waste products. Place crushed ice in a freezer-weight Zip-loc bag. Immediately following a shower (most effective if after a contrast shower), lie down on the floor and prop feet over a bed or couch. Place ice pack under the lumbar spine. Stretch the spine and gently perform lateral (side-to-side) flexion alternated with pulling knees to chest. These actions counteract stiffness resulting from cryotherapy. Spend at least 15 minutes, but no more than 20, on the ice.

A FEW LAST WORDS

To continually gain muscle, you are going to have to continually overload your training.

In exercise physiology, the first principle discussed many times is the principle of overload. The bigger and stronger you get, the more stress you must impose on your body from intense weight training.

Your work capacity will improve and build up over time, but when you first started out, a moderately intense 2-day-a-week full body split added muscle and increased symmetry.

As you evolve to an advanced bodybuilder, you may need 20+ sets per body part and have to use extremely intense bodybuilding methods like drop sets and rest pauses.

This takes a toll. While your recovery will improve, it won't be at the same linear rate as muscle size and strength do.

You can drastically improve this by implementing some of the restorative modalities mentioned in this chapter. Such implementation can help keep you injury free, minimize your pain, and allow you more frequent training sessions; the result, of course, will be a better physique.

Bottom line: The most commonly referenced cause of overtraining is "cumulative microtrauma," cellular damage from an overreaching episode that gets worse and worse over time. (Remember, stress is additive.)

There are two ways to cope with cumulative microtrauma.

You can avoid it, or you can treat it.

If you have to treat it, it's too late!

You avoid all the other stressors in your life that can become problematic to your training efforts, whether they are environmental, psychological, sociological, biochemical, physiological, or anatomical in nature.

So, it all boils down to planning.

This is done not by avoiding lifting or by avoiding a small amount of normal cellular destruction, but instead by not letting microtrauma accumulate.

You do this through sensible, scientific weight training and light-resistance systems of training that employ a carefully devised periodicity or cyclical method and paying careful attention to technique.

Additionally, it is your job, if you want to be the best you can be, to eliminate life stressors that are detrimental to your bodybuilding pursuit.

The take-home point is this: The most important way to ensure proper recovery is through proper planning and periodization.

SOURCES

"Cryotherapy." *Wikipedia.* http://en.wikipedia.org/wiki/Cryotherapy.

Berardi, John. "The Science of Nutrient Timing, Part 1." *Bodybuilding.com* (5 September 2004). http://www.bodybuilding.com/fun/berardi54.htm.

Cressey, Eric, and Mike Robertson. "Self-Myofascial Release: No Doctor Required!" *RossTraining.com* (12 July 2004). http://www.rosstraining.com/forum/viewtopic.php?f=9&t=4136.

Fenton, Reuven. "Bio-Alarm Clocks Set for Perfect Wake-up." *Reuters* (29 August 2007). http://www.reuters.com/article/technologyNews/idUSL0878172320070829.

Francis, Charlie. *The Charlie Francis Training System: The Most Comprehensive Training and Preparation System Available* (14 September 2011). http://www.scribd.com/doc/64993560/The-Charlie-Francis-Training-System. Downloadable PDF.

Greenfield, Russell. "Massage—With Your Genes On." *Alternative Medicine Alert* 15, no. 3 (2012): 35–41.

Guilleminault, Christian, and Martina L. Kreutzer. "Chapter 1. Normal Sleep." Pages 3–10 in *Sleep: Physiology, Investigations, and Medicine*, edited by Michel Billiard (in English). Springer, 30 September 2003. E-book.

Hall, Richard. "Stages of Sleep." *Psychology World* (no volume no.), 1998. PDF. http://web.mst.edu/~psyworld/sleep_stages.htm.

Hatfield, Frederick C. "Finding the Ideal Training Split." *Dr. Squat.* (n.d.). http://www.drsquat.com/content/knowledge-base/finding-ideal-training-split.

Hatfield, Frederick C. *Specialist in Sports Conditioning.* Santa Barbara: International Sports Sciences Association, 2001. (Unpublished manuscript.)

Kern, Mark. "Branched Chain Amino Acids (BCAA)." Pages 20–21 in *CRC Desk Reference on Sports Nutrition.* Boca Raton, FL: CRC Press, Taylor & Francis Group, 2005.

Kirkendall, D. T. "Mechanisms of Peripheral Fatigue." *Medicine & Science in Sports & Exercise* 22, no. 4 (1990): 444–49.

Kraemer, W. J., N. A. Ratamess, J. S. Volek, K. Häkkinen, M. R. Rubin, D. N. French, A. L. Gómez, M. R. McGuigan, T. P. Scheett, R. U. Newton, B. A. Spiering, M. Izquierdo, and F. S. Dioquardi. "The Effects of Amino Acid Supplementation on Hormonal Responses to Resistance Training Overreaching." *Metabolism* 55, no. 3 (2006): 282–91.

Marano Hara Estroff. "How to Get Great Sleep." *Psychology Today* (1 November 2003). http://www.psychologytoday.com/articles/200310/how-get-great-sleep.

Morton, R. "Contrast Water Immersion Hastens Plasma Lactate Decrease After Intense Anaerobic Exercise." *Journal of Science and Medicine in Sport* 10, no. 6 (2007): 467–70.

Petersen, Nicholas, Niels Secher, and Peter Ramussen. "Understanding Central Fatigue: Where to Go?" *Experimental Physiology* 92 (2007): 369–70.

Quinn, Elizabeth. "Does Sports Massage Improve Performance or Recovery?" In *About.com Guide* (updated 3 June 2012). http://sportsmedicine.about.com/od/injuryprevention/a/Sports_Massage.htm.

Richter, Jeffrey. "Foam Rolling for Optimal Performance." *Technique* 32, no. 3 (2012): 24–27.

Robson, David. "The Importance of Sleep." *Bodybuilding.com* (2 April 2004). http://www.bodybuilding.com/fun/drobson5.htm.

Schulz, H. "Rethinking Sleep Analysis." *Journal of Clinical Sleep Medicine 4*, no. 2 (2008): 99–103. http://www.pubmedcentral.nih.gov/articlerender.fcgi?tool=pmcentrez&artid=2335403.

Shih, C. Y., W. L. Lee, C. W. Lee, C. H. Huang, and Y. Z. Wu. "Effect of Time Ratio of Heat to Cold on Brachial Artery Blood Velocity During Contrast Baths." *Physical Therapy* 92, no. 3 (2012): 446–56.

Thibaudeau, Christian. "7 Secrets to Rapid Recovery." *T Nation* (26 January 2005). http://www.t-nation.com/free_online_article/sports_body_training_performance/7_secrets_to_rapid_recovery.

Thiriet, P., D. Gozal, D. Wouassi, T. Oumarou, H. Gelas, and J. R. Lacour. "The Effect of Various Recovery Modalities on Subsequent Performance, in Consecutive Supramaximal Exercise." *Journal of Sports Medicine and Physical Fitness* 33, no. 2 (1993): 118–29.

Wilson, Jacob. "Hippocrates—Was He Hardcore?" *Hyperplasia Magazine* (2003). http://www.abcbodybuilding.com/magazine03/searchanddestroy.htm.

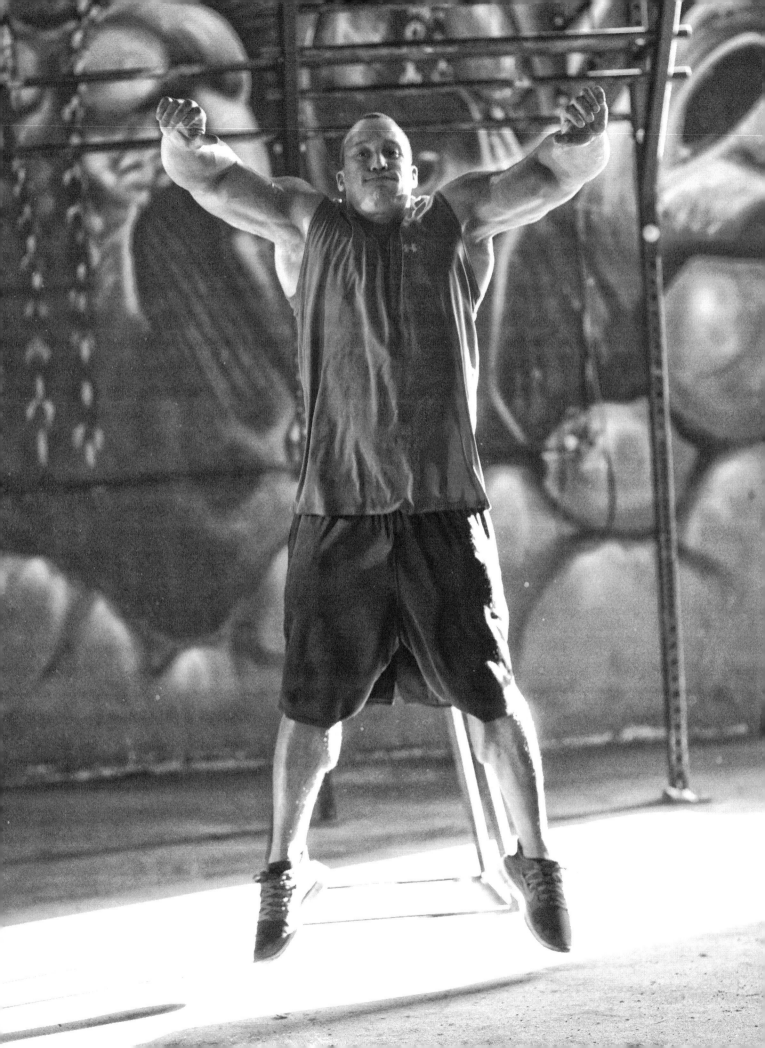

CHAPTER 12.

Stretching

If you want to build as much muscle as possible, you will need to do at least an hour of yoga every day.

Of course, I am kidding. Yet the fact remains some bodybuilders totally ignore flexibility work, and this is not wise.

The stereotype has always been as muscle increases, a person's flexibility decreases. This is gym lore. If anyone is a serious fan of contemporary pro bodybuilding, they'll remember seeing photos of Ronnie Coleman doing the splits on stage. Folks who've seen that are in awe at how someone with so much muscle can have such amazing flexibility.

BILATERAL RANGE OF MOTION (ROM) DEFICITS

Even more worrisome than a range-of-motion deficit is the discovery of a bilateral deficit, in which a joint on one side of the body has a significantly different range of motion than the corresponding joint on the other side of the body.

Take the old-time bodybuilder who can fully extend one arm but not the other. In this case, one side has full ROM and the other side is lacking full ROM, so a bilateral deficit exists. An effective prescription would be not to dump pressing exercises altogether, but just use dumbbells, which, unlike barbells, will not cause overcompensation. Continue trying to regain the lost ROM; in extreme cases, with bone-on-bone blockage, surgery maybe the only viable solution. Significant bilateral deficits can lead to postural erosion and can also impair how much weight you can lift. Even if health is not a consideration, it's important to remember this!

INFLEXIBILITY AND INJURY POTENTIAL

Weight training through full ROM increases flexibility in many instances, or it remains neutral; never does weight training decrease flexibility. However repetitive, limited ROM training over a prolonged period can create shortened muscles. I am not saying never to perform partials, though, as they certainly have a significant place in training.

The old saying, "full range of motion for full development," most certainly holds true when talking about flexibility.

Bodybuilders lifting chronically with a partial range of motion will lose flexibility over time. Countless examples exist whereby inflexibility leads to injury. Most frequently, you will encounter problems caused by shortened hip flexors, overly tight hamstrings, and overly tight quadriceps.

Chronically shortened muscles can be the first step in a series of events leading to injury. Shortened hip flexors, to use the previous example, can lead to a reduction of the normal lordotic curve of the lumbar spine. This can impair the spine's load-bearing and shock absorption capacity; in layman's terms, your squat will suffer because you cannot maintain an adequate arch.

When the spine cannot function normally, a wide range of injuries can result. Overly tight hamstrings have the same effect on the lumbar spine. Watch an overly tight bodybuilder try to perform an Olympic squat; the pelvis will shift forward, which is biomechanically inefficient and invites a back injury.

SPECIFICITY AND FLEXIBILITY

Specificity is obviously of profound importance if training is to be successful. Like all other bio-motor abilities, joint flexibility can be enhanced only if the training methods are specific to the desired result. Flexibility is specific to three criteria:

1. **Joint specificity:** A flexibility training program for the hips, for example, will not improve flexibility in any other joint. The joint-specific nature of flexibility training does not necessarily mean that all joints must be targeted with flexibility exercises. Flexibility training can be prioritized toward joints that are most in need, as a way of maximizing training efficiency.

2. **Speed specificity:** For maximum effectiveness, stretching exercises must be very similar in form and speed to the skill you are trying to improve. Slow, static stretching, for example, will not improve flexibility in fast movements nearly as well as dynamic stretching. Conversely, dynamic stretching methods have limited ability to improve a static skill, such as a split on the floor. In bodybuilding, generally, dynamic stretching will have the best transference.

3. **Resistance training as a contributor to increased joint flexibility:**
   Properly conceived resistance training programs can have a beneficial effect
   on flexibility levels. In fact, whatever your level of flexibility, the primary
   concern is the degree of strength throughout a joint's full range of motion.
   Two key points are to perform resistance exercises through the involved
   joint's full range of motion, and to work antagonistic pairs of muscles equally,
   e.g., biceps and triceps.

How Much Flexibility Is Enough?

This, of course, varies from individual to individual, but it can safely be said that individuals need enough flexibility for any situation they will normally encounter in day-to-day life, plus a little bit more. This "little bit more" is called the flexibility reserve.

The Effect of Body Temperature on Flexibility

Body temperature is an important consideration when attempting to improve joint flexibility. Increased temperature helps to facilitate increases in ROM, while decreased temperature tends to preserve increases in muscle length. Prior to performing stretching exercises, body temperature must be elevated through a warm-up.

The warm-up can be passive, meaning a hot bath or shower, or, preferably, active, meaning a brief session of cardiovascular activity that is classified as your general warm-up. The general warm-up can be 5–10 minutes on the bike or elliptical and, like training, a warm-up goes from general to specific.

Getting more specific is dynamic stretching, and the final part of the warm-up should be performing, at a lower intensity, the activity you are warming up for. If it is chest day and your first exercise is bench press and the first set is with 250 pounds, a specific warm-up would look like this:

   Bar x 6 x 2 sets, 95 x 6 sets, 135 x 5 sets, 185 x 3 sets, 225 x 1 set

It's a warm-up, not a pre-exhaust!

This helps dial in the motor pattern and specifically warm up the muscles you will be using. If the next exercise is incline press, it will require less warm-up; many times a single set will suffice.

Duration

Ideal stretching duration can vary depending on many factors, primarily the type of stretching method being used (described subsequently).

Dynamic stretching for instance, involves several swings that last only a moment or so each. Static-active and contract-relax methods involve longer periods lasting up to a minute or more. Stretching sessions rarely last more than 20 minutes, with each individual muscle normally taking 2–3 minutes at most.

Breathing and Relaxation

During the stretch, breathe normally, and visualize the muscles, tendons and ligaments' lengthening during the stretch. Avoid breath holding, as it can increase blood pressure and general muscular tension.

STRETCHING AS A MEANS OF PREVENTING DELAYED ONSET OF MUSCLE SORENESS (DOMS)

Although research does not confirm this, in the field many swear by the notion that low- to moderate-intensity stretching exercises may be effective in reducing post-exercise muscle soreness (perhaps the best rationale for most people to stretch regularly).

PERIODIZATION OF STRETCHING

Like all training components (including nutrition), stretching exercises should be periodized throughout the training cycle. If you require high levels of ROM, the following points will be helpful when designing your overall training schedule:

- If flexibility is a weak area for you, focus on correcting it in the off season and maintain it during contest prep.

- Excessive flexibility appears to be detrimental to some athletes involved in strength and power sports. For example, too much hip flexibility can weaken the stability of the low position in the squat. Also, track and field throwers often report that a certain level of tightness in the pectoral region can facilitate elastic energy in the final stages of the throw; top bench pressers seem to agree.

- If the objective is to increase ROM, intensive stretching should not be performed every day, as the muscle and connective tissues need time to heal. Consider a schedule where adaptive tension stretching occurs every other day, interspersed with days of light tension stretches.

- When reduction of DOMS is the objective, stretching exercises can be performed every day, or nearly every day. The most effective method involves stretching muscles immediately after they have been resistance trained. If you wish to plan static stretching on a day where no resistance training occurs, perform a low intensity 10–15 minute cardiovascular session (active warm-up) or take a hot shower, steam bath, or Jacuzzi prior to stretching.

Static Stretching

Static stretching is contraindicated prior to resistance training; numerous studies have shown it can temporarily lower strength levels, power output, and speed.

If this is of interest to you, read this study by the University of Texas, Arlington: "Acute Effects of Static and Proprioceptive Neuromuscular Facilitation Stretching on Muscle Strength and Power Output." Power and strength were both adversely affected when PNF or static stretching were performed pre-workout. Some still insist static stretching prior to working out reduces injuries and increases dynamic flexibility in the cage. Not one study has ever shown a reduction in injuries when static stretching was employed pre-workout or competition.

Dynamic Stretching

Used primarily by athletes who need to increase range of motion for sports skills, dynamic stretching involves swinging the arms and or legs in a controlled manner.

Various patterns can be utilized. It is a good idea to do movements similar to that which you will be training for the greatest transference. When stretching dynamically, care must be taken not to exceed the present range of motion for the joint(s) being stretched, or injury could result.

Perform dynamic stretching as described to ensure the safety of this type of stretching.

First, establish an even, controlled rhythm with swinging movements initially well within the current range of motion; then, gradually increase the amplitude of the movement until you are at the desired level of tension at the end-point of the movement.

Please bear in mind that these are specialized movements, and care must be taken with their use. Never do dynamic stretching until a general warm-up of 10 minutes has been performed.

This warm-up is not a rule, but a guideline. Experiment to find what works best for you.

The Warm-up

This warm-up and cool-down routine is adopted from Dr. Robert Wolff's *Bodybuilding 201,* with a few minor changes.

These tips are to enhance performance and decrease the chance of injury.

1. Warm up and stretch before every workout—general warm-up, dynamic warm-up, and specific.
2. Start with 5–10 minutes on the bike, elliptical, or stair master, or even do a light jog; this is the general warm-up.

3. After performing the dynamic warm-up, start out with light warm-up sets and stay with the lighter weights until the body part you are working is fully warmed up.

4. Use good form for each exercise. Repetition is the mother of skill; build great form with light weights.

6 Immediately stop doing any exercise if you feel any twinge, pain, or abnormal workout discomfort. Remember, this not a license to be a wimp; as you gain experience you will learn what is good pain and what is bad pain. When in doubt, shut it down!

The warm-up is really important as it helps raise the core temperature of the body, really gets the blood flowing (helps your muscles perform better and greatly reduces the chance of injury), helps make the muscles elastic, and gets the joints moving, with synovial fluid (think of it like grease for your joints that helps them move easily) lubricating those joints. All of those are great things.

I've found that certain factors will affect not only my workouts and stretching, but warm-up as well.

For one: the temperature.

Colder weather is tough on the body and the colder the weather, the more time you will require to get warmed up for your workout.

Conversely, warmer weather is easier on the body, so it takes less time to "heat things up on the inside," so to speak.

The Pre-Workout Stretch Dynamic Warm-up

1. Finger stretches: Open each hand up and spread the fingers as wide as possible, then close them and do it again and again. Open. Close. Open. Close. 10–20 repetitions.

2. Hand/wrist rotations: Rotate small circles forward and backward 10 times each way.

3. Elbow rotations: Rotate at the elbows in a circular fashion forward and backward 10 times each way.

4. Rotations of the shoulder: Swing the arms in a circular motion forward and backward 10 times each way.

5. Knee-ups: Stand in place and raise one leg up to your waist and then the other. Terrific for warming up not only the knees but the quads as well; 10 repetitions each side will suffice.

6. Lunges around the world: Lunge forward, lunge forward at a 45-degree angle, lunge laterally, and then finally lunge backward; do this to each side. Around the world once is really 8 lunges; 2–3 times will suffice.

7. Standing bodyweight-only calf raises: 20–30 non-stop reps. This really helps stretch and warm up the calves, ankles, and feet.

8. Standing trunk twists with either arm in front of the body or holding a broomstick behind your neck and twisting from side to side for 30–60 seconds, non-stop.

9. Jumping up and down, in place, for 30–60 seconds.

10. Bodyweight squats: 10 repetitions.

11. Neck circles: Rotate the neck in circular manner to the right and left 5–10 reps.

12. Hamstring kicks: Keeping the legs relatively straight, kick up, alternating legs and increase height each kick. Proceed with caution.

Now, it's time for the workout. Always begin each exercise with a "mock" set; go through the exact motions and movement for the exercise you're about to do, but do it without any weights.

The goal is to get the body settled into "the exercise groove" and the mind and body to be in total synch when the weights are used.

You're going to like what this will do for your workouts.

A FEW LAST WORDS

Foam Rolling and static stretching can also be done post workout and on off-days. Please refer to Chapter 11 on recovery, for a full explanation and routine.

Flexibility is not the name of the game in bodybuilding, but you will feel and perform better with adequate flexibility. To be the best, don't neglect any aspect of your training.

SOURCES

benShea, Adam, and Josh Bryant. *ISSA MMA Course*. Santa Barbara: International Sports Sciences Association, 2012.

Hatfield, Frederick C. *Specialist in Sports Conditioning*. Santa Barbara: International Sports Sciences Association, 2001. (Unpublished manuscript.)

Wolff, Robert. *Bodybuilding 201: Everything You Need to Know to Take Your Body to the Next Level*. New York: Contemporary Books, 2004.

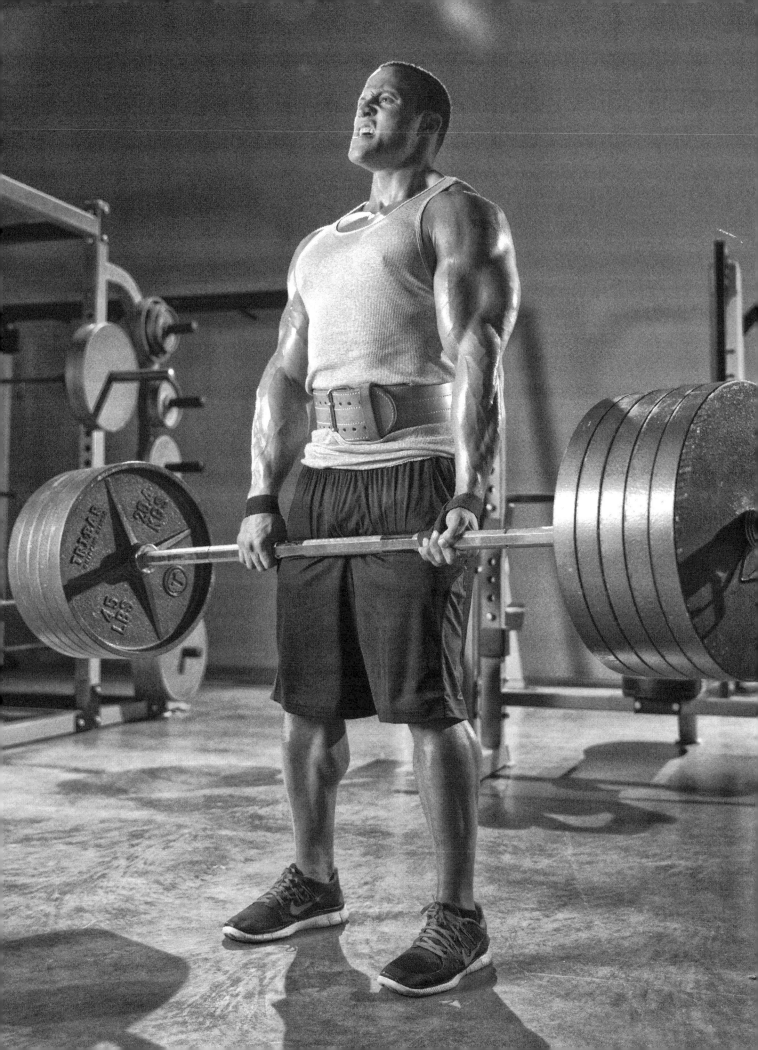

CHAPTER 13.

Testing and Evaluation

ASSESSMENTS FOR BODYBUILDERS

Testing an athlete for performance enhancement is a very common practice in sports such as football, but it is not nearly as common in bodybuilding.

While "big numbers" do not offer a one to one correlation of the status of your physique, testing provides you with valuable information on several levels.

It is all too common today for many bodybuilders' trainers to go by "feel" alone. Having a good feel on level of progress is important; however, bodybuilders will be judged on how they look on stage. As a bodybuilder advances, listening to intuition and having instinctual elements of training become important, but relying only on "feel" can mask the ineffective program.

THE BENEFITS OF TESTING

Testing yields several benefits:

1. **Testing provides information on individual strengths and weaknesses.** A one-size-fits-all training approach does not apply to bodybuilding programs. Testing will provide you with information on some changes that need to be made in regards to the current training program; this will aid in performance needs as well as reduce possible health risks.

Different athletes will have different needs, and those needs should be addressed accordingly. Just think, if you can do leg extensions for reps with 150 pounds with ease but struggle to leg curl 50 pounds, you are setting yourself up not only for asymmetrical imbalances but a greatly enhanced chance of injury.

2. **Testing is motivational**. As a trainer, after a successful evaluation of performance, I can tell an athlete definitively, "You have gotten stronger; your arms have grown by half an inch!" This motivates my athlete and sparks great enthusiasm. Even saying "Your bench press improved by 10%" can generate excitement.

   Whatever the reason for testing and evaluation, it must, above all, serve a purpose. There must be a reason for the test. In addition, it must be properly planned, and it must provide useful data. Testing for the sake of testing (often a result of the athlete or coach's self-gratification) is purposeless and often dangerous.

TESTING PROBLEMS AND CONCERNS

Testing holds many advantages, but it also involves pitfalls. Here are a few:

Validity

Is the test valid? Is it a suitable measure of what is intended to be measured? Obviously, a one-rep max in the bench press does not measure leg strength. However, many popular tests are not valid for the athletic attributes for which the coach believes he is testing.

For example, using 225 pounds for reps in the bench does measure strength. But, what kind of strength is being measured? If the athlete can bench press 450 pounds, then it is certainly not limit strength being measured!

It is absolutely comical that the 225-pounds bench press trial for 350-plus pound linemen is a staple strength test in NFL combines. A consideration of this testing protocol shows that it may need to change to become valid. Just because a multibillion dollar entity like the NFL refuses to change its dated testing procedures does not mean you have to follow suit.

Reliability

Testing must be consistent. In other words, if you repeat the test again and again under the same conditions, will you see the same score? If there is no consistency in measurements, a "measurement error" has occurred. How many times has someone started a workout program and measured their arms accurately at the commencement of the program, then reported gains a month later with a more "friendly" measurement procedure?

Furthermore, the measurement needs to be taken at the same time of day; measuring arms "cold" in the morning, is different than measuring them pumped after a high volume workout that was preceded with a pre-workout supplement that encourages a "pump."

The following lists describes possible reasons for inaccurate data, with a practical example for each:

1. Those who measured the performance(s) did not take accurate measurements. (See arm example above.)

2. The athlete being tested did not perform consistently. (Could range from illness to shoddy equipment to just an "off" day.)

3. The instrument used during testing failed to produce an accurate measurement. (E.g., if testing maximum isometric force and the dynamometer does not register a score.)

4. Standard procedures were not followed. (The first test was a full squat for a one-repetition max, but the next test was a half squat for a one-repetition max)

Objectivity

Objectivity pertains to whether clear instructions have been given during the test. If a test has a high level of objectivity, several testers can administer the same test on the same athlete and obtain nearly the same results.

Validity, reliability, and objectivity are all closely related. If there is no objectivity during the testing process, the test cannot be considered reliable. If a test is unreliable, it clearly is invalid.

However, a test can be reliable and objective and still be invalid. As in the above example, you can have high levels of validity and objectivity using 225 pounds for reps in the bench press. (The repetitions are all according to directions, and all testers counted the same number of repetitions.) You do not, however, have a measure of limit strength, as the test reveals little about how much weight the specific lineman can bench press one time.

SAFETY

To recap from earlier, testing is often an act of maximum performance. However, you must remember you will not win the Olympia or even the "hot body" contest at the local honky tonk bar during a test! While there are several reasons to administer a test, it should never result in an injury, nor should it expose you to increasing the probability of injury.

BODY COMPOSITION TESTING

Practical methods of assessing body composition, such as skinfolds, bioelectrical impedance, DEXA scans, and hydrostatic weighing, are based on the two-component model of body composition, i.e., fat and fat-free weight. Further dividing body fat into essential fat and storage fat leads to the search for the best way to measure storage fat.

The search and research for the most valid, most practical, and most affordable method of body composition testing continues. It is important to know that most methods carry a 3%–4% error factor in their prediction of body fat. The higher the skill of the person taking the measurements, the lower the error rate.

The three most common measurement techniques are hydrostatic weighing, bioelectrical impedance, and skinfold measurement.

Considered the standard, hydrostatic weighing applies Archimedes' Principle that an object immersed in a fluid loses the amount of weight equivalent to the weight of the fluid displaced by the object's volume. Since fat is less dense than muscle, fatter individuals have a lower total body density than their leaner counterparts.

Although for years considered the most accurate, many now believe the DEXA scan is the gold standard. DEXA scans and hydrostatic weighing's greatest disadvantage are their inaccessibility to most gym rats, unless they are in a medical or university setting.

Bioelectrical impedance is based on the fact that the body contains intracellular and extracellular fluids capable of electrical conduction. Since fat-free bodyweight contains much of the body's water and electrolytes, it is a better conductor of the electrical current than fat, which contains very little water. This technique is essentially an index of total body water from which body fat is estimated. If you retain more water than most, you will read higher than you truly are.

Bioelectrical impedance's popularity has increased over the last few years because it is painless, quick, and easy to perform. One drawback is the initial investment cost of the machine, which can run upwards of $3,500. And although bioelectrical impedance is okay for most people, it does tend to overestimate body fat in very lean people and underestimate body fat in obese people.

DEXA scan uses a whole body scanner along with two different low dose x-rays that read soft tissue mass and bone mass. This procedure usually takes about 15 minutes. It is completely painless. This is an expensive assessment, usually around $250.

The skinfold method of determining body fat is practical, affordable, and fairly easy to perform, with practice. This method is done with calipers. These calipers measure the thickness of the outer layer of fat on your body. The measurements are then automatically "plugged" into regression equations to determine percentage of body fat.

Once you have measured the skinfolds at the sites indicated, you can easily compute your percent body fat through the use of a table of norms. There's no math for you to do with these techniques.

The skinfold method is based on the fact that the distribution of subcutaneous fat and internal fat is similar for all individuals. This assumption is not without error, however. Research has shown that older people of the same body density and gender have proportionately less subcutaneous fat than do their younger counterparts. There is considerable variation in regard to age, gender, and degree of fatness. The skinfold equations, however, have been developed to estimate the body fat of men and women varying greatly in age (10–61 years) and body fatness (4%–44%).

The leanest athletes in traditional sports usually carry about 5%–8% body fat for men, and 10%–15% for women. Top bodybuilders will drop even lower than these levels, but only for a short time in the 2%–4% range; during off season, for health reasons and to be able to adequately add muscle and operating in a caloric surplus, these levels will go higher.

As a competitive bodybuilder, "If you do not see the outline of your abs and any veins in your arms or legs, you are getting too fat," to quote Branch Warren in a conversation we had. For a competitive bodybuilder, rarely would it make sense to go above 12% body fat in the off season; generally, more in the 10% range will make the most sense when bulking up. When you get too fat, not only is more aggressive dieting called for (meaning a more intense catabolic state) but so is, generally, a longer time in this state. Since you will struggle so hard to get lean enough, preserving muscle mass will be an afterthought.

Look at the example of top bodybuilder Branch Warren in 2006. At 5 feet 7 inches, he would balloon up to 272 pounds. Then, with a lighter competitive bodyweight in the 230s and now in the 240s, his off-season weight got to the mid-260s.

Since Branch has stayed leaner year round, he has much more efficient contest prep with no crashing, allowing him to train more intensely. While he has used this strategy, he has been a perennial Arnold Classic Champion and had numerous Top 10 Mr. Olympia finishes, including 2nd and 3rd place.

Body-fat testing is important for the bodybuilder; while it makes no guarantees about symmetrical appearance, it is a good way to track data when bulking or cutting.

If you gain 10 pounds but 9 of those pounds are fat, that is not a very efficient bulk; conversely, if you weigh 200 pounds and drop four pounds and your body fat decreases 2%, your cut is spot on.

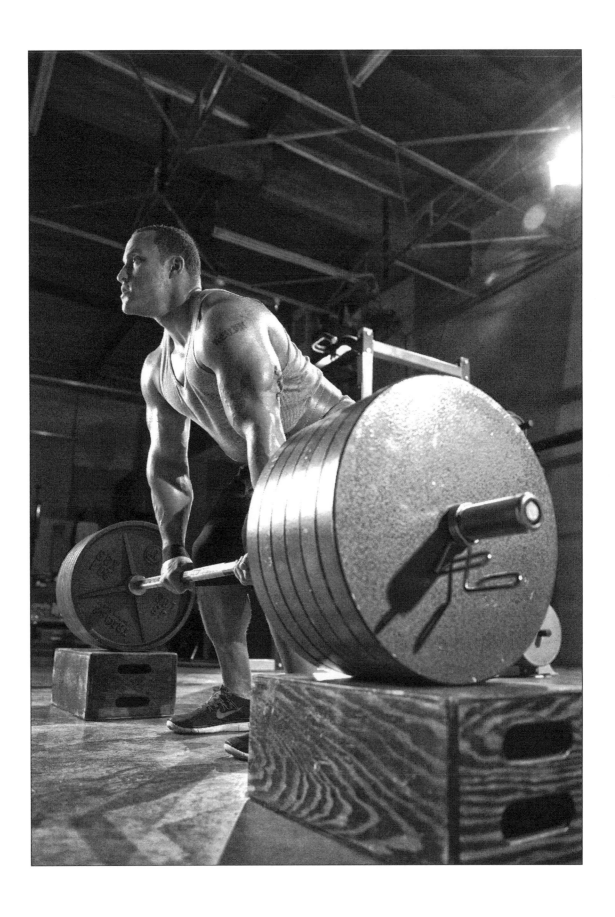

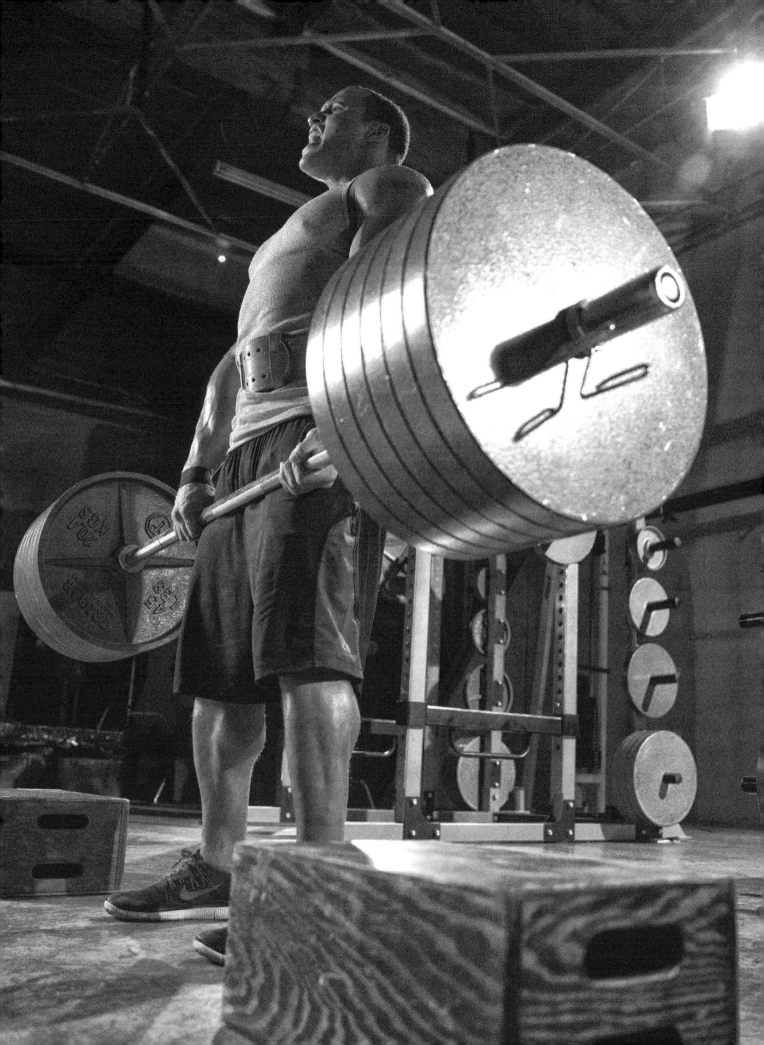

Whether you're a bodybuilder or a fitness enthusiast, the scale doesn't tell the whole story. Body-fat measurements, coupled with scale weight, give a realistic outlook on what is taking place when cutting or bulking.

TESTING FOR LIMIT STRENGTH

Your limit strength, or how much force you can exert for an all-out effort, is obviously going to be different for each muscle or movement. Further, differences in strength exist between men and women of different ages and bodyweights.

As a bodybuilder, this is your base!

Your relative strength is your limit-strength-to-bodyweight ratio, which is extremely important. You should remember that the fatter you are, the lower your relative strength level will be. That's because your ratio of fat to muscle is poor. You can't flex fat. For a quick recap, muscle, not fat, moves weight.

Limit strength is tested by lifting maximal weights. A max-effort movement is classified generally as 1–3 repetitions with greater than 90% of an athlete's one-repetition max.

The most effective measurement of limit strength is powerlifting. In all other sports, limit strength is a component and, as an athlete advances and becomes stronger, decreasing amounts of time are devoted to building his limit-strength base. Powerlifting is limit strength and relative strength; you lift as much weight as possible for a one-repetition max, there is no time limit to lift the weight, and you are compared to competitors within your weight class.

The best way to test limit strength is with a one-repetition max in a core movement. Many people question the safety of this practice, but look at it logically: Form breaks down sometimes with heavy weight, but also with fatigue.

Doing a one-repetition max, you risk some form breakdown. Doing a repetition max with 85–90% of your one-repetition max, you are still lifting heavy weight, but fatigue will manifest its ugly head; this is a surefire way to have form break down.

I have seen more injuries on the last rep of a squat or deadlift than on heavy singles. The mindset for a heavy single is just that, to perform a heavy single. For max reps, there is no true mindset besides one more and push through the pain. Technique from a psychological standpoint is a focus when maxing; it seems to be put on the back burner for rep maxes.

Powerlifting in the off season?

Johnnie Jackson does it, and he won the FIBO Pro Bodybuilding contest in Germany, placed second at the New York Pro, and finished Top 10 in the Mr. Olympia.

During the off season, Johnnie trained "powerbuilding" style with me. Johnnie did a meet and deadlifted 832 pounds raw, one of the best deadlifts in the world!

Johnnie's career in bodybuilding was considered over by most "in the know." His career was resurrected by going back to his roots.

Ronnie Coleman and Branch Warren started off as powerlifters. Even Arnold deadlifted over 700 pounds in a contest. Building limit strength gives the muscle that dense, grainy look when dieted down, creating an imposing prowess that wins shows.

Bodybuilders can do powerlifting meets in the off season; it gives them a goal to measure, knowing their limit-strength feats were performed under the strictest standards. These can be single-lift bench presses or deadlift contests; powerlifting training quantifies limit strength, and training powerlifting style will shock the system and provide psychological stimulation because of the freshness.

If you, as a bodybuilder, decide to powerlift in the off season, follow these guidelines:

1. **Deadlift conventional**—conventional deadlifting is the best posterior chain builder (back side of the body). Sumo deadlifting is legal, but it is a leverage lift; it will do little to enhance muscularity unless specifically focusing on the adductors. As a bodybuilder, you want the increased range of motion, the increased muscle tension, and the increased time under tension. Plus, your objective is to test true strength, not enhance mechanical advantages.

2. **Lift raw**—raw lifting means to lift with the only supportive equipment allowed being a belt, wrist wraps, and sometimes knee wraps. When you hear about world records increasing drastically over the past 20 years, it is because of gear.

   The raw records over the past 8 years have finally started to be broken. Without supportive equipment, the deadlift world record is much higher than the squat; with it, the squat is 300 pounds higher. Without getting into the right and wrong of this, the fact remains the sport is going a majority raw, which means raw meets are easy to find and compete in.

   Compare the best raw powerlifters to the best equipped: The raw powerlifters, even the fat, super heavies, carry much more muscle. The best raw bench pressers in the world right now, Jeremy Hoornstra and Al Davis, look like off-season bodybuilders; the best equipped, many times at first glance, would appear not to work out.

   Supportive powerlifting equipment mechanically assists the lifters; elastic-like energy is stored in the supportive shirts or suits on the eccentric portion of the lift. A spring-loaded, rubber-band-like effect helps catapult the weight back up to the starting position; bench shirts can add 400+ pounds in many instances, squat suits even more, and, generally, deadlift suits will top around 150 pounds of added support.

That's why the suit adds so much less on the deadlift; there is no true eccentric phase. Powerlifting supportive gear does the work of your muscles! For the bodybuilder wearing bench shirts, squat suits, and deadlift suits, in most instances, these add undue stress to the central nervous system and do little to add muscle.

The argument could be made that bodybuilders could use a squat suit to help them out of the bottom portion of the lift, with less and less help given at the top, but this is not needed—you can squat with chains or use a safety bar.

3. **Bench press like a bodybuilder**—the goal is to win on stage. Do not excessively arch and bring the bar to your belly. Chopping the range of motion down and only worrying about going from point A to point B is fine, if your goal is to become a world champion powerlifter.

   As a bodybuilder, you want a full range of motion for full muscular development. I am not saying to become so engulfed with purposeful intention of trying to isolate the pecs. To lift big weights, you have to focus on the movement; don't excessively arch and don't belly bench, and you will be fine.

4. **Don't cut weight**—powerlifting will be done in a bulking phase. Compete to win, but not at the expense of cutting weight. The goals are mass and limit strength; weight cutting is a variable that needs to be eradicated from your mindset in this instance.

5, **Squat to grow**—raw powerlifters will generally squat with a much narrower stance than their equipped counterparts; the idea is to maximize the elasticity of the suit and minimize the range of motion to move the most weight.

   For squatting, even if EMG activity is similar in the quadriceps with a wide or regular stance, much less mechanical work is done when using the wide stance. 400 pounds x 10-inch ROM = 4,000 pounds of mechanical work; if the range of motion is twice that, it would be 8,000 pounds. You can squat shoulder-width or even wider, but just don't get to the point of absurdity; this is generally not an issue, as rarely can someone squat more raw with an excessively wide stance.

Obviously, the easiest and most reliable method for determining limit strength is to perform one repetition for each exercise. Some may prefer to estimate their one-rep max by performing a multiple repetition test.

High school strength coaches are notorious for using special "formulas" to estimate their athletes' one-rep maximums. I have had high school clients be off in their estimated one-rep maxes to their actual ones by over 65 pounds in the bench press; we are talking athletes in the 300-pound bench range, so that is a greater than 20% margin of error.

With that kind of inaccuracy, it might be easier for coaches just to eyeball their athletes and make a guess. These are not "podunk" high school football programs; they are some of the winningest high school programs in the football fabled Lone Star State.

Even some colleges have not divorced themselves from this strength training debauchery; they choose to remain in a self-induced purgatory of true strength assessments.

Formulas do not take into account muscle fiber make-up, training history, training methods being used, or level of psych, desire, and testicular fortitude.

If it is unsafe to lift your max in a core movement, it is probably unsafe to lift 90% of your one-rep max for a maximum number of reps. The total is unknown, and fatigue will potentially show its ugly head, making one more enemy to proper technique.

Review Chapter 4 on Periodization and look at Fred Hatfield's ABC System of Bodybuilding. The inserted chart of how many repetitions an easy gainer can do with 80% of his one-repetition max is a lot different than what a slow gainer can do.

That, folks, is why there is no universal formula for testing one-repetition maxes; at best they are an educated guess, and at worst they are a complete fallacy used by people to inflate their egos and, of course, their maxes.

MEASUREMENTS

As a bodybuilder, it is always important to remember you are judged based on the illusion your physique portrays to the judges. A bodybuilder with 17.5-inch arms may appear to have bigger arms than a bodybuilder with 19 inch arms if his biceps has a better shape when he hits a front dumbbell bicep pose; if this bodybuilder has smaller joints, he will appear to have bigger biceps.

Because of this, the tale of the tape doesn't tell the whole story, but it sure helps in the assessment process. If a bodybuilder is devoting a specific training block to add size, and a specific focus is set on adding size to the arms, the easiest way to measure efficiency is with a tape—assuming body fat does not spiral out of control.

If your arms were 16 inches and now they are 16.5 inches, they have gotten bigger. This is also a great way to track the muscularity illusion as you diet down.

Sure, body fat tells the physiology of what has taken place, but measurements will help evaluate the illusion. If you lose 2 inches off your waist, yet your arms do not drop in size, the illusion is that they have become bigger.

Anyone who has successfully dieted down for bodybuilding has had people say things to them like, "Wow, you look like you're getting huge." It is funny to proclaim, "I have lost ten pounds."

That's the illusion we are after.

Steve Reeves, a bodybuilding pioneer who was known for his symmetry, believed that once a certain amount of mass was surpassed, aesthetics would suffer and symmetry would rapidly disintegrate.

Many who endorse the classical bodybuilding physique still believe in Reeves' ideals. He believed a 6-foot-tall bodybuilder had to weigh less than 200 pounds to be symmetrical; certainly there have been bodybuilders much larger than that in the modern era with beautiful symmetry, but the largest mass monsters usually don't have best symmetry.

Reeves believed that bodybuilders striving for the symmetrical physique should have the proportions listed below.

STEVE REEVES' ULTRA-SYMMETRICAL PHYSIQUE RATIOS
Arm size = 252% of Wrist size
Calf size = 192% of Ankle size
Neck Size = 79% of Head size
Chest Size = 148% of Pelvis size
Waist size = 86% of Pelvis size
Thigh size = 175% of Knee size

Measurement guidelines:

- Take measurements in a relaxed state. Do not flex the muscle you are measuring, and do not measure when the muscles are pumped full of blood. Instead, measure muscles in a natural state at the same time of day each day.

- Don't leave the tape loose; sure, this will give your arms bigger measurements, but not accurate ones, so there will not be a way to quantitatively assess data; most bodybuilders lie about their measurements. For your sanity, your measurements should probably remain between you and whoever is assisting with your contest prep.

- Write down measurements; it is a great way to assess your physique. Bodyweight, body fat, and measurements won't lie.

- Measure in the same spot every time; your thighs, for example, will be bigger if you measure them right above the knee verses at the butt cheek.

A FEW LAST WORDS

If you want to be a competitive bodybuilder, all that matters is the illusion on stage.

To help create the best illusion on stage, the bodybuilder can assess progress in training by the assessments listed. Do assess your training. To be the best, you will need to do more than stare in the mirror and go by "feel."

I also highly encourage you to get a Photobucket account. It's free and allows you to do comparisons of past photos in a slide show setting.

Take pictures from different angles, and save these pictures with the date and your bodyweight; doing the assessments listed and using Photobucket will help make you become the best you can be.

SOURCE

Hatfield, Frederick C. *Specialist in Sports Conditioning*. Santa Barbara: International Sports Sciences Association, 2001. (Unpublished manuscript.)

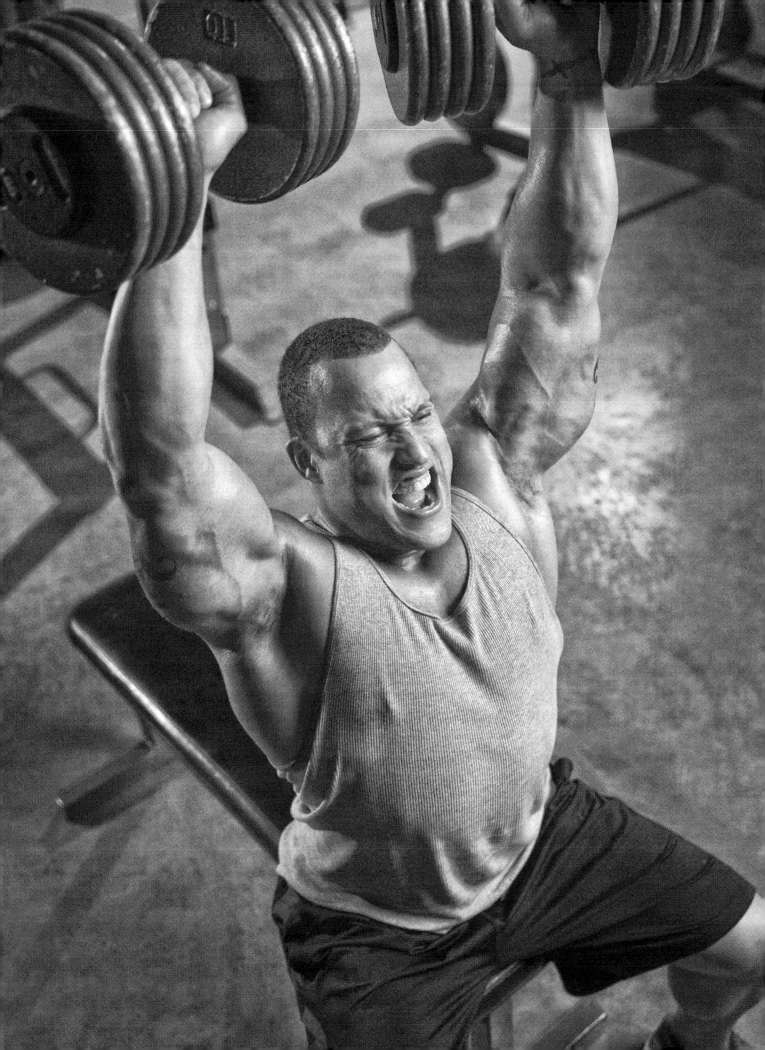

CHAPTER 14.

Top Ten Exercises

EXERCISE SELECTION

Compound movements, isolation movements, bands, chains, barbells, dumbbells, machines… the choices are more numerous than the whisky selection at an Irish Pub. So which do you choose?

Why not choose them all instead of limiting yourself to just one? Just remember that mechanical tension, metabolic stress, and muscle damage are the contributing factors to muscle hypertrophy.

With science as your guide, you can never go wrong.

Mechanical Tension

In spite of not following typical hypertrophy guidelines, powerlifters possess extreme muscular development. At a first glance, this would seem anomalous, but it ratifies science because of the mechanical stress placed on muscles during a heavy powerlifting regimen.

Powerlifters avoid workout fluff because their only objective is to pile more pig iron on the bar.

This has to be done with proper technique or the weight lifted will not count in a contest, where it matters for the powerlifter. Heavy weight through a full range of motion with proper technique epitomizes mechanical stress.

Aha!

It now makes since why powerlifters pack on so much muscle. Even though muscles cannot quantitatively gauge the pig iron they lift in poundage, they know tension. Muscle tension is the result as bar weight increases, assuming proper technique is being used with a full range of motion. Increasing training weights is indispensable, but never at the expense of form.

Metabolic Stress

Metabolic stress caused by moderate repetition ranges has generally been shown to be superior in achieving muscle hypertrophy. This range is generally in the 65%–85% of a one-repetition max, with repetitions ranging from 6 to 15.

Because metabolic stress is the objective for core lifts, rest intervals between sets are in the 1–2-minute range generally, for single-joint movements in the 45–90-second range. Rest intervals for pure strength training range in length from 2 to 5 minutes.

Some advocate that time under tension, rather than the repetition range, is the primary variable determining the hypertrophic response to weight training. The logic is that 12 repetitions performed in a squat, taking 10 seconds, with 40% of your one-repetition max, will invoke a much different adaptation than 12 reps with 70% of your one-repetition max.

As weight increases, bar speed will decrease, so the muscles will be under tension much longer. Time-under-tension advocates generally believe 30–60 seconds is the ideal time to set completion for the best hypertrophic response.

Maximizing limit strength is done with less than 85% of a one-repetition max, generally in the 1–5 repetition range. Fueled by the immediate energy system, the anaerobic glycolysis energy system fuels the intensely performed moderate repetition ranges, or the time under tension in the 30–60 second range, causing a significant buildup of metabolites.

Studies performed on bodybuilders post workout, after performing exercises with moderate rep ranges, show significant decreases in muscle glycogen, ATP, and creatine phosphate. To counter that, blood lactate, intramuscular lactate, and glucose increase and build up, serving as a catalyst for muscle growth.

Intense training in a moderate repetition range will cause a full spectrum muscle hypertrophy across slow and fast twitch fibers, aiding in maximizing development.

Training in this moderate repetition range provides for a great "pump," and this begs the question: Is the pump the end all, or is it just self-indulgence of overzealous, solipsistic muscle heads?

One camp is telling us the pump is all that matters; another counters by exclaiming it's meaningless. So who is right: the "bro science" muscle head or the crypto scientific functional trainer?

The pump is caused by a build-up of metabolic byproducts that cause the cell to swell; cell swelling has been shown to help increase muscle growth. The pump should not be worshipped as the end all of muscle hypertrophy, but it can't be dismissed as feel-good bro science, either.

SELECTING THE RIGHT EXERCISES

Compound exercises that involve multiple joints and multiple muscles have a much greater bang for their buck than single-joint isolation exercises. Leg curls target the hamstrings; deadlifts also provide a great stimulus to the hamstrings, in addition to virtually every other muscle in the body.

Taking a closer look at the reckoning of hypertrophy, the compound-exercise dynasty reigns superior to isolation counterparts. This holds true gauging exercise value thru anabolic hormonal response, calories burned during training and post workout, cardiorespiratory demands, real-world functionality, injury prevention, range of motion, neural adaptations, or even poundage lifted.

Furthermore, as discussed earlier, compound movements are superior for building limit strength, "your base." Odds are, athletes who have squats at the center of their leg development program will have more impressive leg development than athletes who allocate a majority of their energy to leg extensions.

Compound movements, in general, are safer than isolation because forces are spread across multiple joints and muscles. Core lifts, in general, need to remain at the core of the program. Isolation exercises are needed for supernatural development in certain areas and to bring up weaknesses through the overload principle of isolation.

Mechanical Work Performed

"The Veteran," though I never knew his real name, was an older gentleman, a retired bodybuilder who trained at the same gym as I did when I was growing up.

The first time I attempted to squat 405 pounds, I missed it. "The Veteran" saw this and proceeded to scream at me and went on to threaten me with serious bodily harm if I did not come back and squat the weight in 5 minutes. Needless to say, his "encouragement" helped, and I made the weight.

"The Veteran" was crazier than an outhouse rat, but he admittedly had an amazing physique for any age. And he was in his 60s! "The Veteran" had absolutely no filter on his mouth. Anytime someone came in the gym and did an exercise that lacked the proper range of motion, "The Veteran" would bark out, "Full range of motion for full development." While "The Veteran" was not educated in formal exercise science, he was wise indeed!

A lack of range of motion will result in a lack of muscle being built because of the lack of tension throughout the entire range of motion.

A plethora of studies demonstrate that full-range-of-motion exercises eclipse partial movements for inducing hypertrophy, not to mention the fact that the more natural movement pattern of a full-range-of motion movement and the stretch imposed by using the full movement can even cause a subsequent increase in flexibility.

Performing partials requires you to use a much greater load than a full-range-of-motion exercise; less muscle is being worked, but the stress on the central nervous system is exacerbated because of the supramaximal weights being lifted.

More mechanical work will lead to greater metabolic stresses, increased muscle tension, and more muscle damage. Mechanical work is simply the weight lifted, multiplied by the distance it is lifted, multiplied by the number of repetitions.

Hypothetically, you can squat 400 pounds for 5 repetitions and your full squat range of motion is 24 inches. What if you can quarter-squat 600 pounds for 5 repetitions?

Simple arithmetic can determine the amount of work being performed. Full squats would be 400 pounds x 6 repetitions x 24 inches = 57,600 pounds of mechanical work. Quarter squats would be 600 pounds x 6 repetitions x 6 inches = 21,600 pounds of mechanical work.

Even though you are using 200 pounds less, the mechanical work of the full squat is nearly triple that of the quarter squat; and metabolic stress is much greater because time under tension is much greater, due to the increased distance the weight is being moved.

There is certainly a place for some partials in training for overload, and to work specific muscles and ranges of motion, the bulk of your movements should be through a full range of motion.

If you are scratching in disbelief because so many people lift with a limited range motion, the reason is simple… ego!

Never engage in the self-indulgent practice of sacrificing technique for weight if you are serious about your strength goals.

Limiting Factors

For a bodybuilder, deadlifts serve to build the posterior chain and barbell shrugs serve to build the traps. If your grip is the limiting factor in either of these exercises, wear straps. Obviously, you're going to want to build a strong grip, but not at the expense of sacrificing muscular development.

If an exercise has a limiting factor that sacrifices the work the muscle performs, eliminate this factor (in this example, wear straps) or find a new exercise.

This is why BOSU ball squats belong in a Coney Island side show, not as part of the serious muscle building process. The take-home point is simple: Let the muscles you are training limit the weight you use in training if hypertrophy is the desired result.

Nevertheless, there are a number of ways to select the right exercises for you, taking into account the variables that have been outlined.

There are plenty of great exercises out there. Here are some of my favorite go-to, results-producing exercises.

TOP TEN EXERCISES FOR LEGS

Nothing looks sillier than a pair of chicken legs coupled with a massive upper body. More and more emphasis is being placed on lower body development in today's contests. Size, separation, and even striated glutes have become the norm in high-level contests.

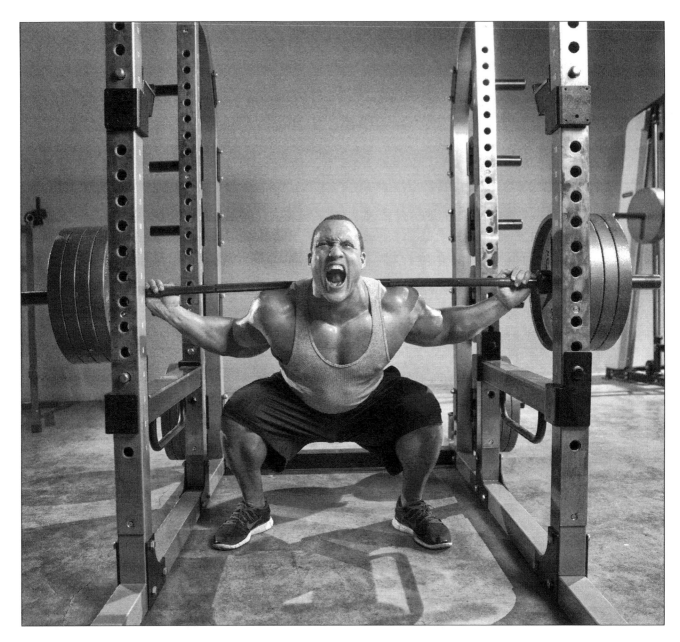

Squats (Front and Back)

"There is simply no other exercise, and certainly no machine, that produces the level of central nervous system activity, improved balance and coordination, skeletal loading and bone density enhancement, muscular stimulation and growth, connective tissue stress and strength, psychological demand and toughness, and overall systemic conditioning than the correctly performed full squat," said strength coach Mark Rippetoe.

He was right.

Squats are king.

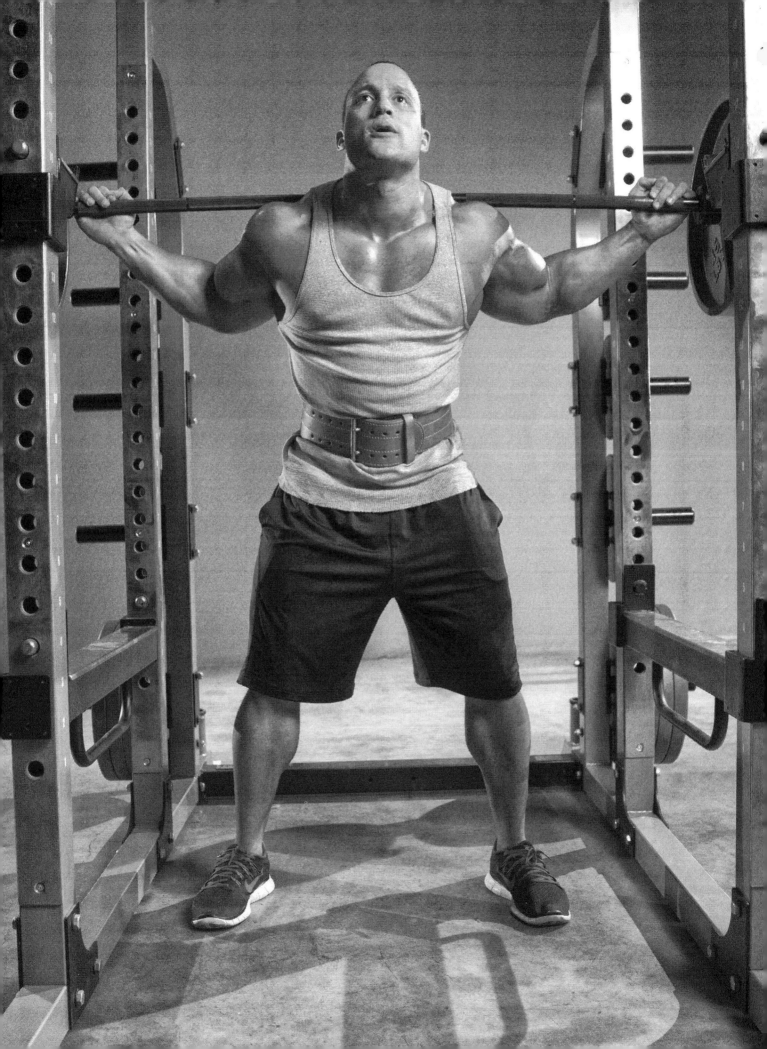

How to correctly perform a back squat:

- Place a barbell on top of the posterior deltoids
- Un-rack the barbell and step back one leg at a time to a shoulder-width or wider stance
- Keep your chest up and shoulder blades retracted
- Initiate movement by pushing your hips back (don't bend at the knees first)
- Make sure to push your knees out on the descent and ascent
- Squat down below parallel
- Return to the starting position

Safety squats with a safety bar will allow you to squat with more weight, maintain a more upright position, and pull yourself through sticking points, ceasing assistance at points where leverage is advantageous—where you are the strongest.

Unfortunately, most gyms do not have safety bars. Regular back squats can be performed with additional bands or chains. Total band or chain weight should be somewhere between 10% and 25% of bar weight.

If you are squatting 300 pounds of bar weight, this means an additional 30–75 pounds of total band and chain weight can be added to the bar. Bands can also be tied to the top of the rack in a reverse-band style using the same guidelines.

Important note: When performing heavy squats, breathe before the initial descent and between reps. When squatting, perform the Valsalva Maneuver. This is done by exhaling against a closed glottis; this increases intra-abdominal pressure and allows you to have a more rigid torso and produce more force. There is not one shred of evidence of ill health effects in healthy adults performing this maneuver. Quite the contrary: This is an injury-prevention and strength-enhancing movement. Those with high blood pressure should avoid the Valsalva Maneuver and heavy squats, period.

How to correctly perform a front squat:

- Front squat technical cues are pretty similar to those of back squats.
- Place the barbell on your shoulders; it should be very close to your neck
- Un-rack the bar with a clean grip or a bodybuilder "California Style" cross grip
- Keep your arms crossed in front of you and at parallel position to the floor to prevent the barbell from rolling forward and away from your neck

- Keep your chest up throughout the entire movement
- Initiate movement by pushing your hips back (don't bend at the knees first)
- Make sure to push your knees out on the descent and ascent
- Squat down to the position of at least parallel or below parallel
- Return to the starting position

Advantages of the front squat:

1. Front squats are more quad dominant. Don't worry if your front squat poundages are less than what you use for the back squat. You will see and feel the front-squat difference!

2. Front squats are easier on your back because your torso is more erect and, obviously, less weight is being handled

3. If you go forward on a front squat, you lose the weight; so it's impossible to lean forward too excessively

4. Front squats are also a good tool to teach someone to back squat with an erect torso

5. Front squats offer great transference to jerks, push presses, and Olympic lifts; more core stabilization is required than for back squats

Important note: Like back squats, front squats should be performed with the Valsalva Maneuver. Front squat harnesses are now available, and those who use them swear by them, making the holding-in-the-rack position a non issue. I recommend not front squatting above 8 reps because your rhomboids will fatigue before your thighs, so you will start to gain a hunchback-like posture. Front squats can be done with chains; against bands they feel quite awkward.

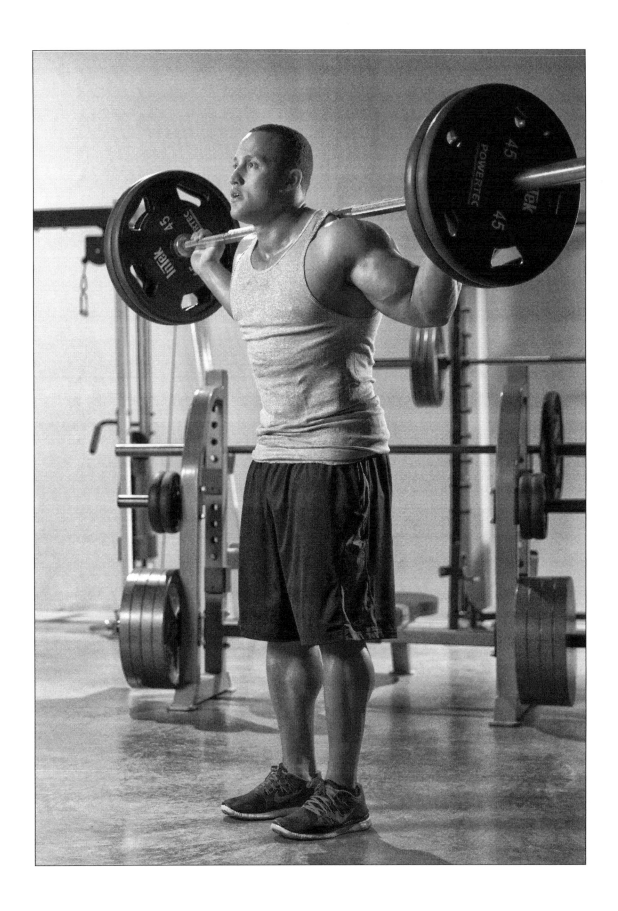

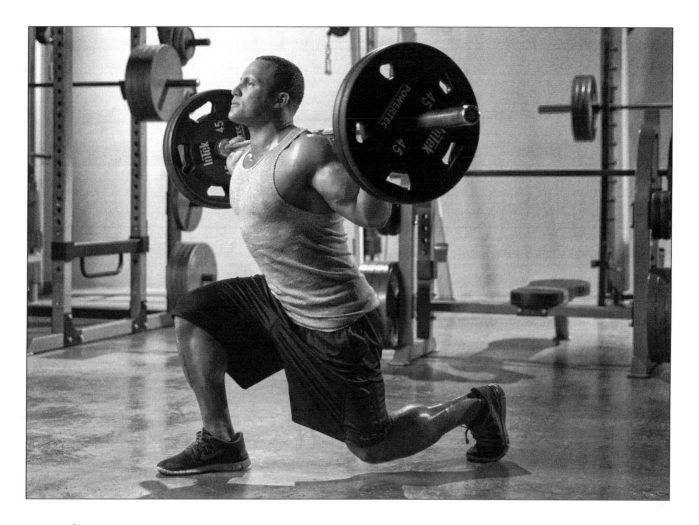

Lunges

How to correctly perform a lunge:

- Hold a dumbbell in each hand or place a barbell on your back
- Step forward with one leg, keeping your torso upright
- Make a 90-degree angle with the leg that is in front
- Be careful not to let your knee go over your toe
- Return to starting position

Important note: Lunges can also be done in a reverse style or even laterally. Walking lunges were a favorite of eight-time Mr. Olympia, Ronnie Coleman.

In Ronnie Coleman's prime, he did walking lunges 405 pounds for a 50-yard lunge! Quoting Brian Dobson, "The walking lunge has now become standard for upper leg separation and glute/ham tie-in." Lunge variations not only assist in total leg development but also strengthen the core and increase stability in heavy squatting.

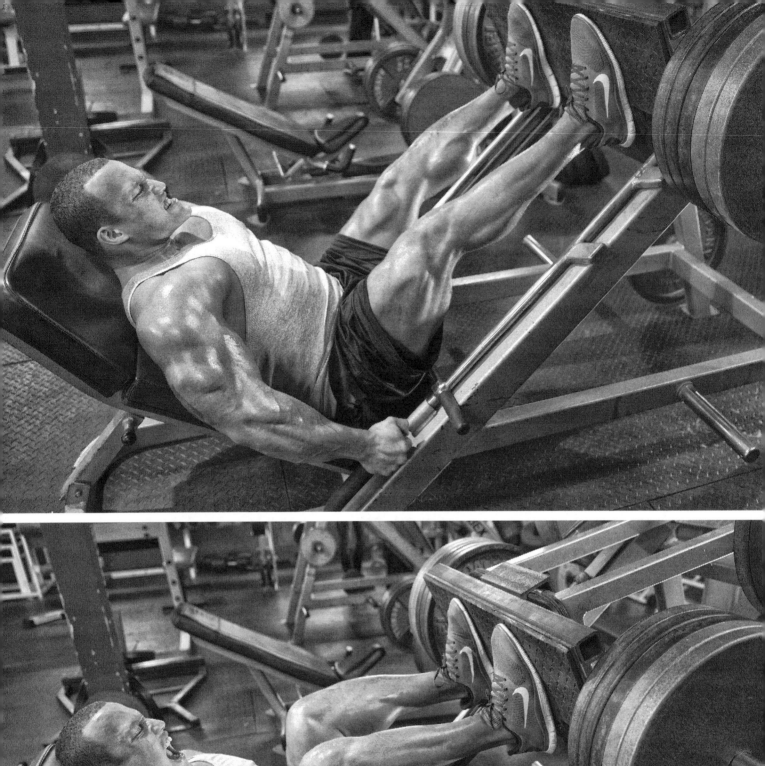
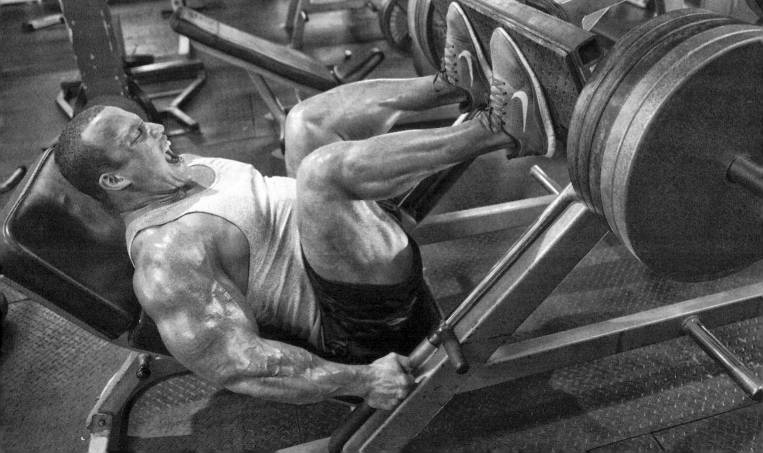

Angled Leg Press

The leg press, while it is an excellent exercise, is not a substitute for the king of all leg exercises, the squat.

How to correctly perform an angled leg press:

- Sit on the machine with your head and back against the padded support
- With your feet on the platform, tighten your abdominals
- Push the platform away from your body by extending your knees and pushing your hips back into the pad
- Make sure your heels remain flat on the footplate
- Do not lift your lower back or butt off the platform
- Bring the weight down so your knees are past 90 degrees
- Push the weight back up to starting position

Important note: The lower you place your feet on the platform, the more intensely you hit the quads. By putting your feet higher on the platform and farther apart, you will more directly hit your glutes and hamstrings.

This is a huge ego lift for many folks; do not fall into this trap by loading hundreds of pounds onto the leg press and moving it just a couple of inches.

Because of the lack of stabilization required to perform the leg press and the fantastic leverage, you can use a lot of weight, which could potentially be harmful because of the fixed motor pattern and the amount of weight your joints have to handle.

Ronnie Coleman, Johnnie Jackson, and Branch Warren all feel they get the most out of this exercise with high reps. Bodybuilding guru and Metroflex owner, Brian Dobson, preaches the same and has been known to do a 4-set routine of leg presses of 50, 40, 30, 20 repetitions.

No one cares how much you can leg press, and it isn't a valid test of limit strength. This movement should be used correctly to build your thighs, not your ego.

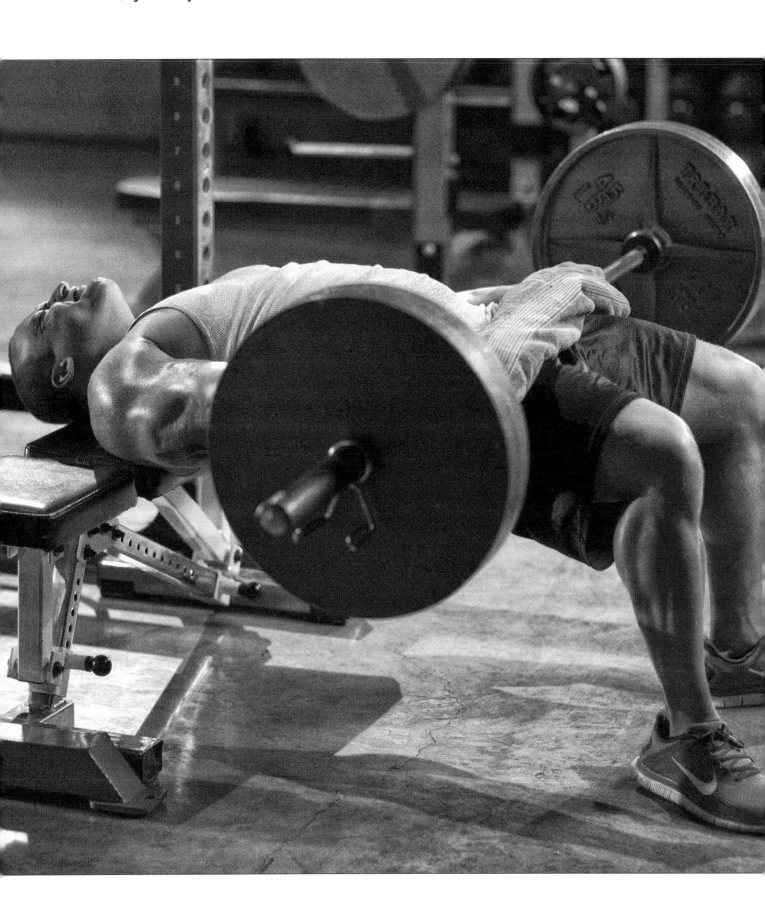

Barbell Hip Thrusts

Glute development, unlike past eras, is essential to win the big shows. One of the best exercises for the glutes is the barbell hip thrust.

I learned of this exercise from Bret Contreras. It directly targets the glutes, and heavy weight can be used. From a strength standpoint, this will enhance the deadlift lockout or any hip thrusting motion.

How to correctly perform a barbell hip thrust:

- Start with your body seated on the ground, with your back rested upon a bench
- Make sure the bench won't move
- Place a weighted barbell on your hips
- If you have large hips, plates can be stacked under the loaded weights to give you extra room
- From here, lean your shoulders back against the bench with your shoulders resting on top of the bench
- Forcefully push your hips up vertically, keeping the bar rested in your pelvis region
- Hold this top position briefly
- Return to starting position

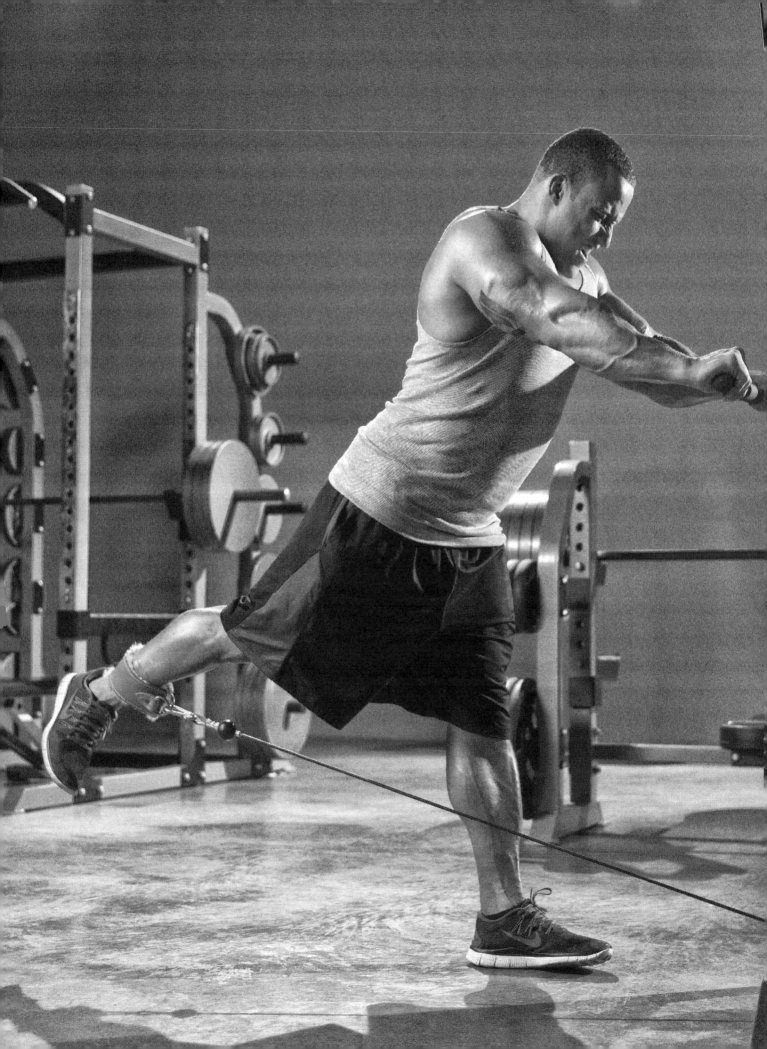

Single Leg Cable Kickbacks

This isolation exercise is very effective for targeting the glutes.

How to correctly perform single leg cable kickbacks:

- Hook a cuff around the ankle (you can use ab straps or even free motion handles)
- Face the weight stack and stand approximately 2–3 feet from it
- Hold the steel supports to balance yourself
- Slightly bend your knees and tighten your abdominals
- Using the leg that has the cuff, kick back as far as you can
- Hold your leg at that position for a second to get a good peak contraction
- Return to the starting position

Important note: This exercise can also be done with resistance bands. Bodybuilders will spend hours trying to isolate the biceps, but glutes deserve a high priority too.

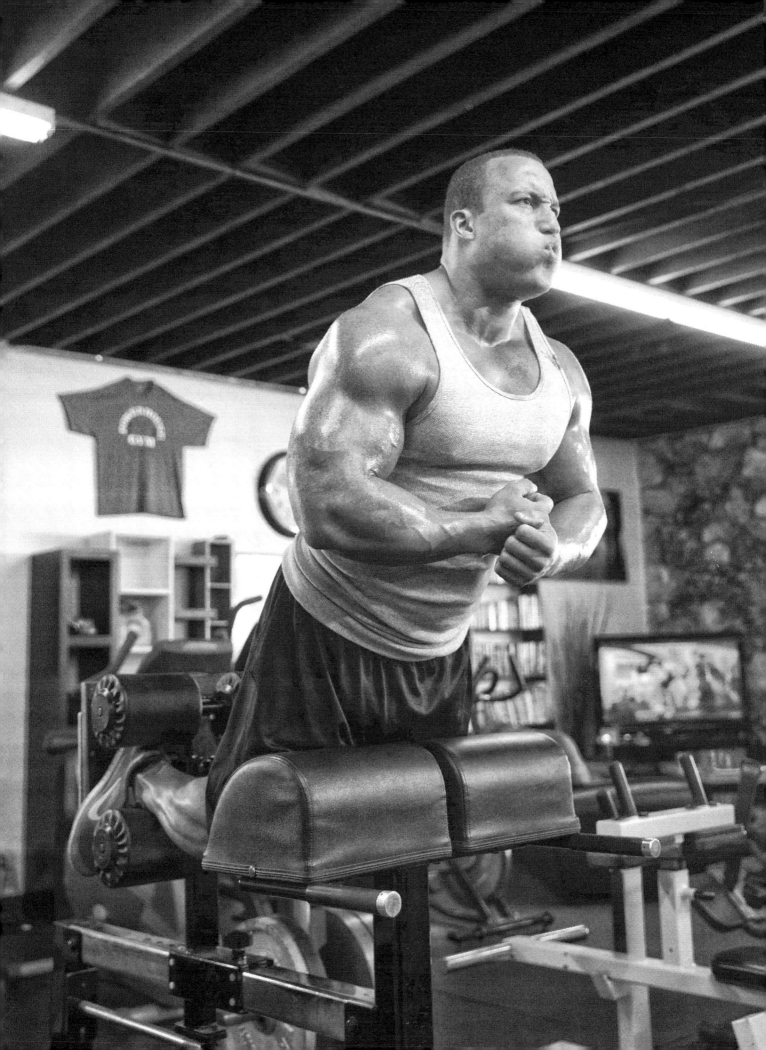

Glute Ham Raises

Glute ham raises are a favorite of those in strength sports for performance increases in pulls and squats. Bodybuilders need to get on board! This compound movement is one of the most effective ways to target the glutes and hamstrings.

How to correctly perform a glute ham raise:

- Place the ankles between the roller pads; your feet should be on the vertical platform

- If you are sweaty, place a towel on the platform to prevent slipping

- Your knees will be on the pad, and the lower portion of your thighs will be wedged against the large arc-shaped pad

- Initiate the movement by lifting your torso with your hamstrings and extending your hips with your glutes

- Keep raising your body by flexing your knees until your torso is upright

- Lower yourself in the opposite manner

Important note: This movement is like a compound leg curl that highly engages the glutes. It is a compound movement because knee flexion and hip extension both take place.

Initially, your bodyweight will be difficult, and many will not be able to do their bodyweight. In this case, you can do them band-assisted, working up to your bodyweight.

When you become proficient, you can add resistance by placing a barbell behind your shoulders like a squat, holding a weight or going against resistance bands. Originally, this machine was called the glute-ham-gastroc machine because it evens hits the calves.

Believe the hype—it works!

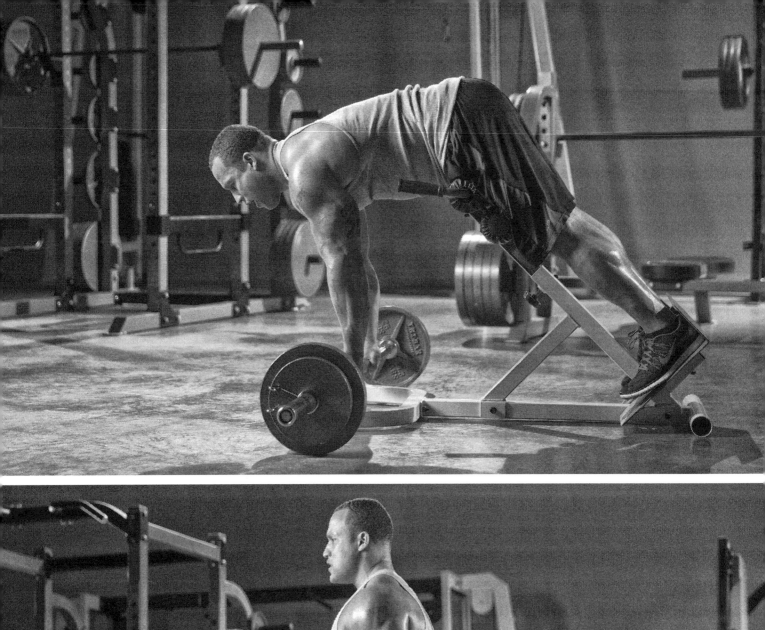
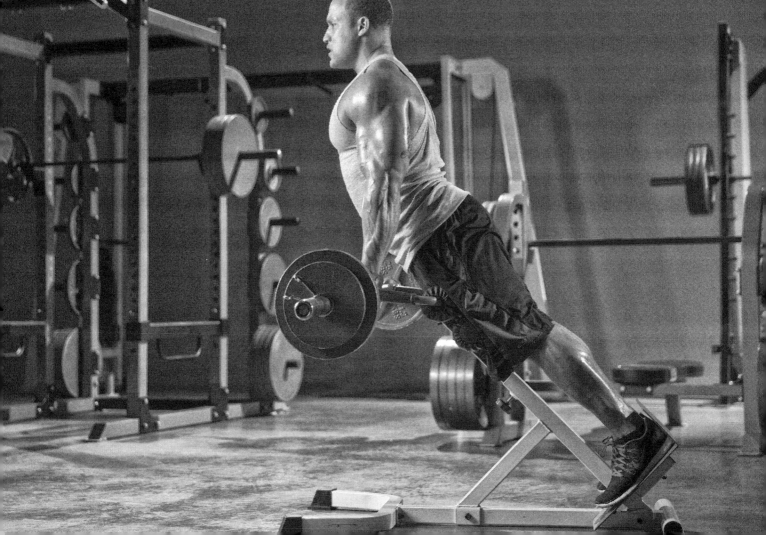

Deadlift Hyper

This movement could be classified as a back movement, as even the glutes play an important assisting role. This is one of the most effective exercises to build and strengthen the hamstrings.

How to correctly perform a deadlift hyper:

- On a 45-degree hyper bench, place your thighs face down on the padding
- Your feet should be flat on the bottom support platform
- Place the barbell or dumbbells in your hands, keeping your back flat throughout the entirety of the movement
- Lift your body upward until your hips are extended, squeezing your glutes as you lock-out the weight
- Lower the weight back to the floor

Important note: If you are unable to get a full range of motion because your hyper bench is too low to the ground, use small plates. Instead of a 45-pound plate on each side, use a 25-pound plate, with 2 tens or even 4 tens and 1 five.

Many with lower back problems have used non-weighted hypers with excellent results. However, those with a history of back problems should either avoid the movement or, if they choose to do it, be careful and use a limited range of motion that *gradually* increases as they get stronger.

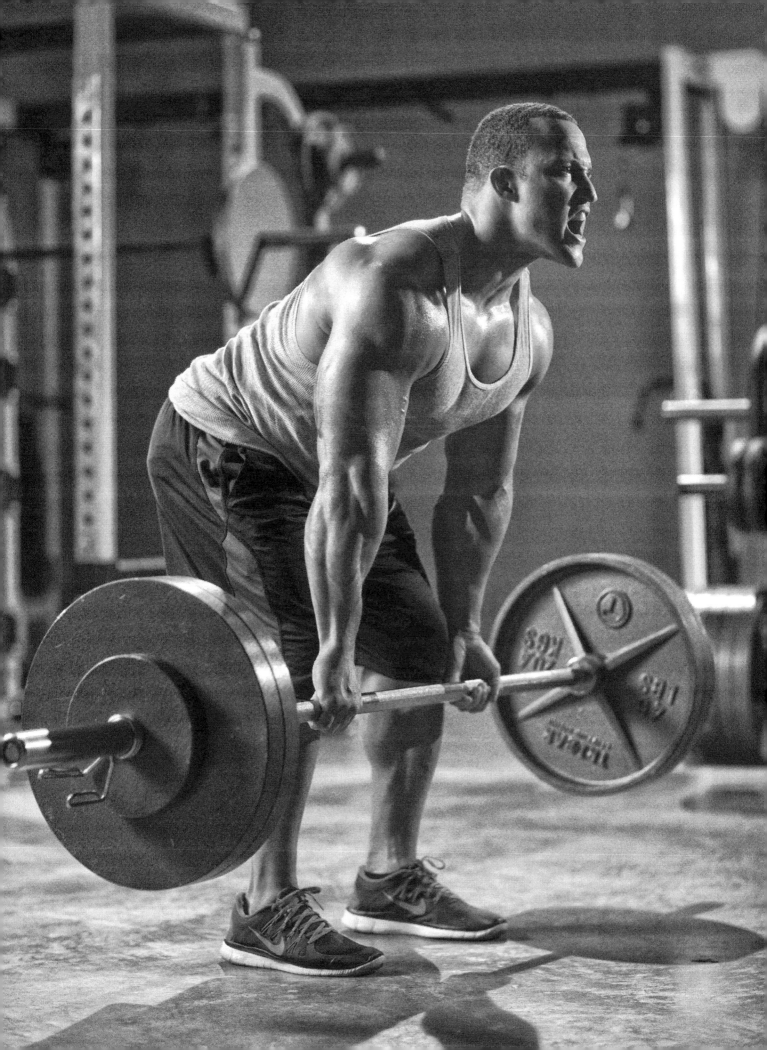

Romanian Deadlifts

How to correctly perform a Romanian deadlift:

- Start this movement standing upright

- The barbell can be picked up off of a power rack; if that is not available, deadlift the weight conventionally off of the floor

- Taking a stance between hip and shoulder width; place your hands right outside of your thighs

- Use a pronated grip (straps are okay)

- Slightly bend your knees, and keep your back arched and flat

- Lower the bar, keeping your chest up by pushing your hips back and purposely putting tension on the hamstrings

- Lower the bar to mid-shin level (your torso should be parallel to the floor)

- Lift the weight to the starting position by extending the hips

- Keep the bar in close to your body; the further it drifts away from you, the more stress will be put on your lower back

Important note: This movement can also be performed with dumbbells. If you want to try something different, try the single-leg version of this movement. Besides the typical unilateral benefits, it will build balance. The single-leg version smokes the hamstrings and can be done with dumbbells or a barbell. If you have a history of lower back problems, avoid this movement.

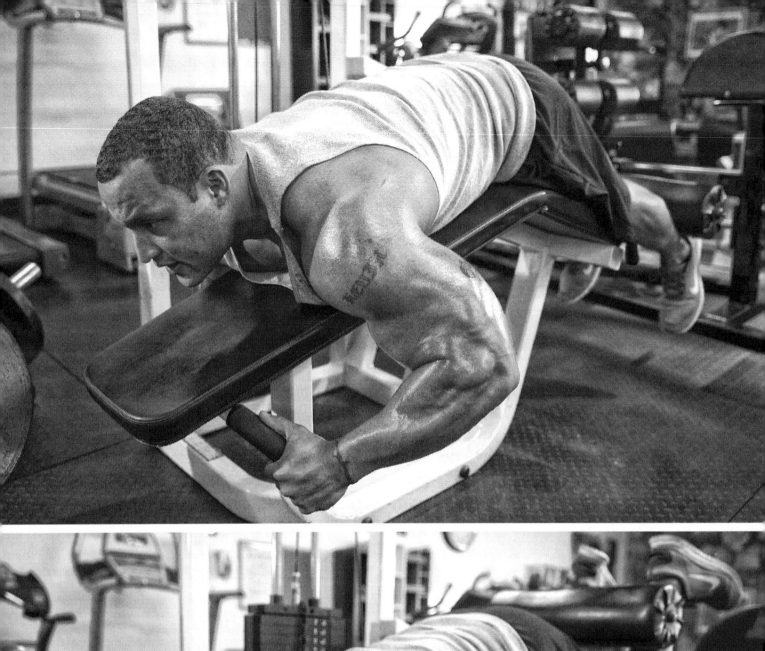
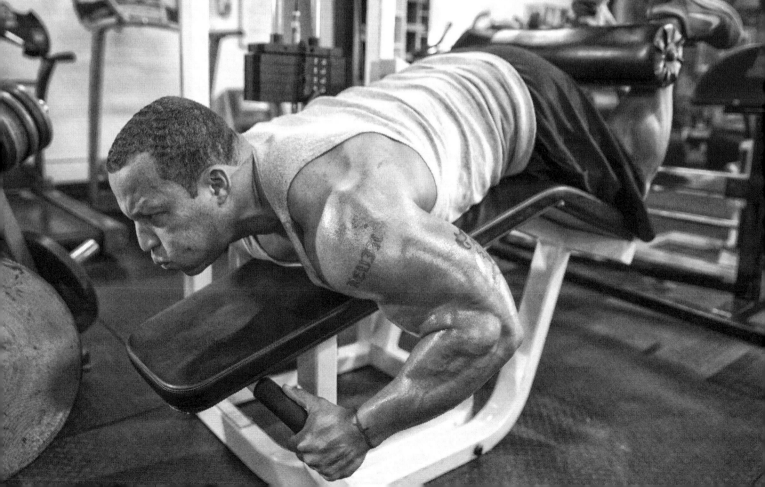

Leg Curls

The hamstrings have two functions: flexion of the knee and extension of the knee. Romanian deadlifts work primarily hip extension, glute ham raises work both, and leg curls work knee flexion.

Hamstrings and their assisting role in hip extension are much more important to strength athletes than knee flexion. Bodybuilders have to work the entire hamstrings. It is impossible to have great leg development or strength without good hamstrings.

How to correctly perform a leg curl:

- Lie face down on the leg curl; adjust it to fit your body
- Put the pad of the lever slightly below your calves
- Keep your torso flat on the bench
- Grasp handles on the side of the machine
- Make sure your legs are fully stretched and curl your legs up as far as possible
- Hold briefly at the top
- Return to the starting position

Important note: Leg curls need to be strict and for a full range of motion. The purpose of the movement is to isolate knee flexion and not perform a pseudo-compound movement.

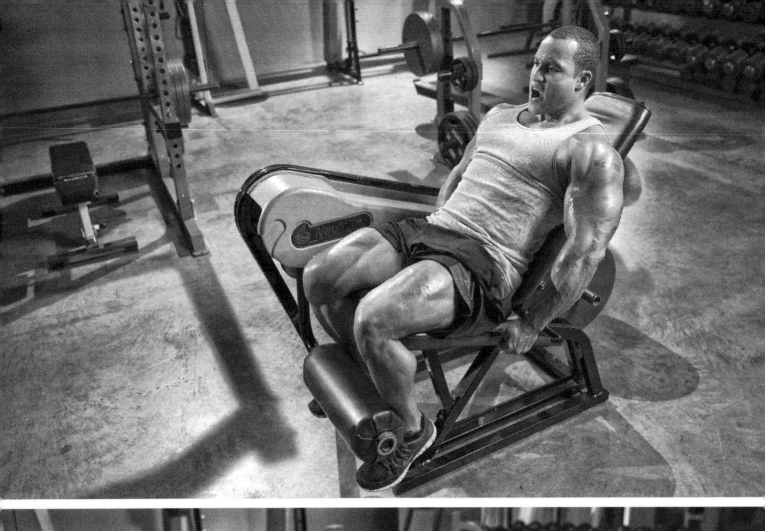

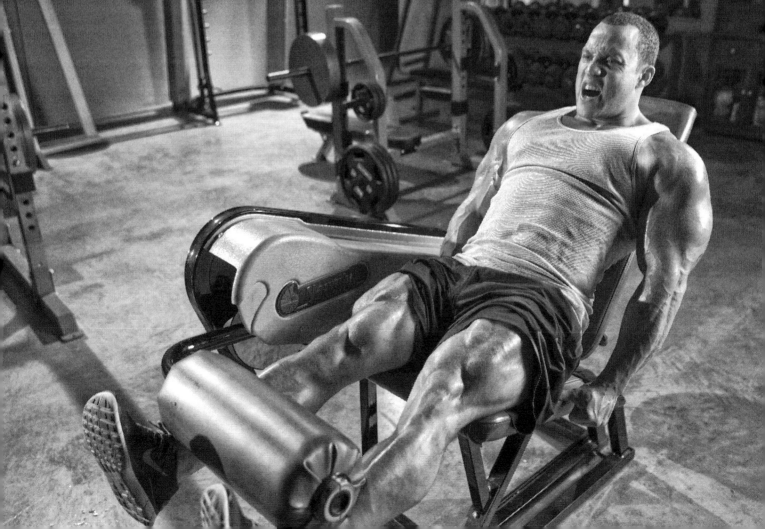

Leg Extensions

Leg extensions directly target the quadriceps. Walking, running and everyday movements require muscles of the leg to work together. Leg extensions isolate the quadriceps, so it is a very unnatural movement. Because of this, it operates on the overload principle of isolation. Having a well-developed "sweep" and "teardrop" are essential to your bodybuilding success.

How to correctly perform a leg extension:

- Sit on a leg extension machine with your back against the padded support
- Place your shins under the padded lever
- Grab the handles for support
- Extend your knees until your legs are straight
- Hold at the top briefly
- Return to the original position

Important note: This is an isolation movement, not an ego lift. Make sure you are getting a full range of motion. Because it is unnatural, using too much weight by cheating puts you at a high risk for injury. Like leg curls, this movement can be done unilaterally.

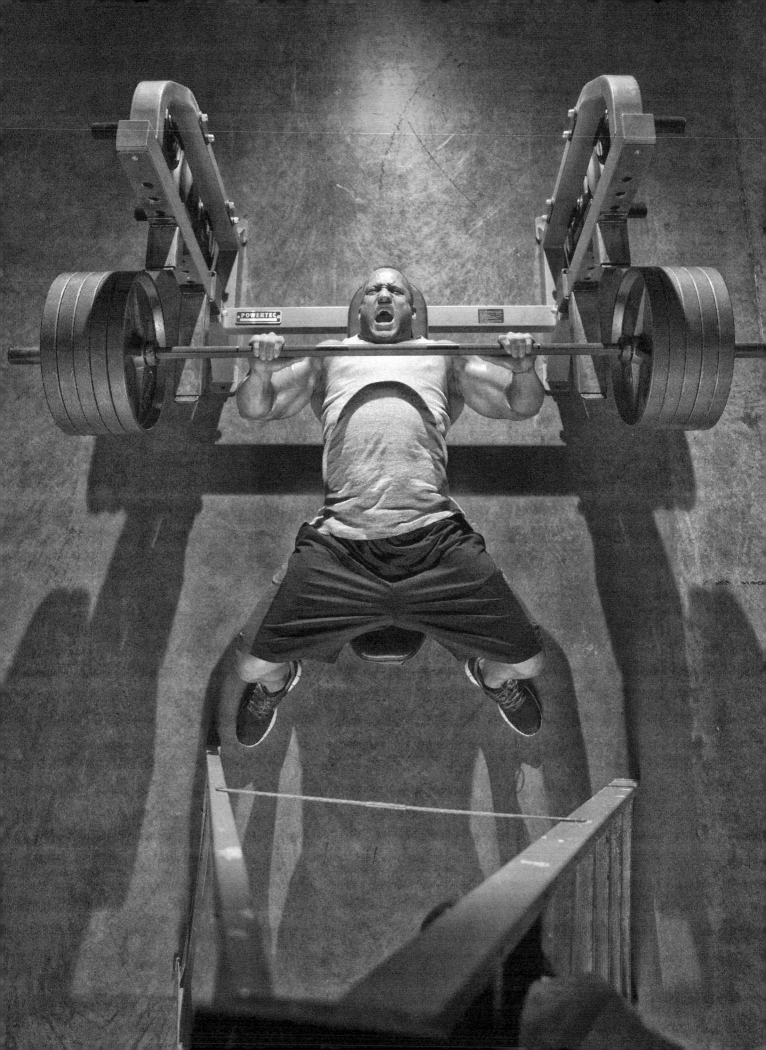

TOP TEN EXERCISES FOR CHEST

Bench Press

This is the no-frills, blue-collar chest builder. Lifting maximum weights in the bench press is a favorite upper-body limit-strength assessment, and it is the lift everyone in the Western world associates with weightlifting.

When experts talk about the bench press, it is hard not to think that personal pride might jade their judgment. Usually, those who are not good at the lift are the first to scream about its being ineffective.

The two best chests of all time are Ronnie Coleman and Arnold Schwarzenegger. Both had powerlifting backgrounds, and both had the bench press at the center of their respective programs.

"Everybody wants to be a bodybuilder, but no one wants to lift no heavy ass weight," to quote Ronnie Coleman.

Heavy bench presses are the go-to lift to develop massive pecs. The bench press allows you to lift more weight than any other free-weight exercise.

Look at some of the best raw bench pressers of all time, like Big Jim Williams, Bill Kazmaier, and Doug Young; they had some of the most muscular chests of all time, and these guys had way more muscle on their frame than bodybuilders of the same era. Arnold was rumored to have consulted with Doug Young for mass building methods long before personal training was a recognized profession.

How to correctly perform a bench press:

- Lie flat on a bench
- Un-rack the barbell at arms extension over your chest
- Grasp the bar with a pronated grip and slightly wider-than-shoulder-width grip
- Keep your upper back tight
- Make sure your feet are flat throughout the entire movement
- Grip the barbell tightly and lower the barbell under control to nipple line or slightly below
- Forcefully push the bar back to arms extension
- Dismount barbell from rack over your chest

Important note: This is a compound movement; and when you use the proper technique, more weight equals more growth.

The bench press is used primarily for chest development, but the shoulders and triceps will experience growth; many other synergist muscles contribute to heavy bench presses. Bands and chains can both be used for bench presses. Generally, stick to 10%–25% of bar weight for the added accommodated resistance.

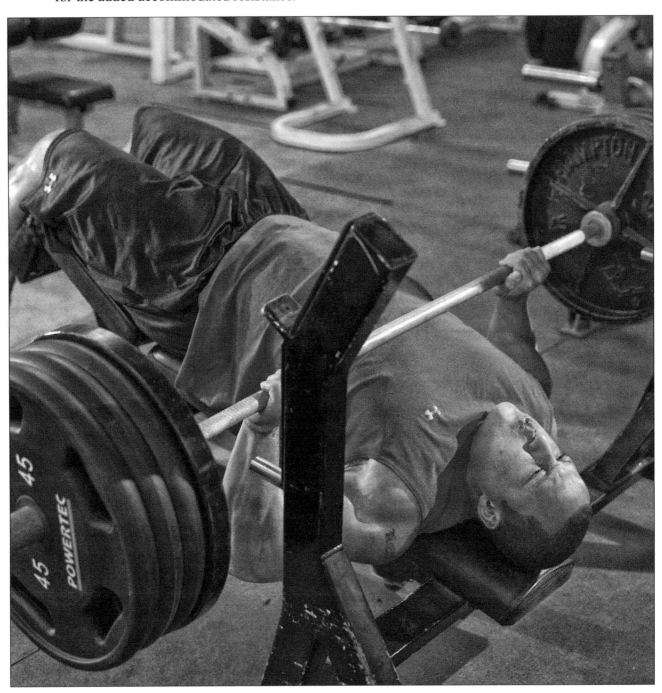

Decline Bench Press

Dorian Yates is a big believer in the decline bench press. He has said the pectoral muscles have two actions: flexion and adduction of your upper arm. Both of these happen during the upward phase of a decline bench press. There is no doubt that decline bench presses target muscle fiber of the lower chest, but they do actually hit the entire chest.

Many people are even able to lift more weight on a slight decline than on a bench press. Decline bench press should be 15–30 degrees declined. Some people with shoulder issues report less pain with decline bench presses because it forces you to keep your elbows tucked in and removes some of the involvement of the shoulder joint.

How to correctly perform a decline bench press:

- Lie on the decline bench press with your feet under the leg brace
- Lift the barbell from the rack with a slightly wider-than-shoulder-width grip
- Lower the weight to your chest
- Press the weight back to full extension

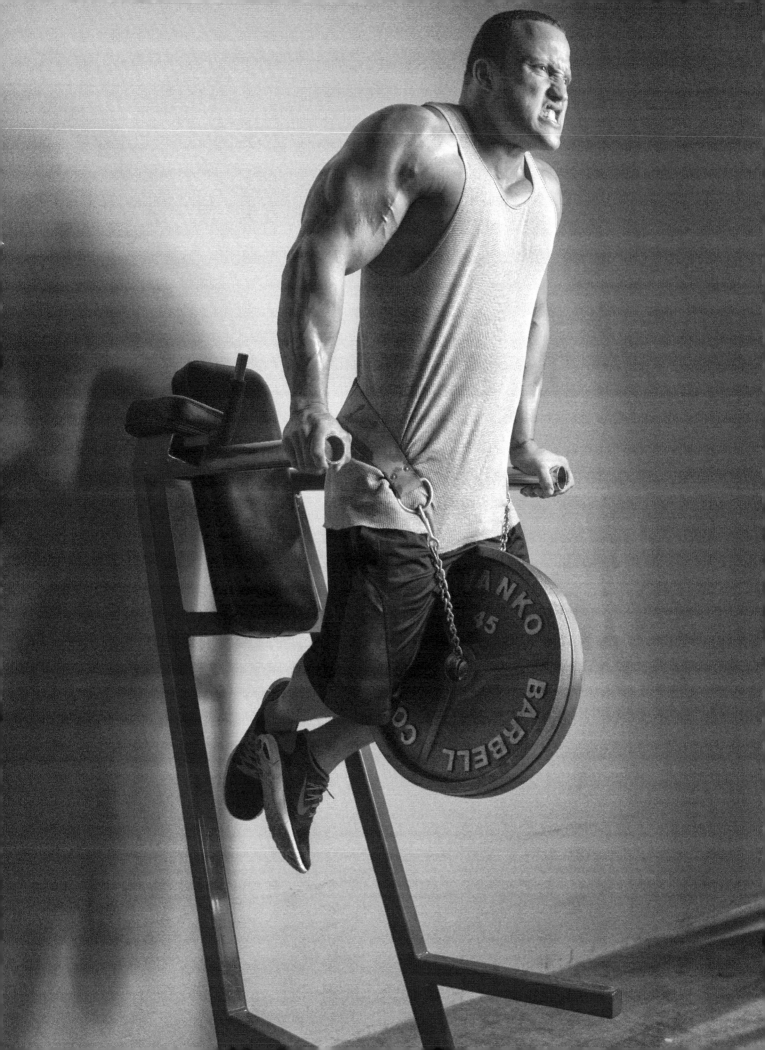

Weighted Dips

These were a staple strength-training movement before modern machines and gimmicks. Weighted dips have a place in a wide spectrum of programs that serve a wide range of goals. They build barrel chests and triceps that fill out shirtsleeves. I have included them because weighted dips force you to handle your bodyweight plus an additional load.

Many will refer to weighted dips as the "king" for the chest and the triceps. How many exercises claim this kind of monopoly on two different muscle groups?

Dips build strength in functional activities and in strength tests. Pat Casey, the first man to bench press 600 pounds, had weighted dips at the core of his program.

Want to bench big? Try dips!

Besides, they offer great transference to overhead presses.

Bodybuilders with shoulder or elbow injuries may find dips to be a good substitute for bench pressing. Most importantly, dips have been the staple of many great physique athletes like Branch Warren, Johnnie Jackson, and Ronnie Coleman, to name just a few.

How to correctly perform a weighted dip:

- Start dips with arms in extension on the dip bar
- Lower your body until your arms are parallel to the floor
- Return to the starting point

Important note: Unlike bench presses, dips are a closed kinetic chain exercise, meaning you push your body through the air instead of using an external resistance object like barbells, dumbbells, or a machine.

This is a more natural movement pattern.

Weighted dips with a forward lean were a favorite of late iron guru, Vince Gironda. In order to shift more emphasis on the pecs, keep the elbows out, tucking the chin to the chest and leaning forward.

A more upright posture with elbows in will shift more of the emphasis to the triceps. Extra weight can be attached by way of adding plates or a dumbbell to a dipping belt; or, if you are lucky enough to have a Nautilus dip machine at your gym, it is much easier to use.

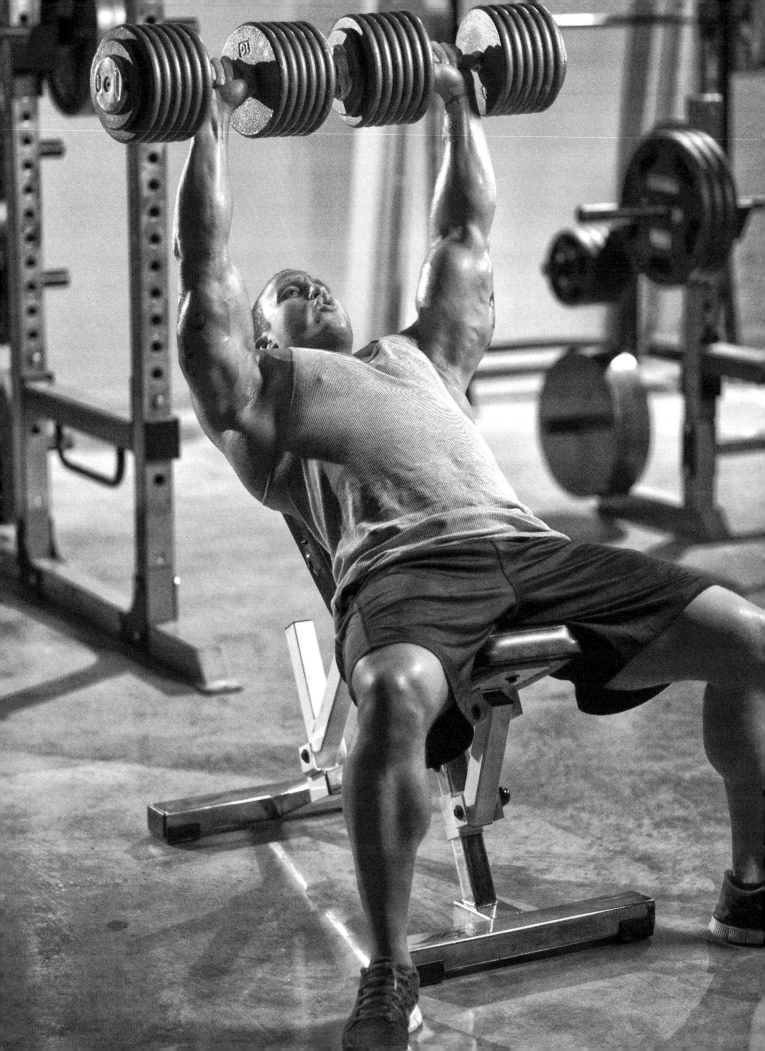

Dumbbell Incline Press

For decades, inclines have been a favorite of bodybuilders to hit the upper portion (clavicular) of the chest. This movement can also be performed against band resistance by placing the band around your back. Barbell variations can also be used.

How to correctly perform a dumbbell incline press:

- Sit down on the incline bench, resting the dumbbells on your thighs
- Kick the weights to your shoulders and lean back (if the weight is really heavy, get a partner to help you)
- Position the dumbbells to the sides of your chest
- Press the dumbbells up until your arms are extended
- Lower the weight back to starting position

Important note: This movement, as shown in EMG studies, also targets the deltoids. Triceps also play an important assisting role. For a fun variation, try the incline dumbbell or barbell press with a reverse grip.

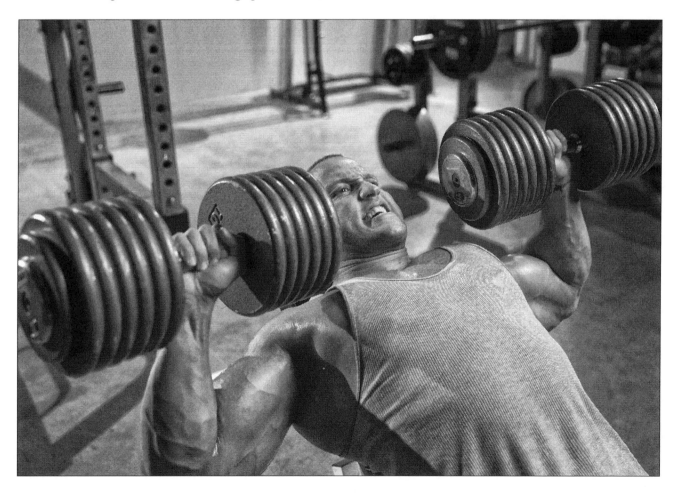

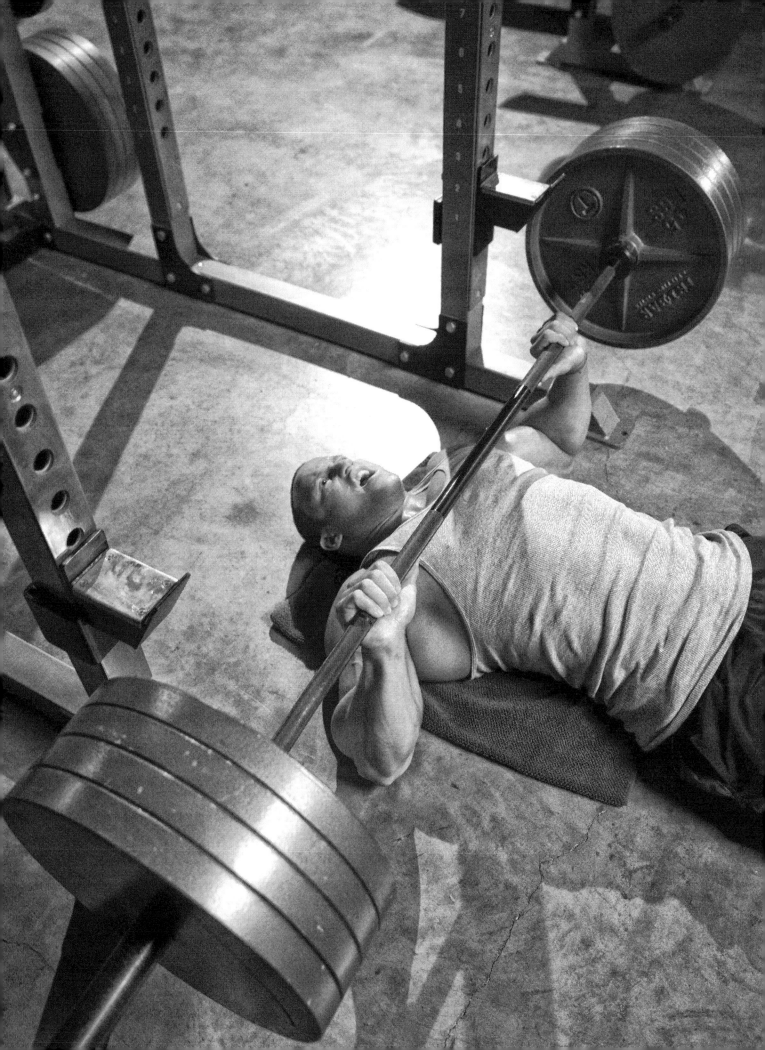

Floor Press

The floor press has two basic variations. The barbell floor press and the dumbbell floor press perform with a neutral grip. It is important to mix in neutral-grip-pressing exercises with dumbbells because it not only hits the muscle at a different angle but prevents wear and tear.

> ### *How to correctly perform a floor press:*
>
> - The floor press is essentially a bench press lying on the floor
> - Set the barbell in supports on the power rack
> - Un-rack it like a normal bench press
> - Lower the weight until your triceps hit the floor
> - Pause for a split second at the bottom
> - Press the weight back up to starting position

Important note: This exercise works very well with the addition of chains.

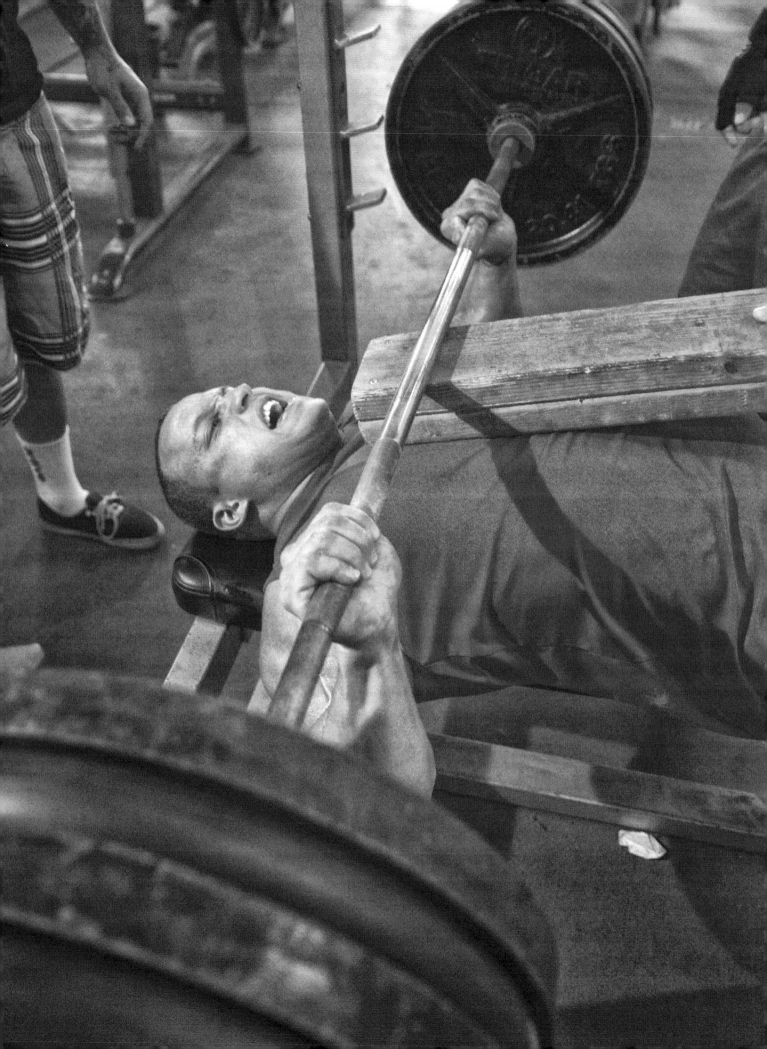

Bench Press with Weight Releasers

As we all know, you can handle more weight on an eccentric than a concentric. To maximize muscularity, bodybuilders have to include eccentrics in their training.

How to correctly perform a bench press with weight releaser:

- Attach the weight releasers to the bar
- Lower the bar like a normal bench press
- As the bar touches your chest, the weight releasers release; therefore, you push up only the bar weight
- Return to the starting position and repeat reps without weight releasers

Important note: Anywhere from about 5%–30% of the bar weight can be used on the releasers. These can be done for a drawn-out eccentric or at a traditional tempo. If done without purposefully slowing the eccentric, the positive portion of the rep will potentially feel much more powerful because of the overload of the stretch shortening cycle.

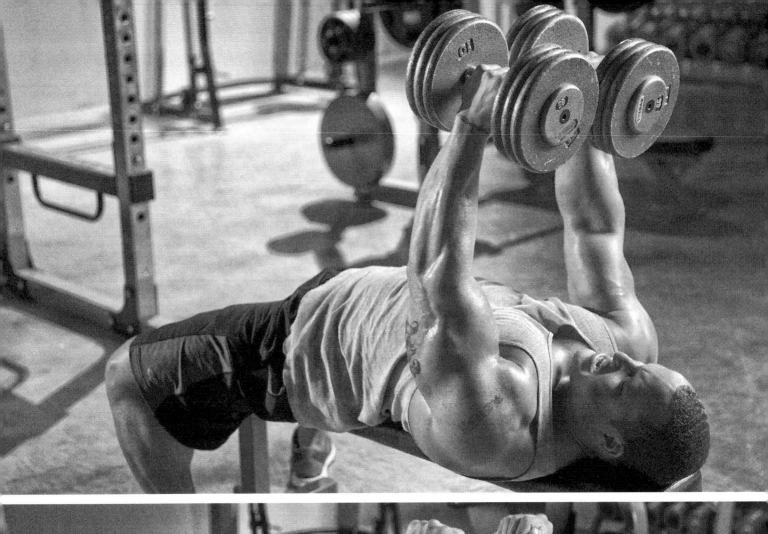
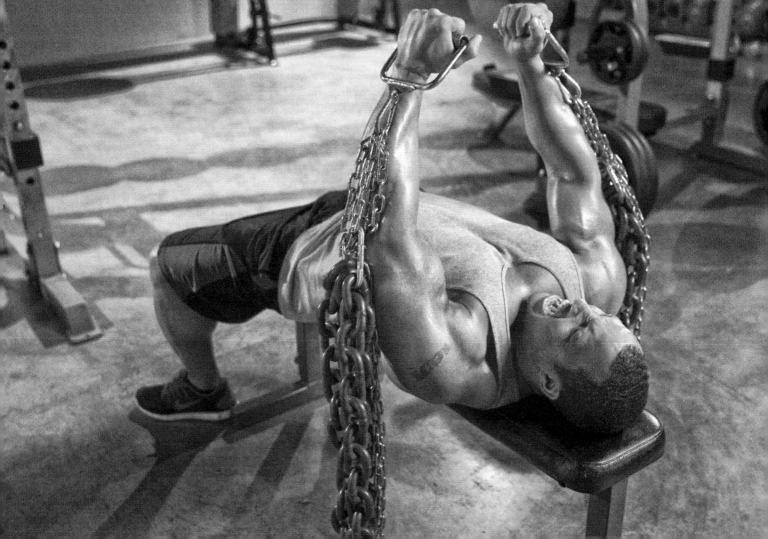

Dumbbell Flyes

This has been a favorite of bodybuilders and top raw bench pressers for decades. This was a staple in Arnold's regimen.

How to correctly perform dumbbell flyes:

- Lie flat on a bench
- Lift the dumbbells above your chest with arms in a slightly bent position (your arms never straighten out throughout the entire movement)
- Lower dumbbells to the side until your chest muscles are stretched
- Bring the dumbbells together in a giant bear hugging-like motion
- Hold the dumbbells together at the top for a brief moment
- Return to starting position

Important note: Remember, this movement is not a press or an extension. Think of it like a giant hug. Once your elbows are bent 10–15 degrees, keep them in this fixed position. Concentrate on the squeeze.

This movement is very effective against resistance bands by putting the bands around your back and holding them in your hands. This not only makes it a great stretch exercise but also adds a peak-contraction element of constant tension throughout the entire movement. This can also be done on an incline or decline. If you have a history of shoulder problems, you will want to avoid this movement.

Chain Flyes

Chain flyes are a great substitute if you have shoulder pain or if you want to put less stress on your shoulders in general.

How to correctly perform chain flyes:

- Attach a single handle attachment with a carabineer to a chain
- Perform the movement the same way as dumbbell flyes

Important note: "I feel this in every muscle fiber in my chest!" screamed Johnnie Jackson after a difficult set of chain flyes. At the bottom of the movement, the chain unloads on the floor so it is not nearly as much weight in the more vulnerable position, but you still get a stretch. As you squeeze the weight up, link-by-link the chain comes off the floor. So, where the movement would be easiest, intensity increases.

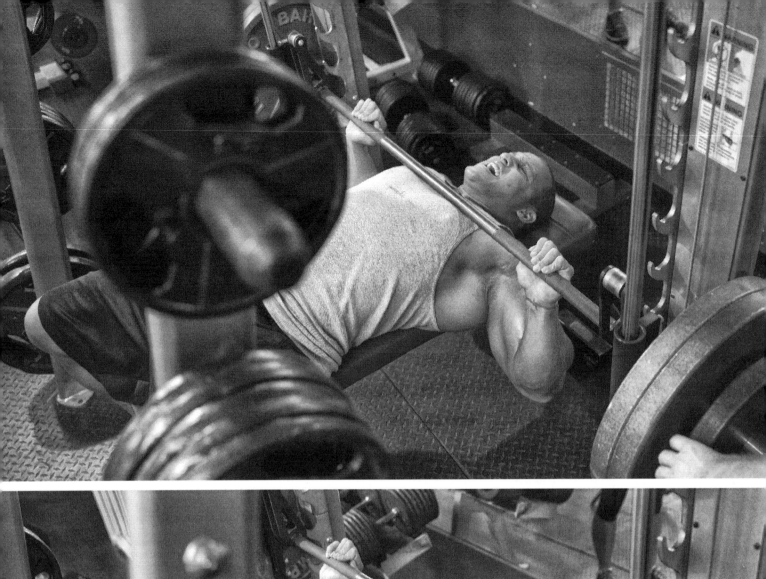
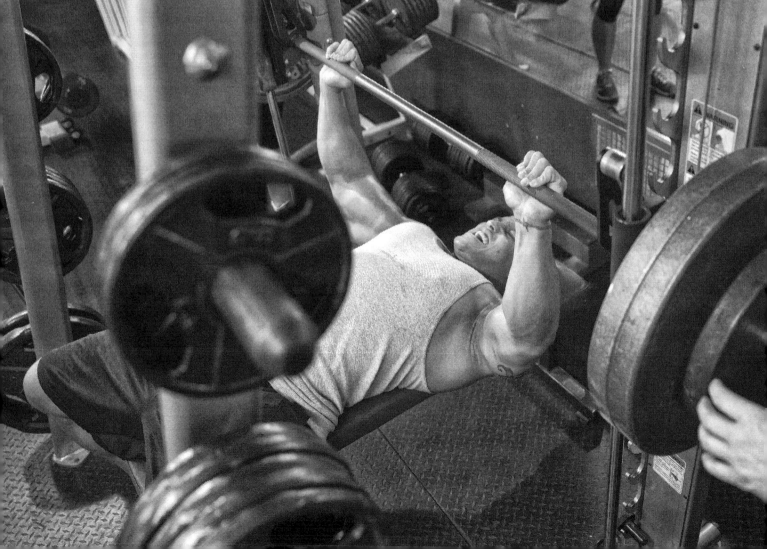

Smith Machine Negative Overload Bench Press

Smith machine negative overloads provide another way to eccentrically overload your pecs. This movement is performed with a Smith Machine and will require two partners.

How to correctly perform a Smith Machine negative overload bench press:

- Lie flat on a bench placed under a Smith Machine (the bar should be directly above your chest)
- Load the bar with 10%–25% extra weight on the outside of the bar sleeves
- Lower the weight to your chest
- At chest level, have a partner on each side pull the extra weight off the bar
- Forcefully press the weight back to starting position
- Then have the partners add the weight back to the bar
- Repeat for necessary reps

Important note: This exercise works best drawing out eccentrics, so take 5–6 seconds to lower the bar, then forcefully press it back up. A good routine is to do that tempo for as many reps as possible. Once you can no longer complete a rep, pull the additional weight off and do as many reps as possible at normal speed.

This is a highly advanced technique and should be used only with caution. Like other intense eccentric and accommodated resistance techniques, avoid them on deloads.

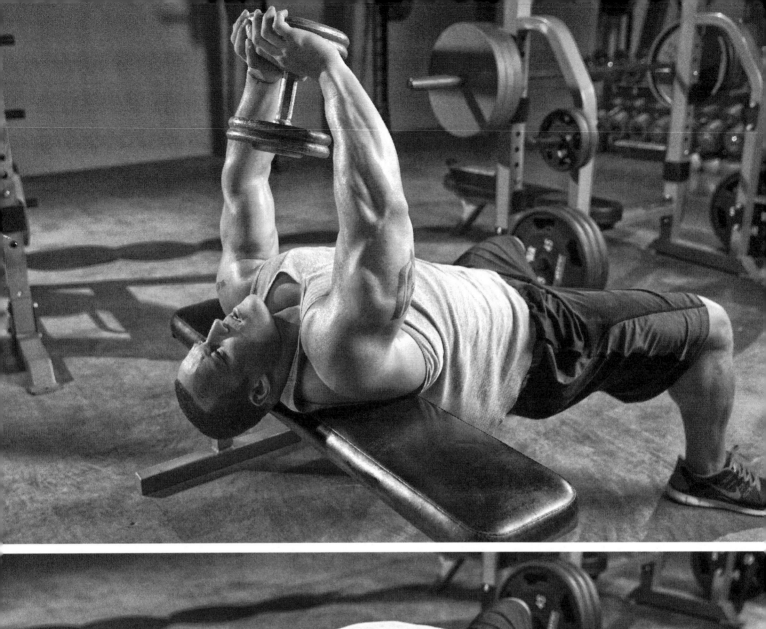
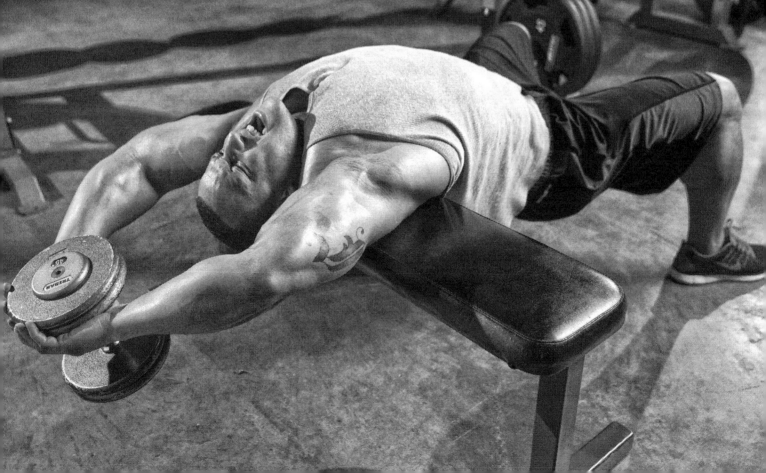

Dumbbell Pullovers

"You will not believe the ache in the sternum that this movement will produce! It literally forces your chest apart and forces it into new growth," said Arnold Schwarzenegger in regards to the dumbbell pullover.

The dumbbell pullover was a favorite of some of the greatest chests of all time like Arnold Schwarzenegger, Reg Park, and virtually any old-timer. This exercise works not only the chest but also the lats and the intercostal serratus anterior (the muscles of the ribcage).

Maximally developed intercostal muscles will give the illusion of a bigger rib cage when taking a deep breath and holding a pose because the ribs are pulled up by the intercostal muscles. I believe one of the reasons chest development hasn't caught up with other body part development is because of the elimination of any pullover variations.

How to correctly perform a dumbbell pullover:

- Lie perpendicular to the bench press, with only your shoulders supported
- Your feet should be flat on the floor, shoulder width apart
- Your head and neck should hang over the bench
- Your hips should ideally be at a slightly lower angle than your shoulders
- Place the dumbbell between your hands that should be in a diamond shape using your thumbs and pointer fingers (palms should be facing the ceiling)
- The movement starts with the dumbbell over your chest, elbows bent 10–15 degrees (maintain this angle throughout the entire movement)
- Slowly lower the weight backward over your head until the upper arms are in line with the torso
- The weight travels in an arc-like motion toward the floor
- Pull the dumbbell back over your chest, purposely squeezing the chest
- Hold for a second, and then repeat the exercise

Important note: If you have a history of shoulder problems, be careful when introducing this exercise. You may need to avoid it.

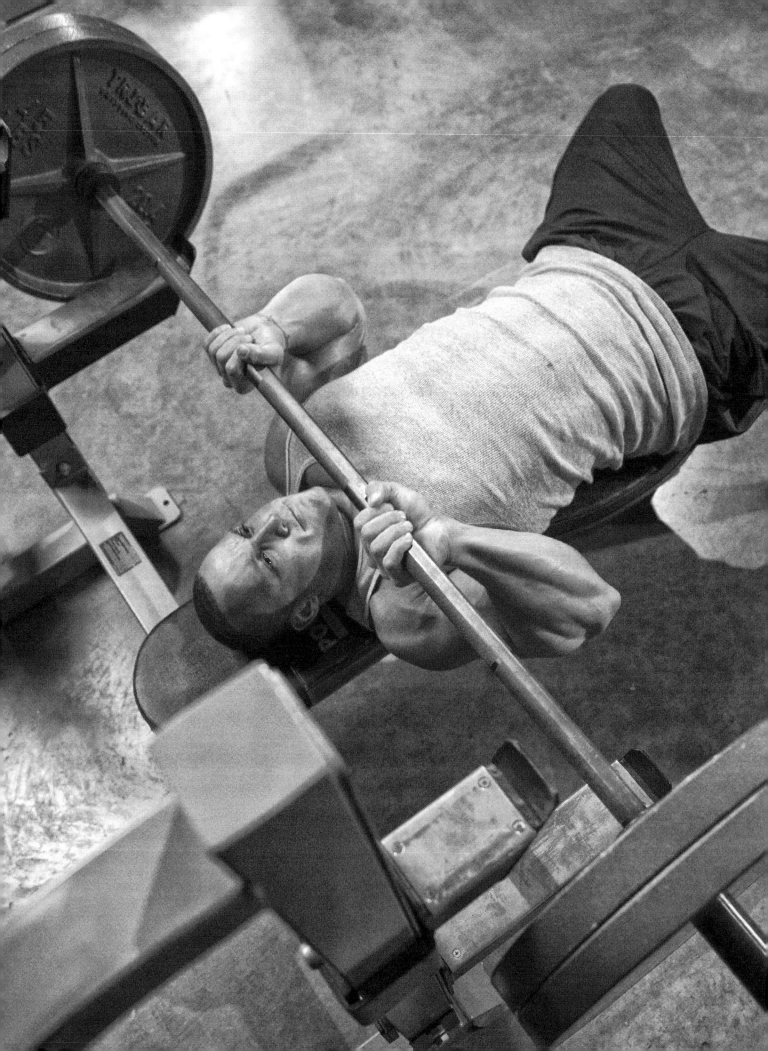

TOP TEN EXERCISES FOR ARMS

JM Press

This is a huge triceps builder that allows you to handle heavy weights. It is a hybrid between a close grip bench press and skull crusher.

How to correctly perform a JM press:

- Lie face up on a bench press
- Grab the bar with a shoulder-width or slightly closer grip
- Un-rack the bar at arms extension
- Start the bar above your upper pecs with arms extended
- As you lower the bar toward your chest, allow your elbows to move slightly forward so they are forward from the wrist
- Stop about 5 inches off your chest, pause for a moment, and then push back to starting position

Important note: With this movement, the bar is not moving straight up and down. Instead, it moves in an arc-like pattern. Make sure you keep your elbows close to your body during the exercise to maximize triceps activation.

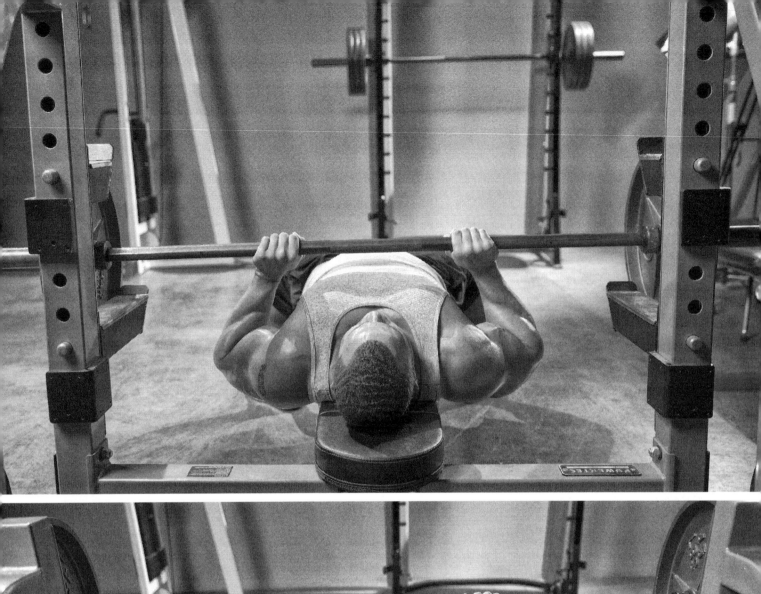
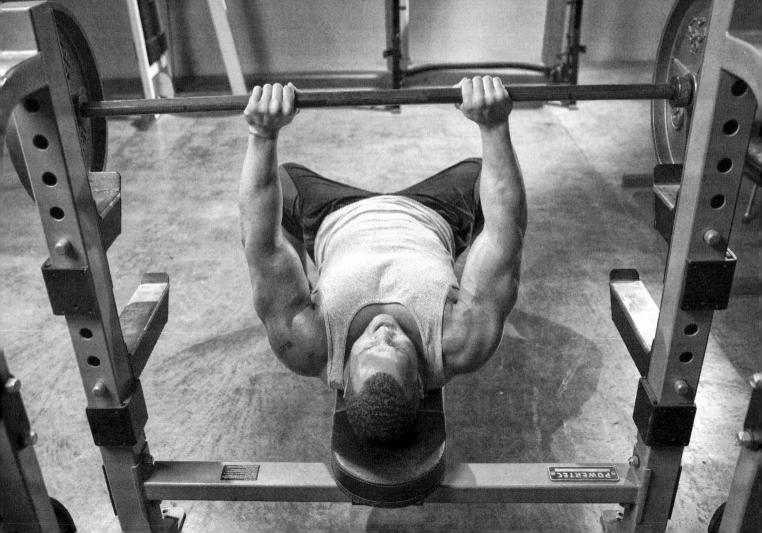

Dicks Press

This triceps movement was developed by legendary powerlifter, Paul Dicks. It is a favorite among bodybuilders I train for slapping slabs of meat on the triceps.

How to correctly perform a Dicks press:

- Lie face up on a bench press
- Grab the bar with a shoulder-width or slightly closer grip
- Un-rack the bar at arms extension
- Start the bar above your upper pecs with arms extended
- Lower the weight to approximately 1 inch above your chest
- Push your elbows up and shift the bar toward your chin
- Maintaining this position, press the weight back up to arms extension, leading with your fists

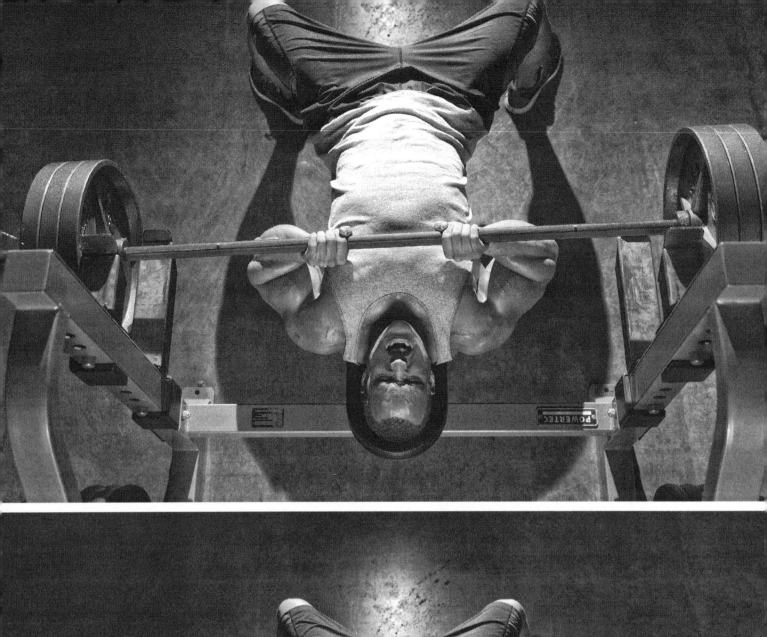

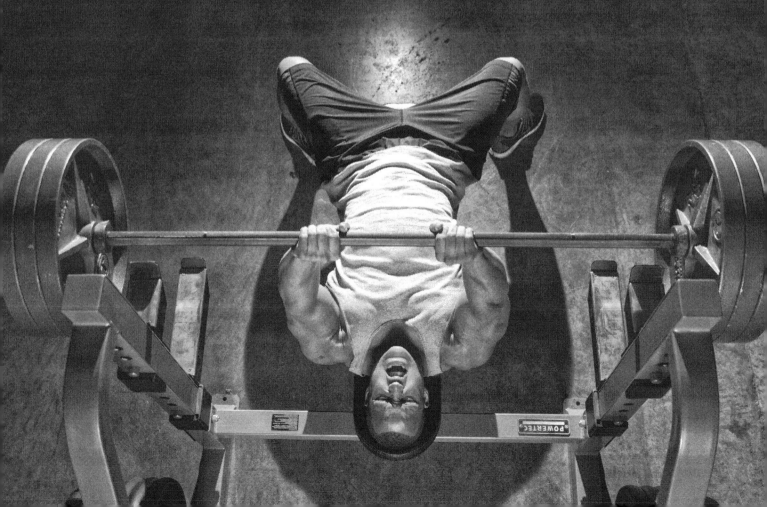

Close-Grip Bench Press

How to correctly perform a close-grip bench press:

- Lie flat on a bench

- Un-rack the barbell at arms extension over your chest

- Grasp the bar with a pronated grip and approximately shoulder width (about 3 inches closer than your regular grip)

- Keep your upper back tight

- Make sure your feet are flat throughout the entire movement

- Grip the barbell tightly and lower the barbell under control to nipple line or slightly below

- Forcefully push the bar back to arms extension

- Dismount the barbell from the rack over your chest

Important note: During close-grip bench presses, try to keep your elbows in for maximized triceps activation. For a variation, you can place 2x4s on your chest, held by a partner. These are called board presses. The number of 2x4s on your chest would be the origin of the name of the exercise. For example: Four 2x4s stacked on your chest would be a 4-board press.

Generally, to overload the triceps, 3–5 boards are used. This will allow you to use a much heavier weight. Also, if you want to further overload the triceps and remove stress from shoulders and pecs, you can use a slingshot device.

One close-grip burn-out workout for your triceps is to complete 5 full-range-of-motion, close-grip bench presses. Then, without racking the bar, have a partner immediately place 1 board on your chest. Perform 5 reps. Then, without racking, have a partner place 2 boards on your chest and complete 5 reps. Then, without racking, have a partner place 3 boards on your chest and complete 5 reps.

Do this again with 4 boards. By the end, you've done 25 repetitions. As you fatigue, leverage improves, providing a killer triceps workout. Close-grip bench presses and board presses can also be done with bands and chains.

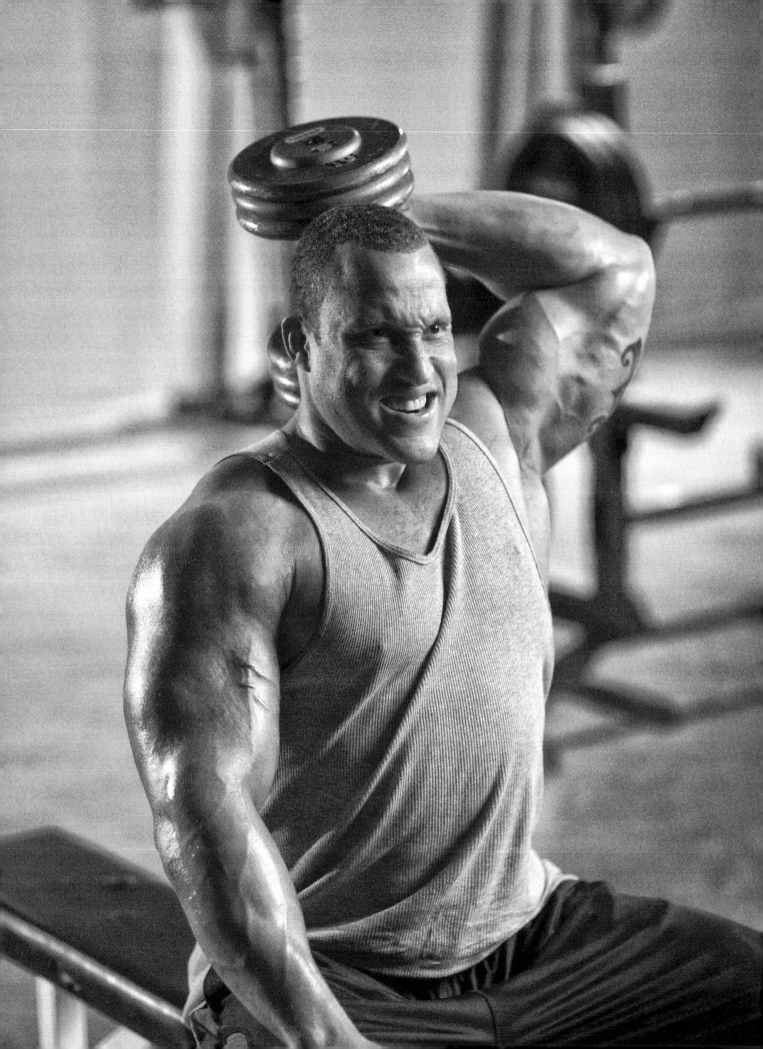

One-Arm Dumbbell Triceps Extension

This is a basic triceps isolation movement. It does not matter how much weight you do. The goal is to provide maximum tension to the triceps through the overload principle of isolation. This can be done sitting or standing.

How to correctly perform a one-arm dumbbell triceps extension:

- Position the dumbbell over your head or slightly back
- Lower the dumbbell behind your head while keeping the upper arms vertical
- Lower the dumbbell until your triceps are fully stretched
- All action should be at the elbow
- Return to starting position

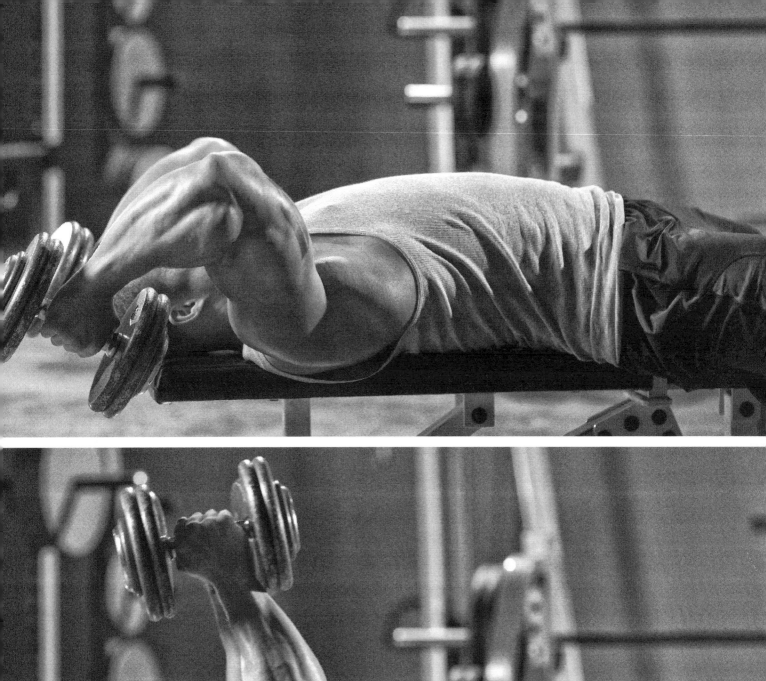
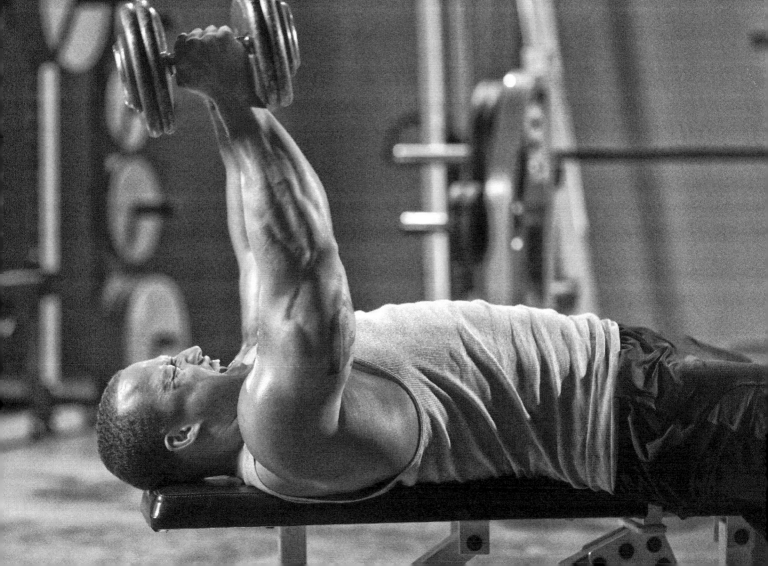

The Tri-Tri Set

I was introduced to this exercise by Joe Giandonato, MS. Joe is a strength coach at one of the top high school sports programs in Pennsylvania and works with a number of college athletes in their off seasons.

How to correctly perform a tri-tri set:

- Grab a pair of dumbbells; Joe recommends 35% of the load you could use on dumbbell bench presses for 10 reps (e.g., if you could do 100s, use 35s)

- Lie down on the bench

- Perform a neutral-grip dumbbell bench press

- From that top locked-out position, lower your dumbbells, hinging at the elbows, to the side of your head

- Extend back to the locked out position

- From the locked out position, lower the dumbbells behind your head

- Then extend at the elbow to the starting position

- That is one rep

Important note: The 35% load was for 5 reps. If you're doing more reps, obviously you may have to lighten the load a little bit.

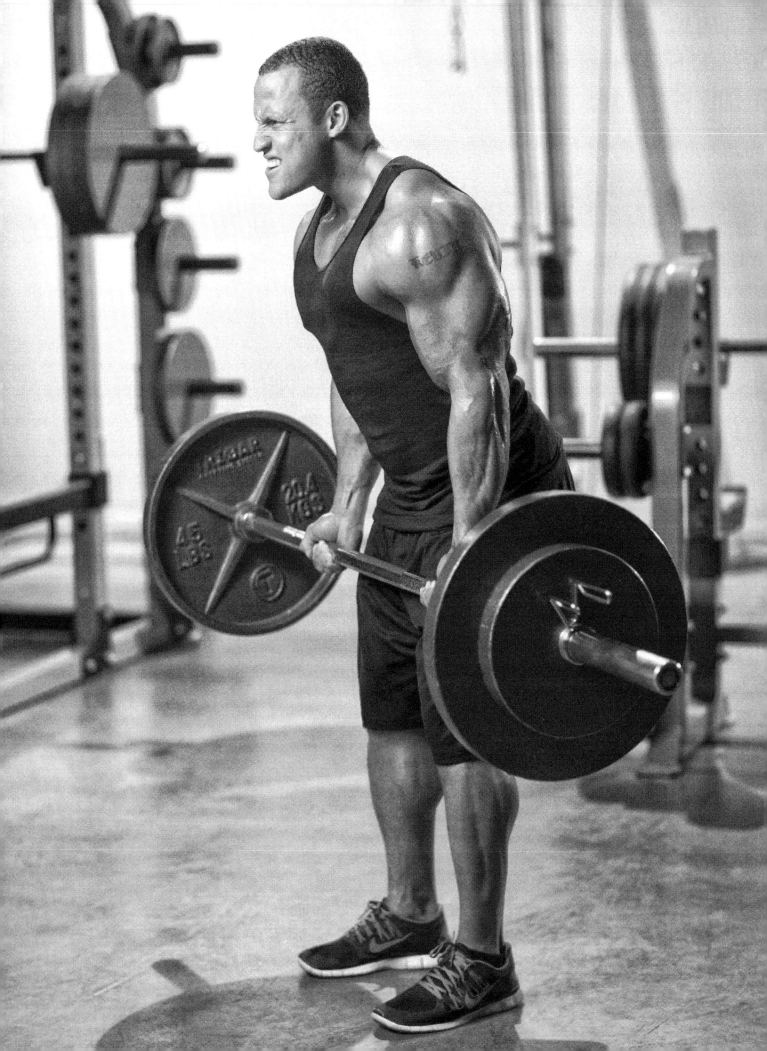

Cheat Curls

This exercise has gotten some bad press. Arnold Schwarzenegger, Ronnie Coleman, and many other legends have had cheat curls as a major part of their biceps training regimen.

Brian Dobson, owner of Metroflex Gym, says, "Generally, if you walk into Pansy-ass Fitness, some trainer with 12-inch arms will tell you cheat curls have no value. My observations say otherwise."

Cheat curls are not recklessly heaving a barbell. They are done to help you get through a sticking point. Generally, you will use anywhere from 10%–25% more weight than you would on a regular curl.

How to correctly perform cheat curls:

- Keep your feet flat
- Stand holding the barbell or EZ curl bar with hands shoulder width apart
- Curl the weight up using your shoulders and hips to help get you past the sticking point
- Hold at the top
- Control the eccentric on the way down, taking 2–5 seconds to lower the weight

Important note: When done correctly, this movement provides a huge eccentric overload. If you are rising up on your toes, you're using too much weight.

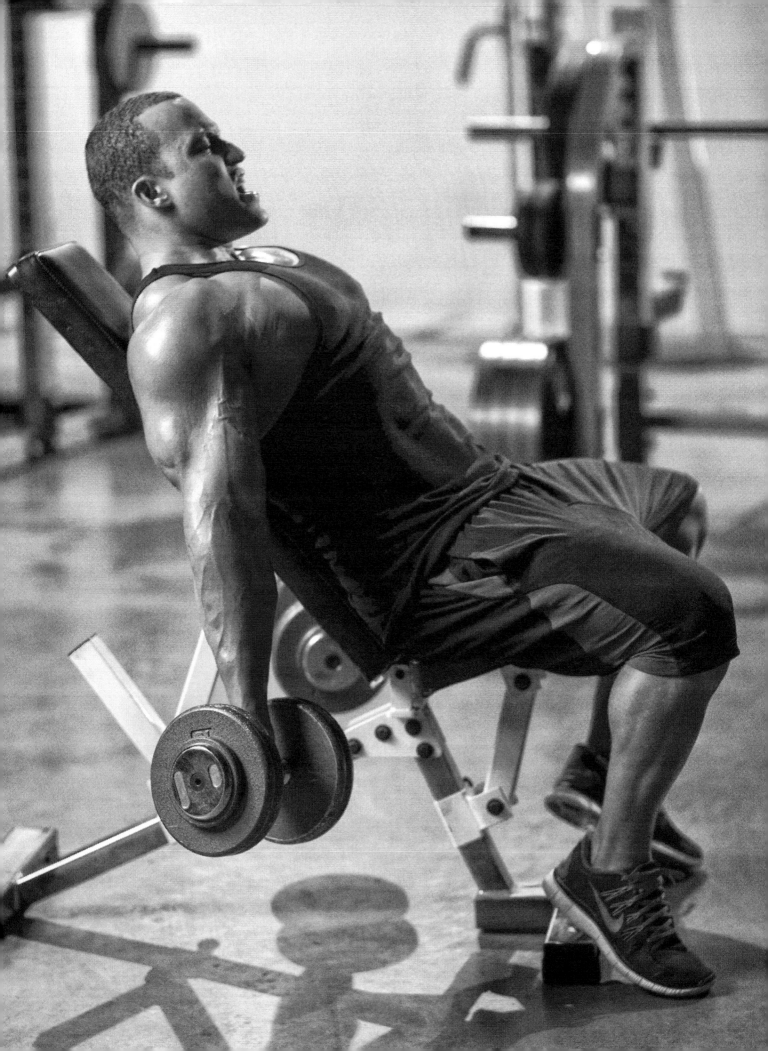

Incline Dumbbell Curls

How to correctly perform incline dumbbell curls:

- Lie back on a 45-degree bench
- Keep your palms supinated the entire time
- Your arms should hang straight down to the floor, fully extended
- Your arms are angled behind your body, so this requires a larger range of motion than a normal curl; it's a great stretch movement
- Keeping your arms stationary, curl both arms up toward your shoulders or as high as you can go
- Lower the weight to starting position, then repeat

Important note: This movement is meant to increase your range of motion. Do not shorten it. It is important to keep your palms supinated the entire time. This movement can also be done in an alternating fashion.

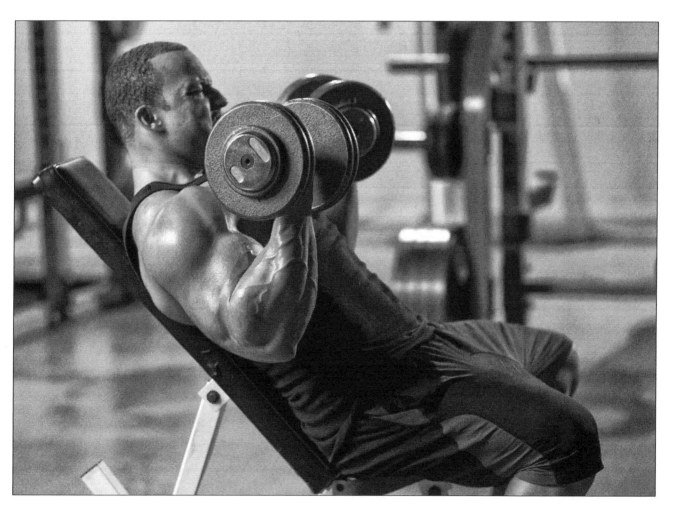

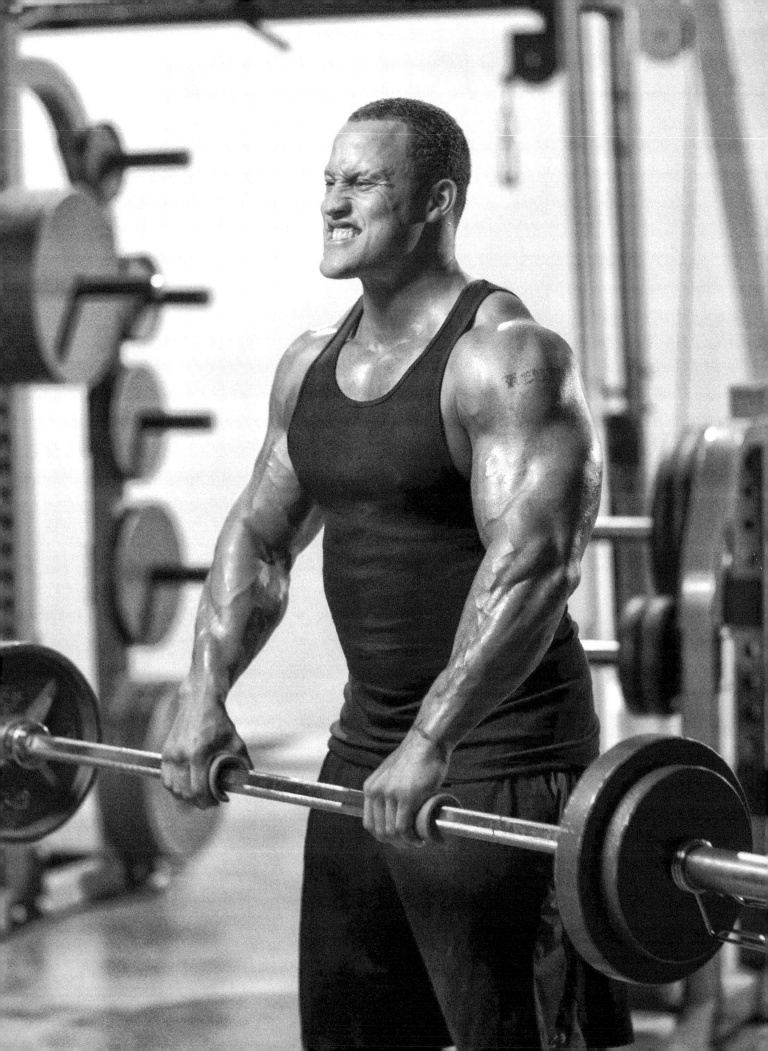

Reverse Fat Bar Curls

Because of the increased diameter of the bar, this movement really works the forearms hard. If you do not have a fat bar, you can order Fat Gripz from EliteFTS.com or just wrap a towel around the bar.

How to correctly perform a reverse fat bar curl:

- Perform this movement standing
- Feet should be shoulder width apart
- Arms should be straight when you start with an overhand grip
- Keeping your back straight, curl the weight up to the front of your chest
- Stop briefly at the top
- Lower the weight back to starting position

Important note: You won't be able to lift as much weight this way. Don't worry if your poundages are down. Make sure you keep your elbows tucked in to your sides throughout the entire movement. For a fun variation, do this movement to failure, follow by traditional curls to failure.

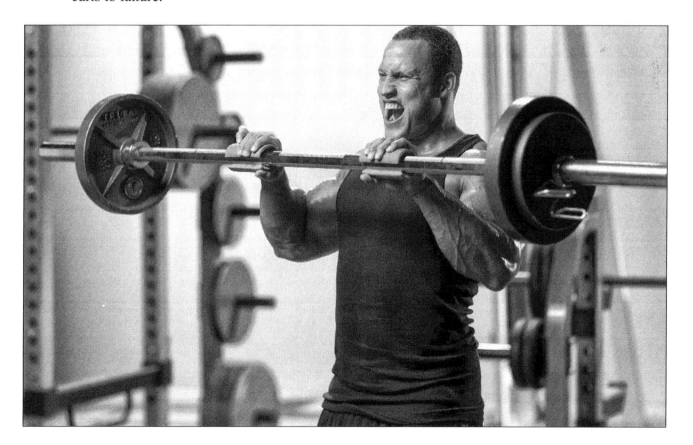

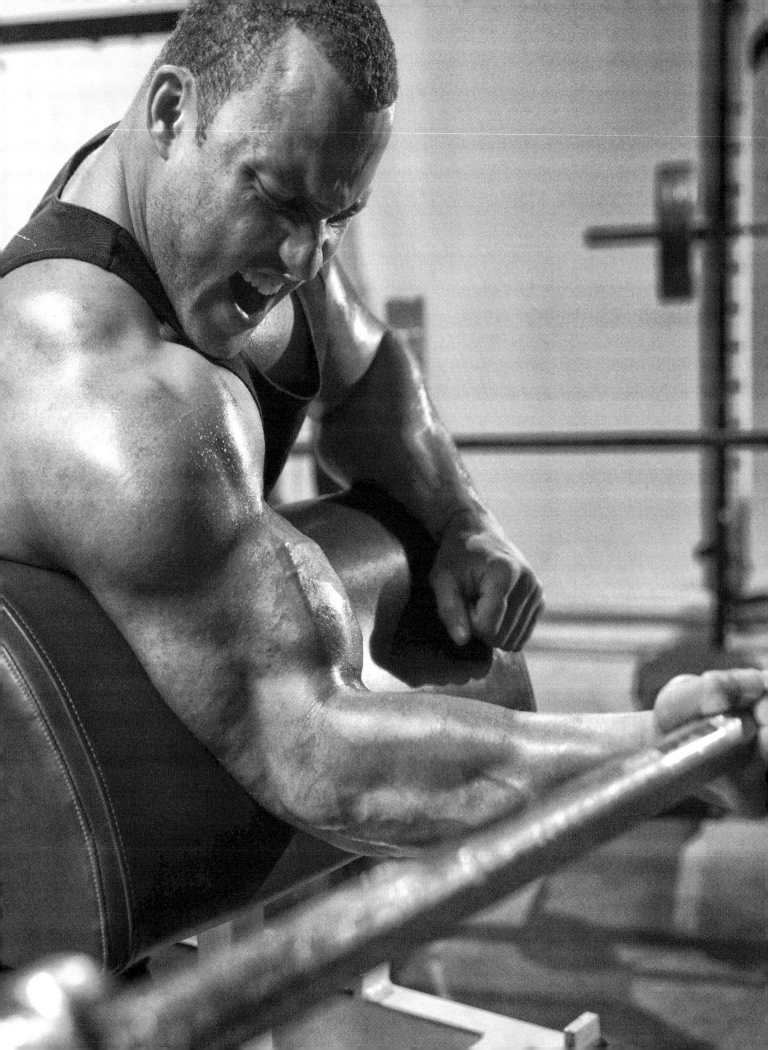

One Arm Eccentric Barbell Curls

How to correctly perform a one-arm eccentric barbell curl:

- Sit or stand behind a preacher curl station

- Rest your upper arm on the pad in front of you, arms supinated

- Start at the top position of the curl

- Slowly lower the bar for a count of 8 seconds to full extension

- Pause briefly at the bottom

- If you have a training partner, have him help you back up. If not, self-spot with the other hand

Important note: Since your arm is supinated the entire time and you have to balance an Olympic sized barbell with one hand, your supinated muscles are forced to work overtime. Remember, the concentric portion of the lift is not what we are emphasizing.

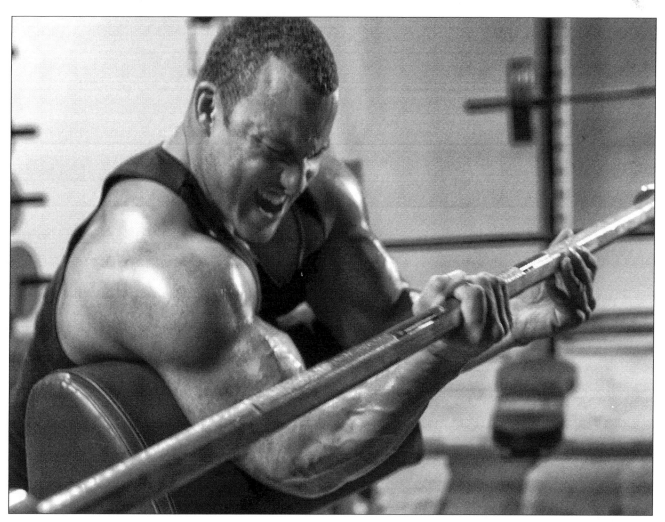

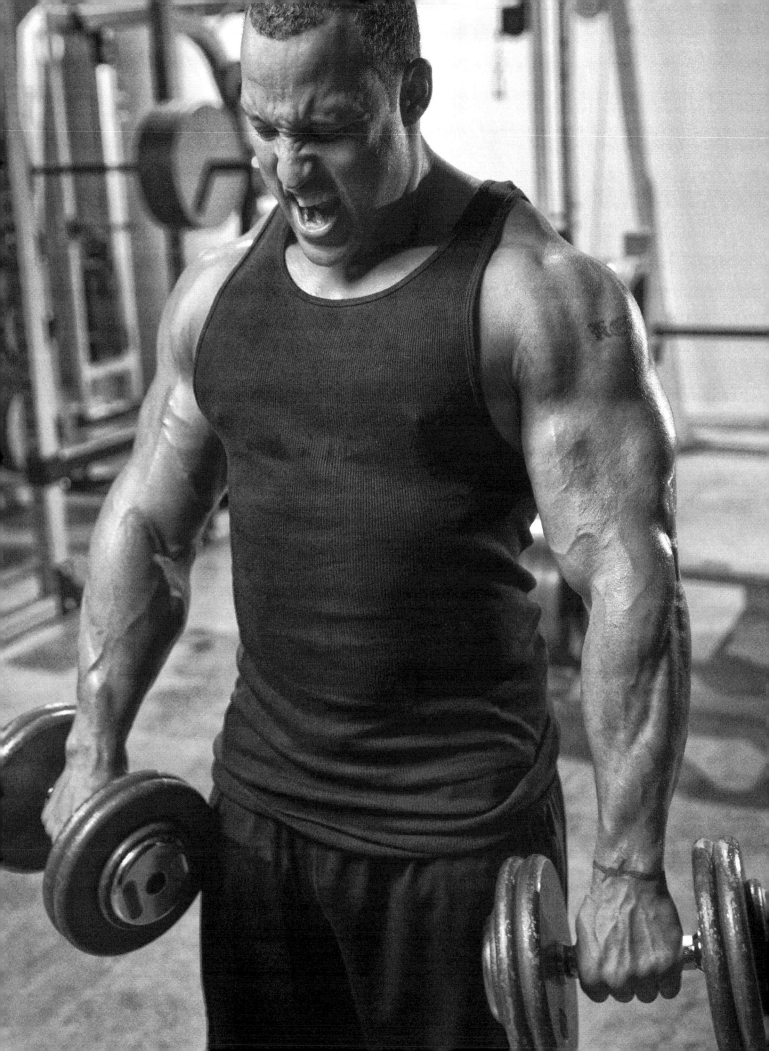

Zottman Curls

How to correctly perform a Zottman curl:

- Hold dumbbells in each hand, palms facing forward
- Stand up straight with your elbows close to your torso
- Curl the weight up to your shoulders
- At the top, rotate your wrists with palms facing forward again
- Then lower the weight with a pronated grip
- At the bottom, rotate your wrists again with palms facing forward
- Repeat

Important note: This exercise, on the negative phase, hits your forearms really hard.

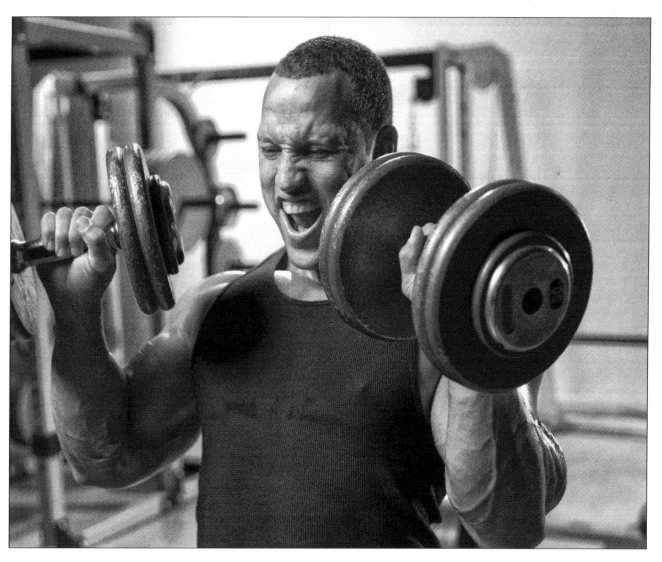

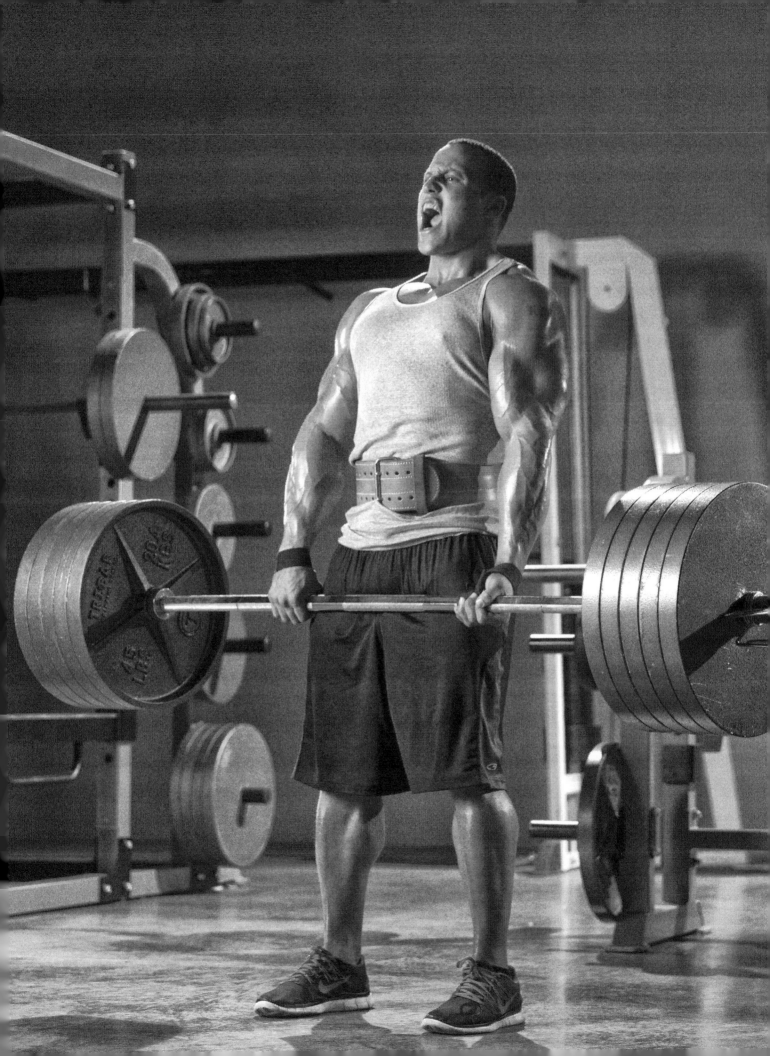

TOP TEN EXERCISES FOR BACK

Deadlift

The deadlift is probably the oldest strength training movement in existence. Most strength training movements took some creative thinking to conceive. Deadlift is as basic as picking up a heavy object off the floor. If we could only choose one movement to train with, it would come down to deadlift or squat.

For a long time, there was a lot of anti-deadlift literature floating around that had absolutely no scientific basis. Thankfully, there has been a deadlift enlightenment lately, and this movement is getting the respect it deserves. Many bodybuilders today lack lower back development, but those who deadlift do not.

How to correctly perform a deadlift:

- Face the bar with your feet approximately hip to shoulder width apart
- Bend your knees
- Grab the bar with an alternating grip, hands right outside your thighs
- In a half-squat position, with your back flat, keep the bar close to your body
- Lift the weight from the floor to a fully upright position
- Lower the weight to the floor
- Remember, the closer the bar is to your body, the lighter the weight is and the safer the movement is

Some reminders for proper deadlift technique:

- Push through your heels
- The middle of the foot should be directly under the bar
- Shins should touch the bar
- The back is in extension; don't round it
- The shoulder blades should be directly over the bar, and shoulders will be slightly in front
- The elbows must remain in full extension throughout the entire movement
- Lower the bar in the opposite way the bar was lifted, in terms of hip and knee angles

Important note: Biceps tears can occur with deadlifts on the underhand grip, so bodybuilders may want to consider doing deadlifts double-overhand grip with straps. This will prevent potential asymmetrical development and lessen the likelihood of injury.

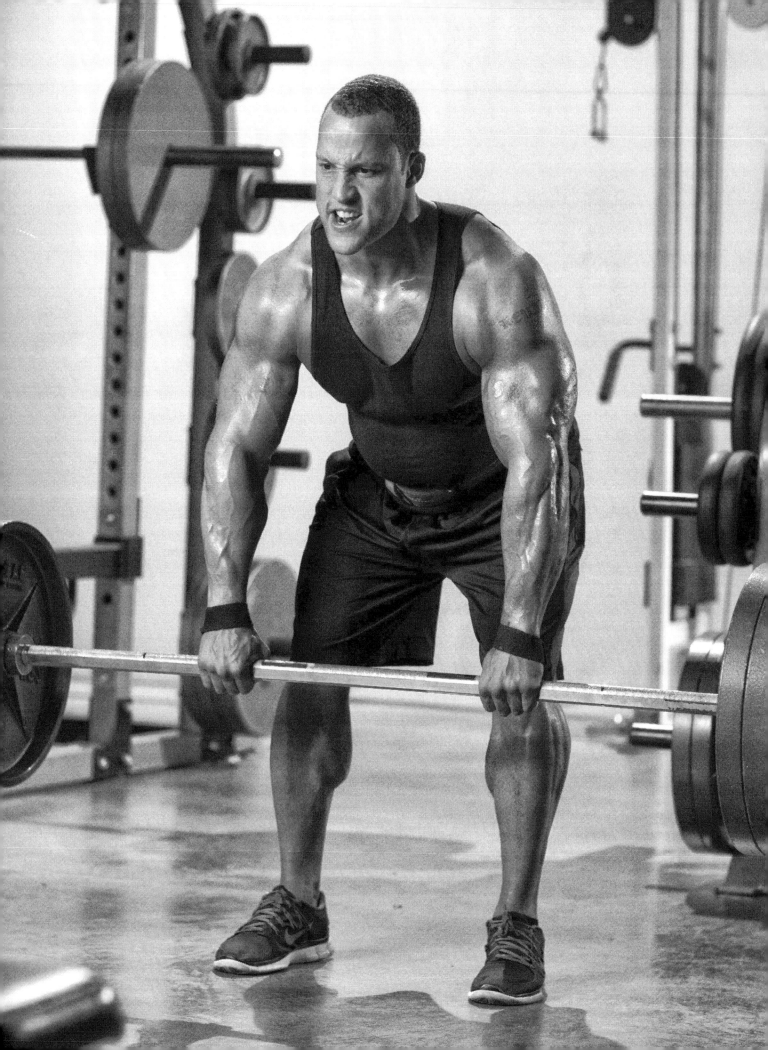

Bent-Over Row

The bent-over row is one of the greatest ways to build upper back thickness.

How to correctly perform a bent-over row:

- Stand behind the barbell with your deadlift stance
- Grab the bar with an overhand grip
- Lift the barbell off the floor to your stomach
- Your torso should be slightly above parallel throughout the entire movement

Important note: You should keep your back flat and have a slight bend in your knees. For a variation, you can perform this movement with your torso at 45 degrees. This way, you could pick it up off a rack instead of the floor and will be able to use more weight.

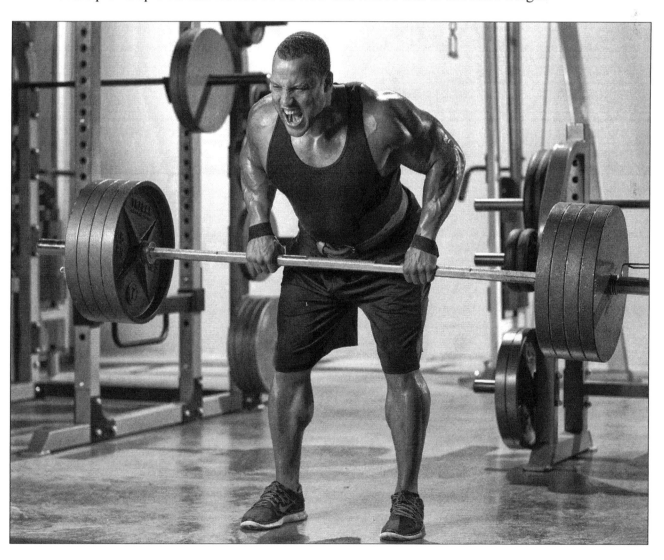

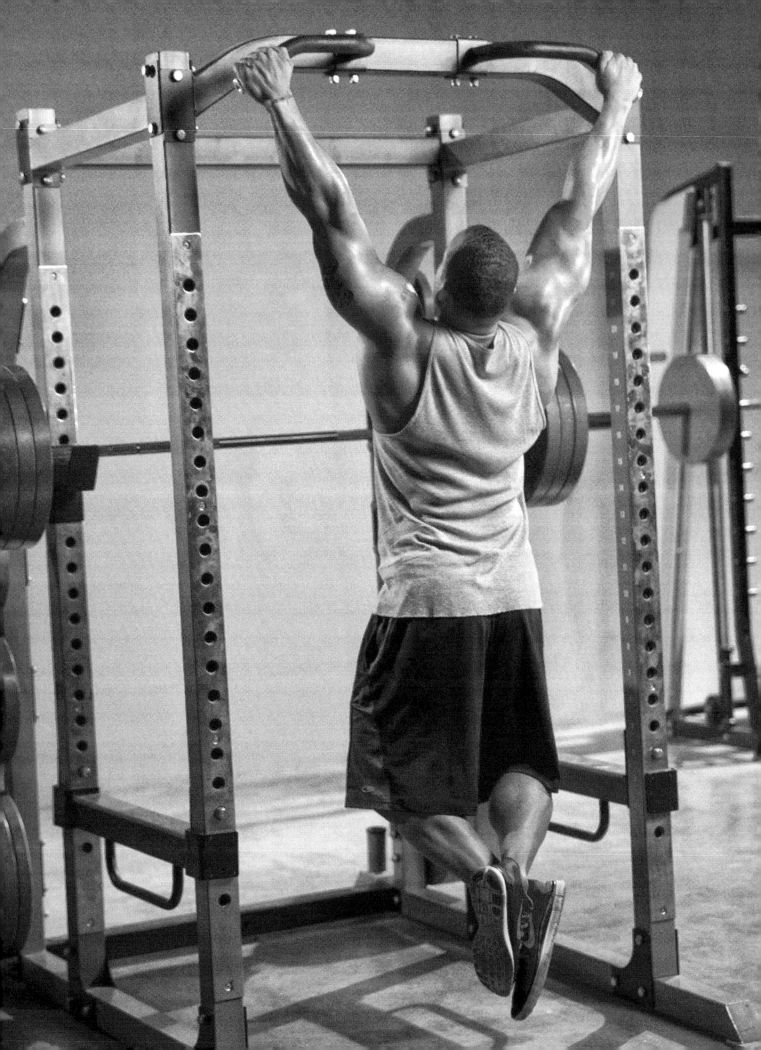

Pull-up/Chin-up Variations

Nothing builds a wide back like pull-up and chin-up variations. These include narrow grips, wide grips, overhand, underhand, and neutral grip. I suggest making these variations a staple in your back-training routine.

Almost all bodybuilders with great back development have included some sort of "chinning" in their routine. If you are unable to do a pull-up/chin-up, instead of using a machine that assists you, opt for resistance bands. You just wrap the band around the bar at the top and put your knees through the other end.

Other exercises to help you get used to handling your weight are negatives, where you start in a chin-up position and purposefully lower yourself slowly. Another way to gain strength is to perform a flexed arm hang for as long as possible.

How to correctly perform a pull-up/chin-up:

- Grab the bar with the grip of your choice
- Hang at arms extension
- Keep your chest up
- Lead the movement with your chest up and shoulders back
- Cross your feet behind you
- Look up as you pull yourself up
- Pull your chin over the bar
- Some heavily muscled bodybuilders will not be able to get their chins over the bar; in this case, just go as high as possible
- Lower yourself under control to the starting position

Important note: You need to include pull-up/chin-up variations in your training. You should mix up what type you use. Not only will this exercise aid in building a broad, powerful-looking back, but it will help you get stronger and improve shoulder health.

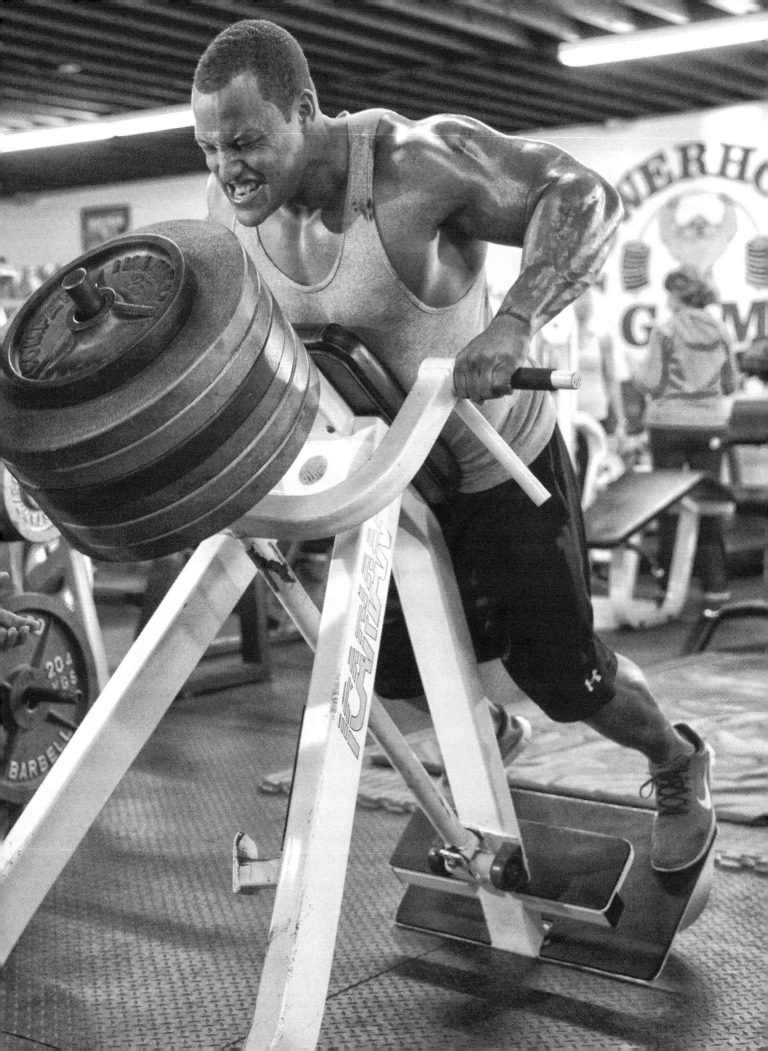

Chest Supported T-Bar Row Eccentric Overload

This exercise has long been a favorite of many top bodybuilders to work their back. This is an eccentric overload variation that is going to make you sore. For most people, the first time they do this with high intensity, they are sore for a week.

How to correctly perform a chest supported T-bar row eccentric overload:

- Load up the T-bar row machine with approximately 25% more than you usually use for 6–8 reps (if you can use more weight, great)

- Your upper chest needs to be on top of the pad

- Lie face down on the pad and grab the handles

- Various grips may be used

- Have a partner help you lift the bar off the rack

- Extend your arms in front of you (this will be where you start)

- Normally, this is the point where you pull the weight up; but now you will pull the weight up, with the assistance of a partner

- From the top of the movement, lower the weight for 5–8 seconds to the starting point

- Make sure that, at the bottom of the movement, your arms are fully extended and you feel a deep stretch in your lats

Important note: This is a very intense movement. Usually, when people do it for the first time, they will feel like their lats are automatically flared out for a few days and feel a severe, deep soreness in their lats. As long as they are performing the movement with maximum intensity and getting a full stretch at the bottom, they will experience the extreme soreness.

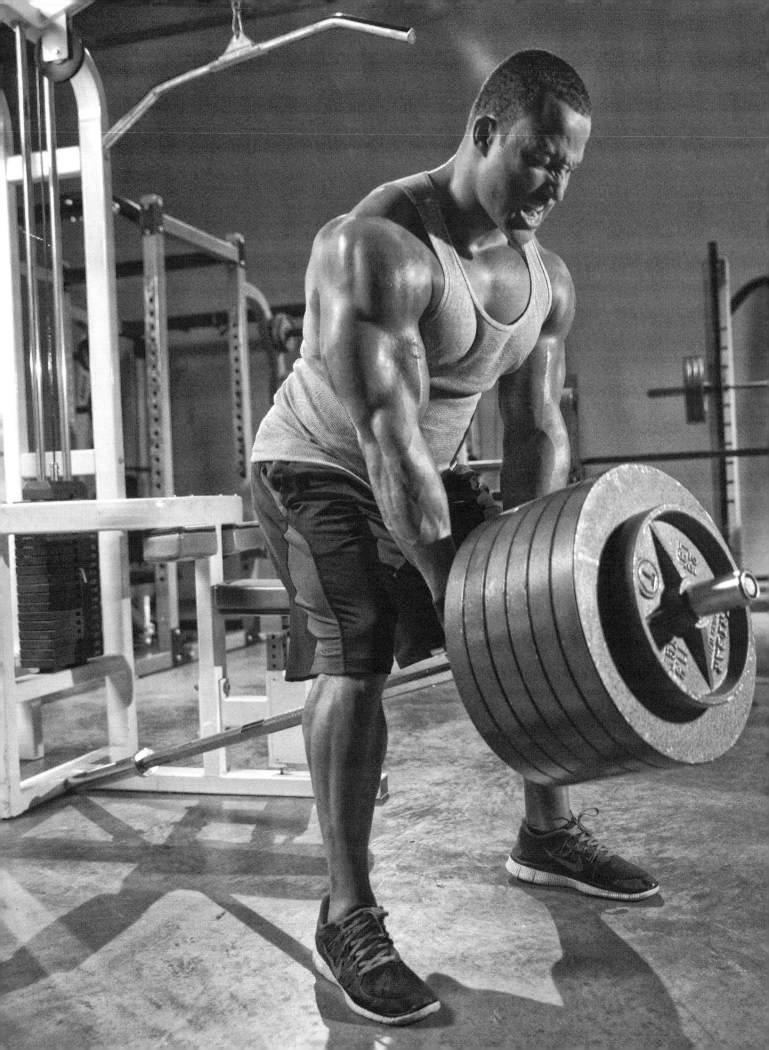

T-Bar Prison Rows

This movement has been used by Arnold Schwarzenegger, Jay Cutler, Branch Warren, Johnnie Jackson, and Ronnie Coleman, to name a few. Many machines have tried to duplicate the prison row, but nothing seems to beat the bare-bones original.

How to correctly perform a T-bar prison row:

- Load one side of the barbell with weight
- Place the opposing side in a corner space in the gym
- Place your feet shoulder width apart and stand over the bar right behind the plates
- Put a close grip handle under the bar and grab it with both hands
- Keep your back flat and arched and have a slight bend in your knees
- Pull the bar up toward your chest, squeezing at the top of the movement
- Lower the weight along the same path
- You should feel a good stretch in the lats at the bottom of the movement

Important note: You should keep your elbows in close to your sides to place more emphasis on the lower lats. Some slight cheating is okay on this movement, but you don't want to be standing upright. This is one of those great exercises that have been passed on from bodybuilding generation to generation.

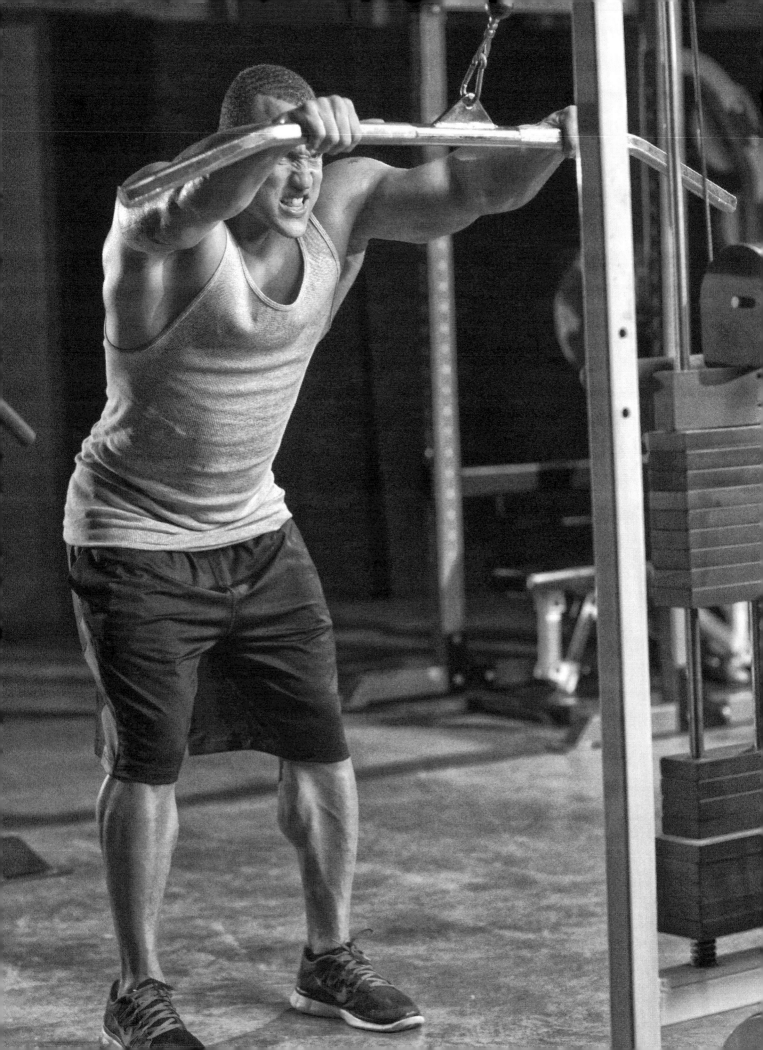

Straight-Arm Pull-down

In some pulling movements, the limiting factor is the biceps. Because they are involved and they fatigue before the back, one isolation movement that is great for back width is the straight-arm pull-down.

How to correctly perform a straight-arm pull-down:

- Grab a straight bar or rope attachment on a pulling machine
- Step backward about 2 feet facing the machine
- Fully extend your arms
- Bend your torso slightly forward
- Tighten your lats
- Pull the bar down using your lats until your hands are down to your thighs
- Make sure you keep this movement strict; if you start to cheat, it becomes ineffective
- Return to starting position, always staying under control

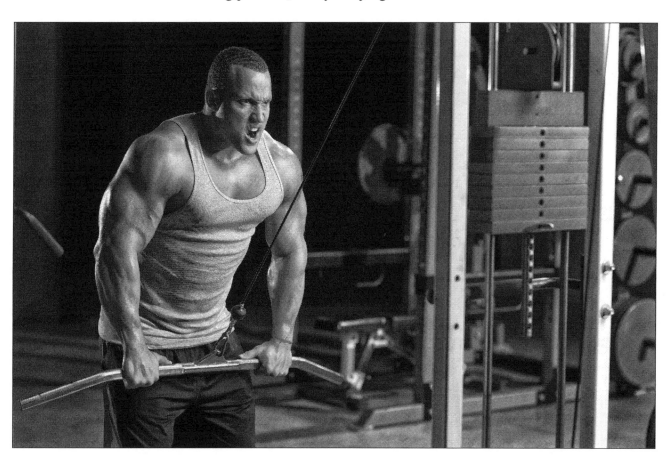

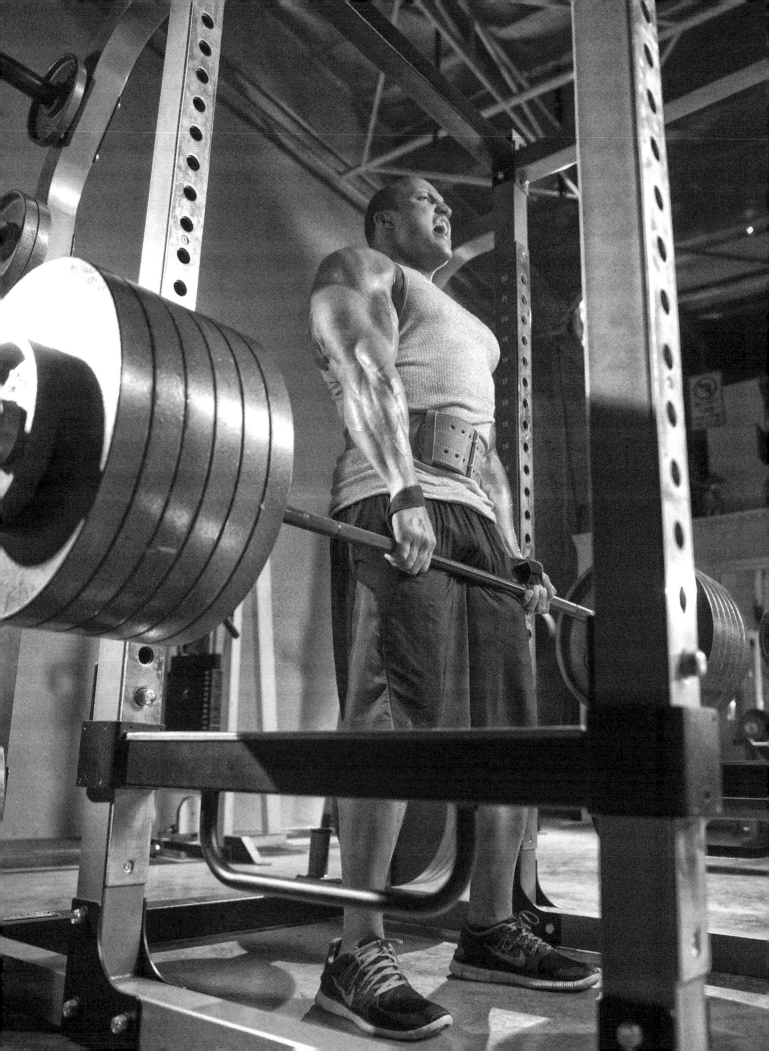

Rack Pulls

Rack pulls are a partial deadlift. They can be used as an overload because you can handle more weight than you can on a full-range–of-motion deadlift. They work extremely well for developing a thick back.

> *How to correctly perform rack pulls:*
>
> - Place a barbell in a squat rack
> - Stand in the squat rack using a normal deadlift stance
> - The bar can be anywhere from 2 inches above the knee to 2 inches below the knee
> - Bend your knees slightly
> - With your arms fully extended, grab the bar with your deadlift grip
> - Extend your hips and lock the weight out
> - Lower the bar back to the starting point

Important note: Rack pulls not only develop your back but also target your hamstrings and glutes very effectively. Some bodybuilders with lower back problems who have trouble doing regular deadlifts may still be able to perform heavy rack pulls.

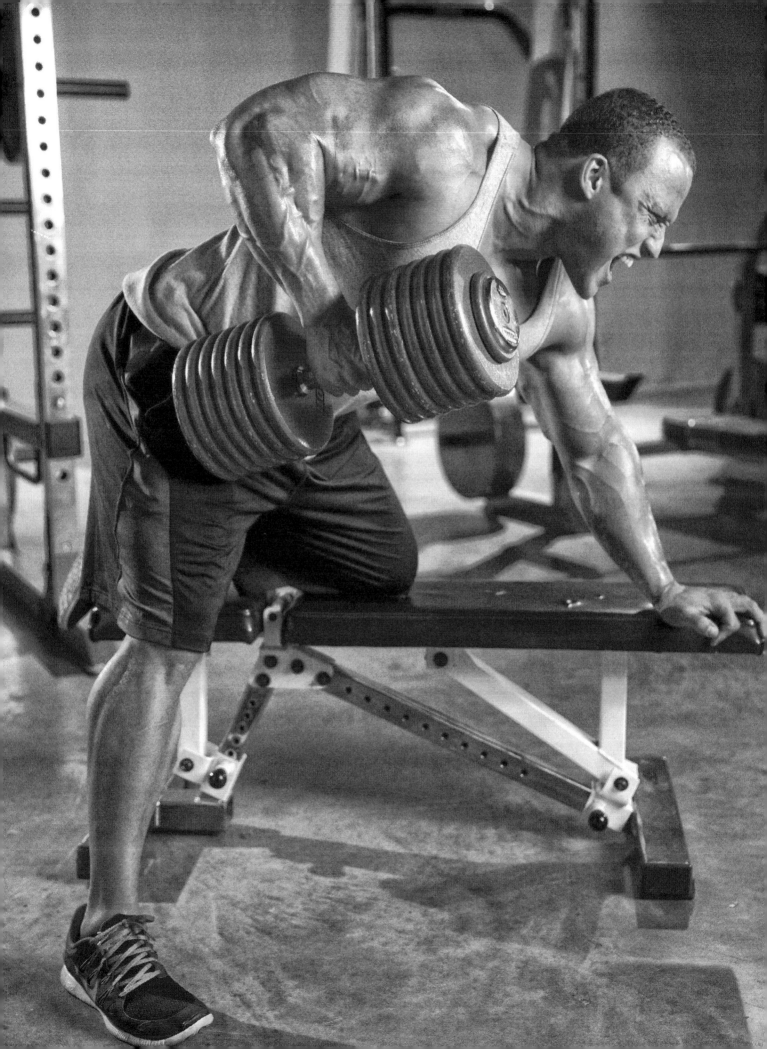

One-Armed Dumbbell Rows

How to correctly perform a one-armed dumbbell row:

- These can be done standing with your hand placed on a rack at approximately waist height

- If you're doing your right side, your left hand would be on the rack

- Place your left foot forward and your right foot back with a staggered stance

- Keep your back close to parallel to the floor

- Grab the dumbbell with your right hand and drive your elbow up toward the ceiling, keeping the dumbbell at your side with a neutral grip

- Concentrate on pulling the dumbbell up using your back rather than your biceps (in the long run, you'll do more weight this way and get the desired result)

- Pull the weight up forcefully, but keep control of the dumbbell during the negative portion of the lift

- At the bottom of the movement, not only return to full arm extension but go beyond this and actually feel the stretch in your lat

Important note: You can do this movement heavy. You're not doing it for your grip, so don't be afraid to throw on straps. If you have a bad lower back, an alternative is to put one arm and the corresponding knee on a bench. This will release pressure from your lower back.

Johnnie Jackson, who had the best back in the 2012 Mr. Olympia contest, did a 250-pound dumbbell for reps consecutively for 30 seconds on both his right and left side. I recommend starting this movement with your weaker side.

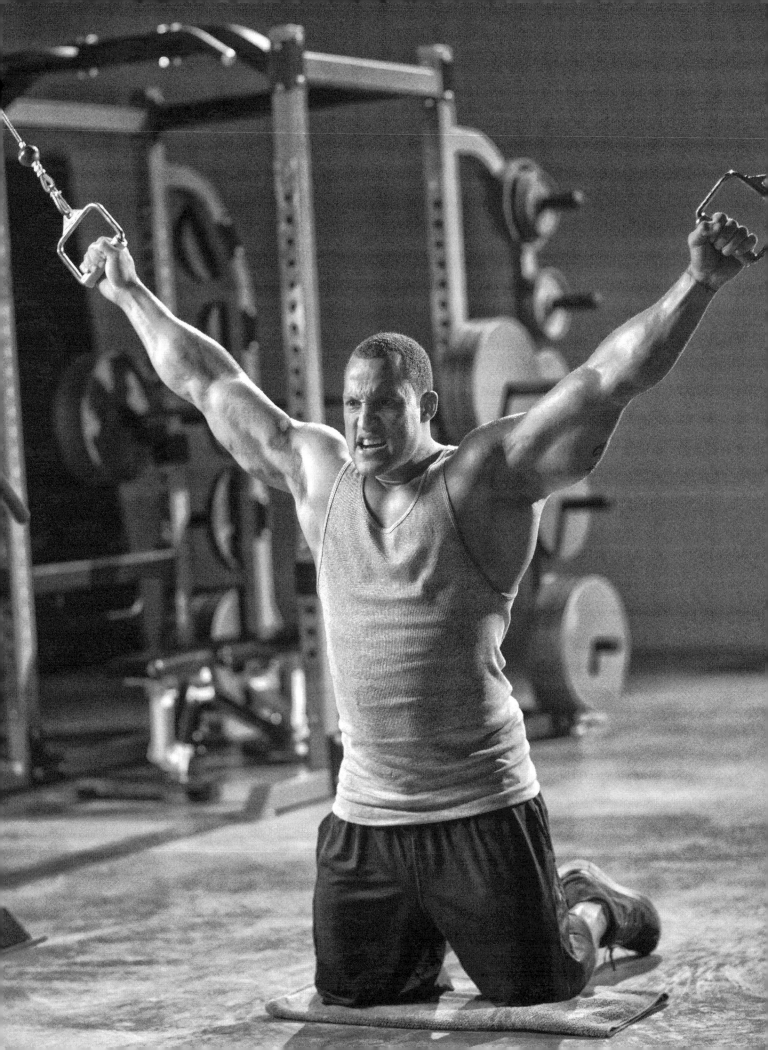

Lat Pull-downs on Your Knees

A great lat isolation exercise is the lat pull-down. One variation that sticks out is performed on the knees with a cable in each hand. The advantage is that both limbs operate independently of one another.

How to correctly perform lat pull-downs on your knees:

- Get on your knees in the center of a cable station
- Grab each handle, making sure your arms are at full extension and you feel a good stretch in your lats
- Pull the weights down to your side
- Squeeze your lats together at the bottom
- Hold this position for a half second (0.5 second)
- Return to the starting position

Important note: This exercise needs to be performed very strictly.

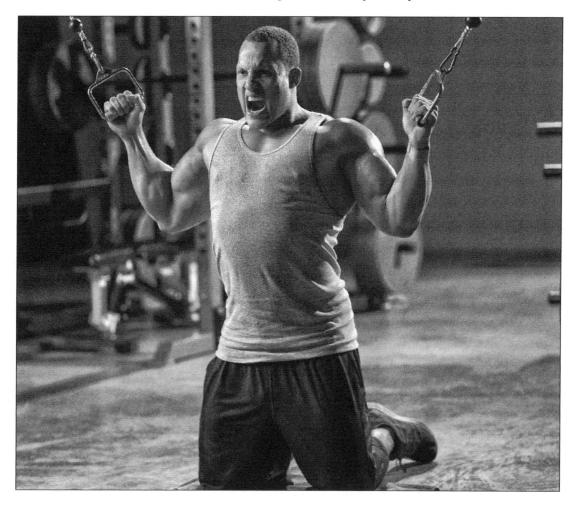

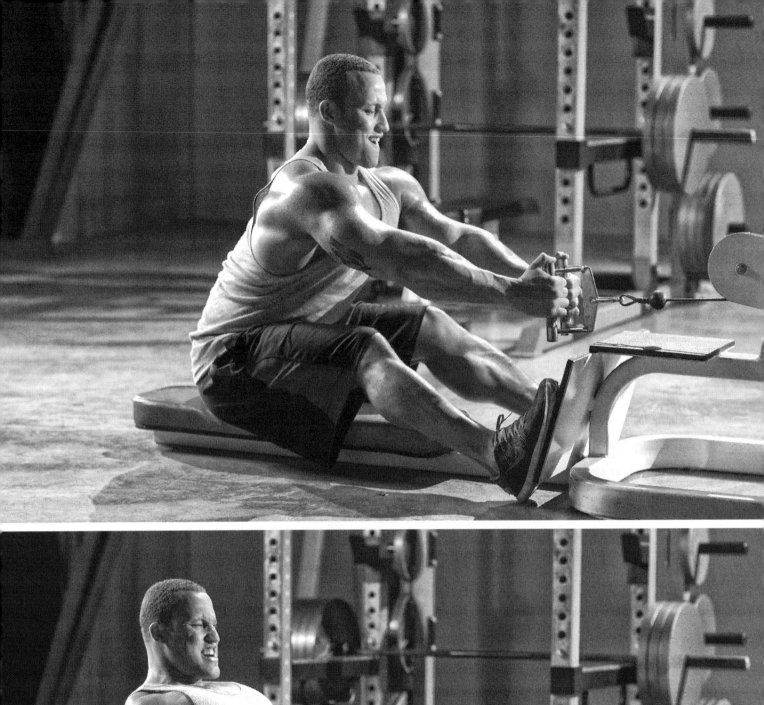
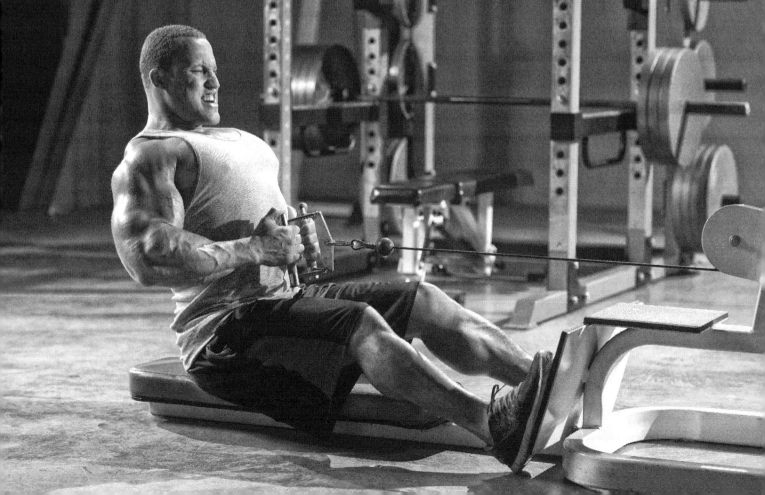

Seated Cable Rows

Seated cable rows have been used by bodybuilders and strength athletes for overall back development for decades.

How to correctly perform a seated cable row:

- Using a low-row neutral grip attachment (looks a V or U), grasp the handle with both hands

- Keeping your elbows in, pull the weight to your stomach

- As the weight touches your stomach, keep your chest up and squeeze your upper back together

- Your legs can be slightly bent

- After a brief hold, return to the starting position with your arms in full extension, feeling a mild stretch in your lats

Important note: A fun variation to this exercise is the eccentric overload version. You begin this exercise the same way, pulling it to your stomach and squeezing your back, but as you release the weight, you will let go with one hand and lower the weight with one arm. You can obviously handle way more weight on the eccentric. Eccentric overloads are very important for bodybuilders to induce satellite cell proliferation, which will help maximize muscle growth.

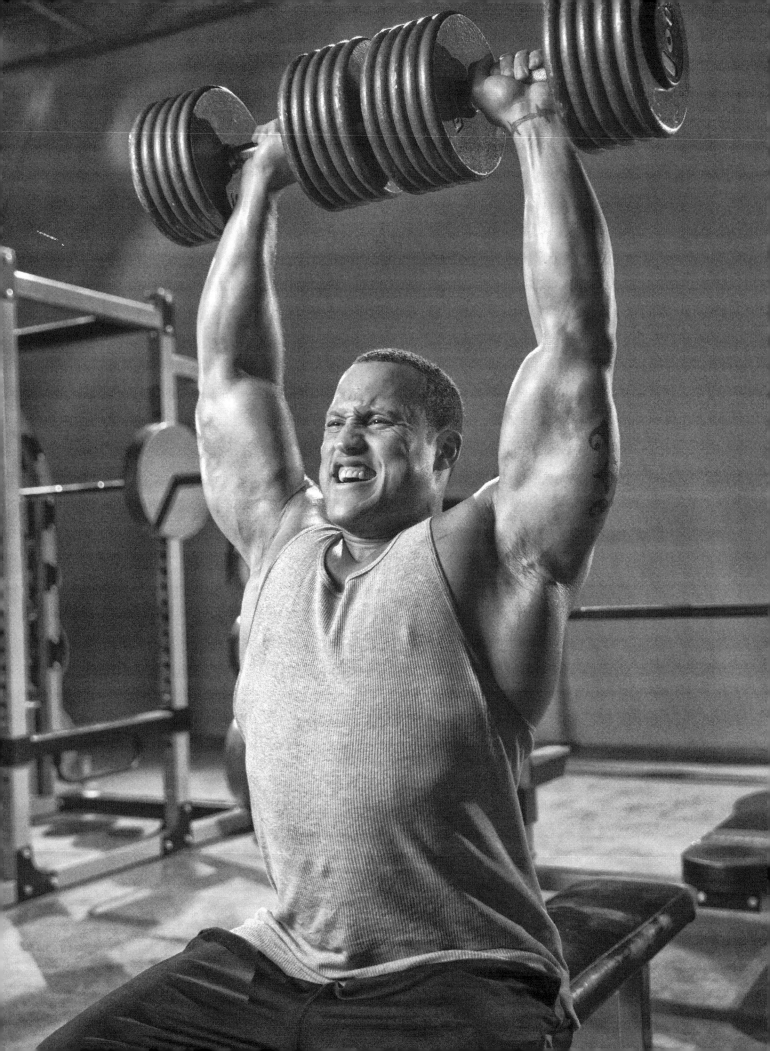

TOP TEN EXERCISES FOR SHOULDERS

Dumbbell Military Presses

The standing military press was an Olympic lift until 1972. Not only does this version work the entire shoulder, unlike most pressing variations, but it is also huge for building core stabilization.

Core lifts are the foundation of a solid bodybuilding program. Doing seated dumbbell military presses allows you to focus on pressing the weight, rather than balancing, because of the support of the pad. Furthermore, dumbbells allow you a better stretch at the bottom of the movement.

Many bodybuilders opt for seated military presses with a barbell over the dumbbell variation. This is fine, but one potential error I see being made too frequently is that the lifter is not completely seated against the pad. His torso is closer to a 45-degree angle than a 90-degree angle, turning the lift into more of an incline press.

> *How to correctly perform a dumbbell military press:*
>
> - Position the dumbbells to each side of your shoulders; if they are heavy, you can get a partner to help you
> - From this position, push the dumbbells upward until the arms are extended overhead
> - A pronated or neutral grip can be used
> - From the extended position, control the negative and lower to the starting position
> - Repeat

Important note: For a variation of this exercise, instead of locking the weights all the way out at the top, try ¾ reps to further overload the deltoids and take some of the triceps involvement out of the movement.

Another fun variation, one that will increase time under tension, is to perform the press by holding the off arm in extension while performing the exercise with the other arm in an alternate fashion.

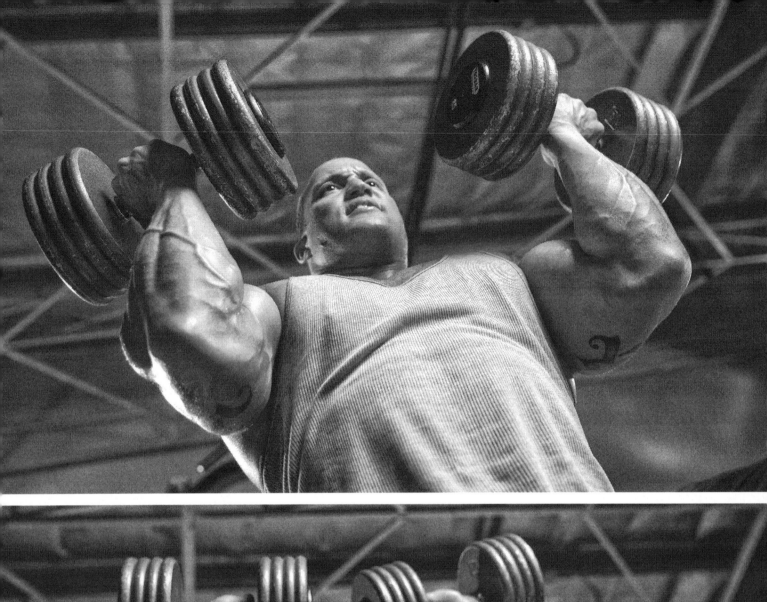
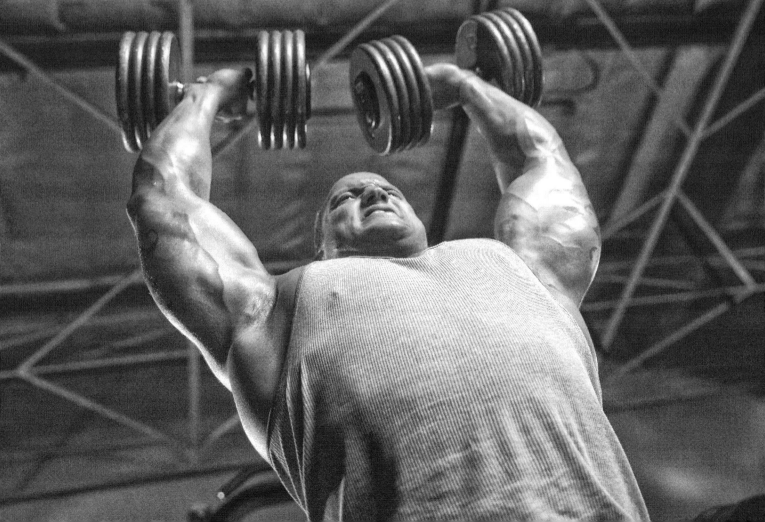

Arnold Presses

The Arnold Press is a great shoulder exercise. I bet you can't figure out who it's named after.

How to correctly perform an Arnold press:

- This can be performed standing or seated
- Stand with two dumbbells positioned in front of your shoulders with your palms facing your body and your elbows under your wrists
- From this position, rotate your shoulders out to the sides
- Continue as you press the dumbbells upward and then to full extension, rotating your palms facing outward
- Lower in the opposite pattern with a controlled negative

Important note: This is a compound pressing exercise. However, because of the shoulder rotation outward (abduction), special emphasis is placed on the middle deltoid.

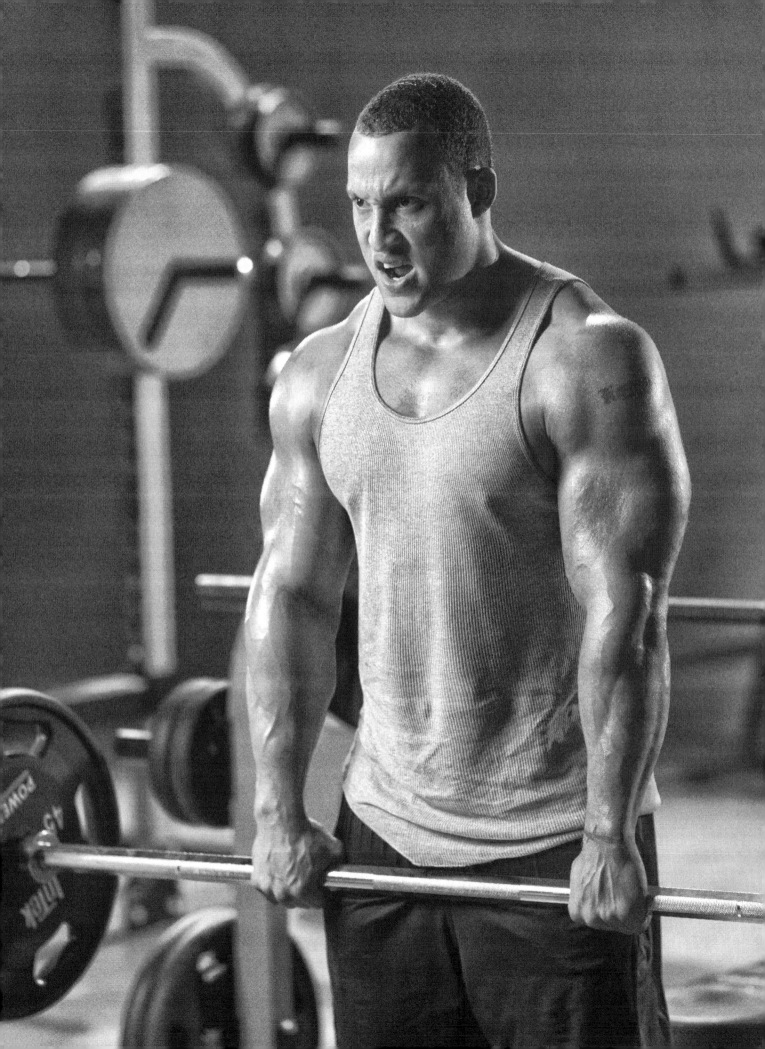

Upright Rows

The upright row is a compound movement. It primarily works the upper traps and the deltoids. Many smaller muscles are also used.

How to correctly perform an upright row:

- Stand with your feet shoulder width apart
- Grasp a barbell with a narrow grip, with palms facing your body
- Pull your shoulders back, lift up your chest, and arch your lower back
- Initiate the movement with your elbows and pull the bar up toward your chin
- Your elbows should remain above the bar the entire time
- Keep this movement strict

Important note: If you have a history of shoulder problems, avoid this movement. Full range of motion is advised; however, limit that range of motion as soon as you start feeling any pain or discomfort.

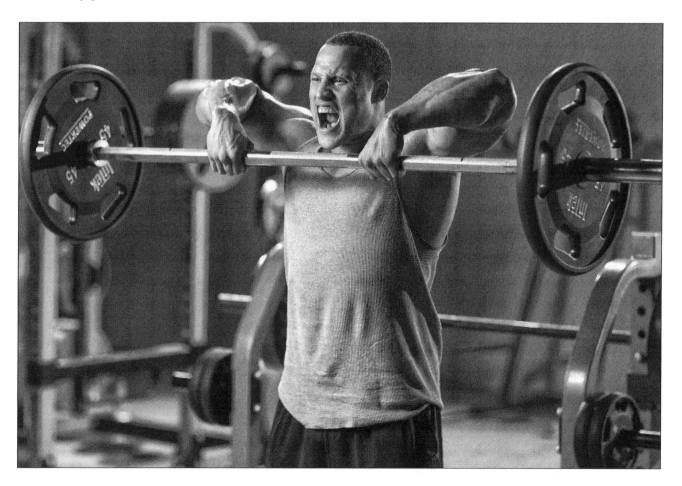

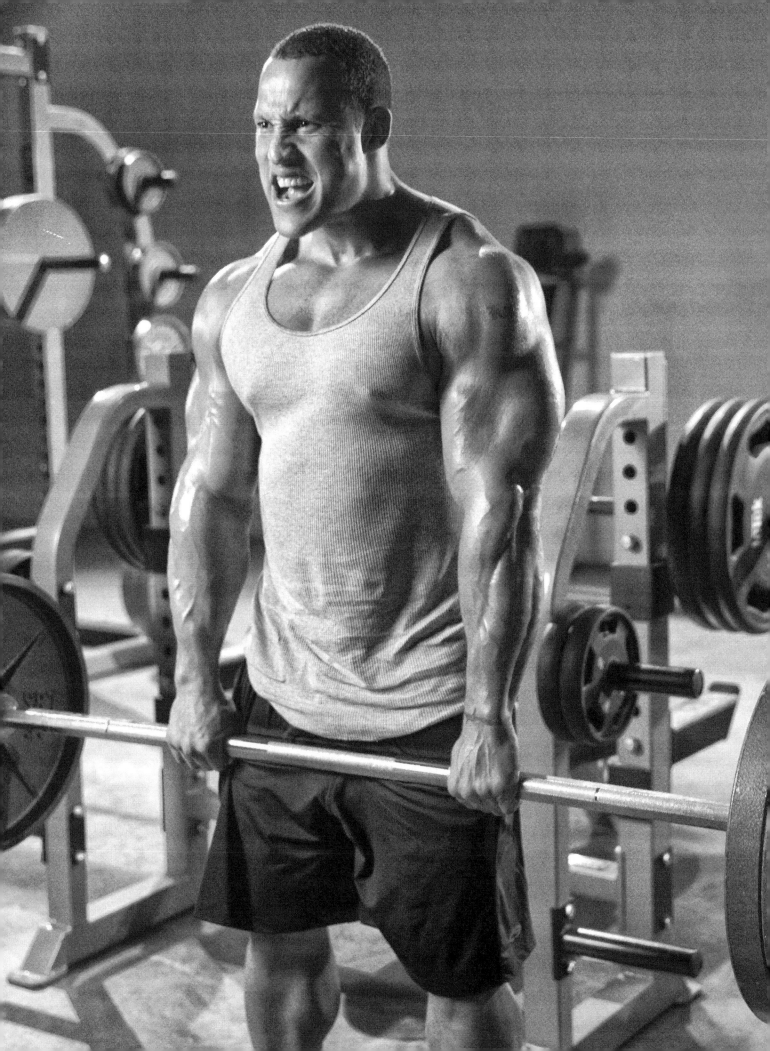

Barbell Shrugs

We are choosing to include shrugs with the shoulder work, but they could have been included with back work. Large traps exemplify an intimidating, masculine physique. Some bodybuilders do have to be careful because overly developed traps can make the shoulders appear narrower. Shrugs are the bread-and-butter trap exercise.

How to correctly perform a barbell shrug:

- Stand in front of a barbell and pick it up off the rack, with your feet hip width apart and your hands approximately shoulder width apart

- Grab the bar with an overhand grip

- Use straps

- With your arms remaining in full extension throughout the entire movement, elevate your shoulders as high as possible

- Lower the weight and repeat

Important note: These can be done explosively or by holding at the top. Explosive shrugs will transfer better to strength lifts and build more overall size. Shrugs done with the peak contraction style are more of an isolation movement.

Repetitively doing heavy shrugs can potentially lead to poor posture because of the heavy weight with the bar in front of you. Therefore, cycle in shrugs with dumbbells as well. These are performed the same way except the dumbbells are held to the side of your body. This can also be done with a trap bar, if you have access to one.

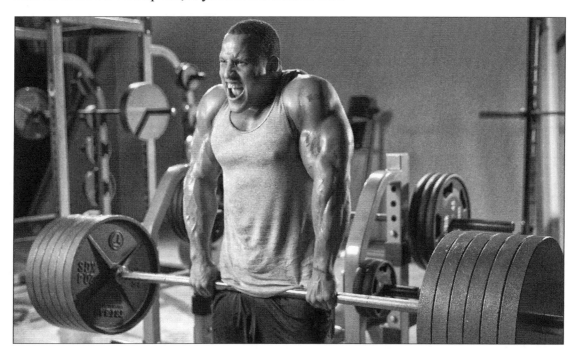

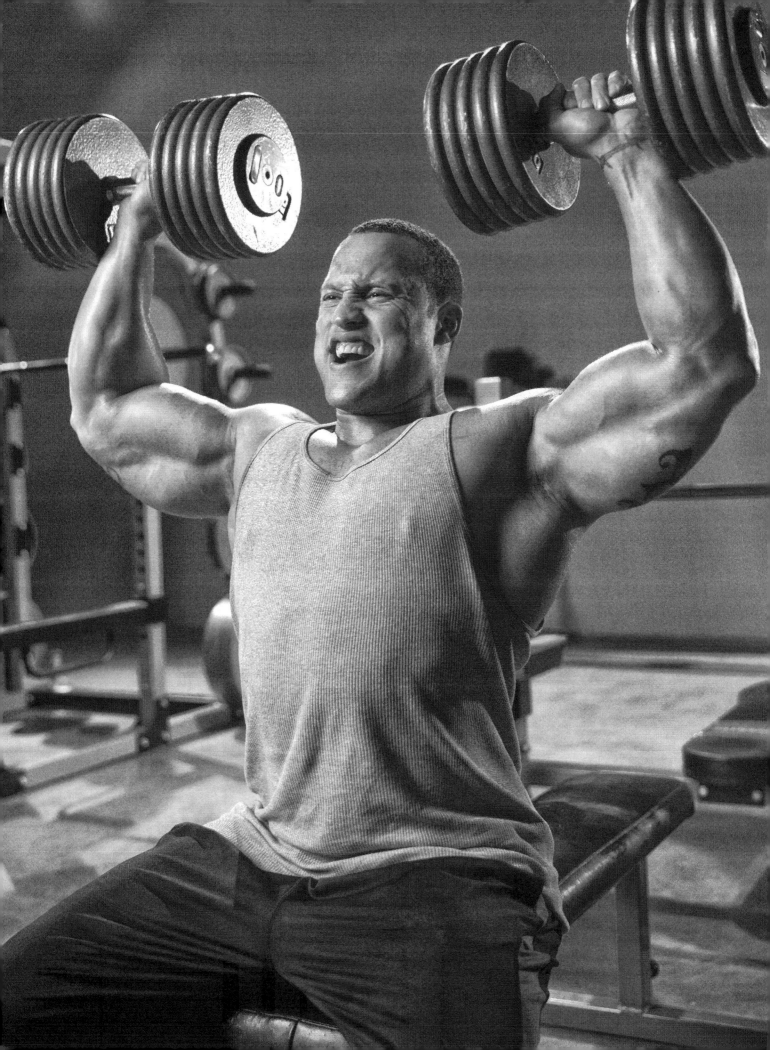

Half-Half Full Dumbbell Presses

This could have been included as a variation of the traditional dumbbell press, but it is simply too effective not to get its own special place.

With this movement, focus on controlling the negative and exploding on the positive. This really stresses the deltoids and greatly increases time under tension.

How to correctly perform the half-half full dumbbell press:

- Start off seated on a seated military bench
- Rest the dumbbells on your shoulders to start
- Push the weight halfway up
- Return to the starting position
- Push the weight halfway up again
- Return to the starting position
- Now push the weight all the way up
- Return to starting position

Important note: This could also be completed with a barbell.

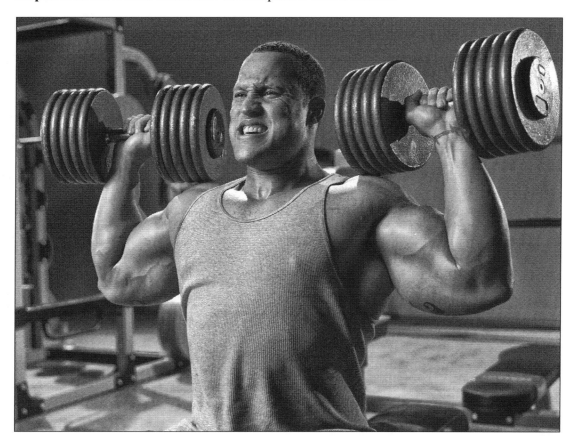

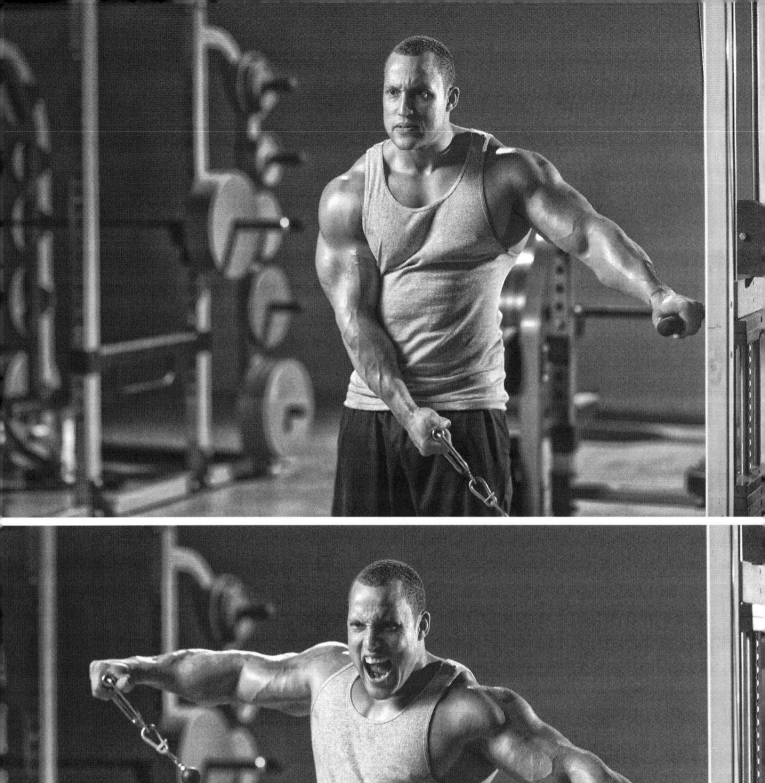
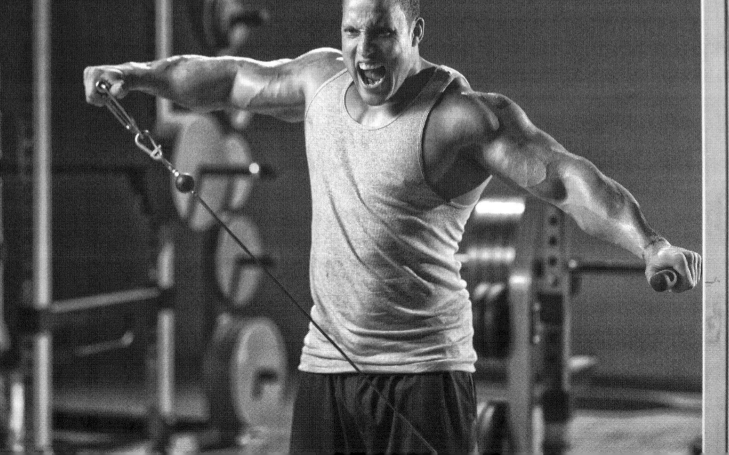

Cable Lateral Raises

The cable lateral raise is one of the best ways to directly stress the medial head of the deltoid. That's the part of the deltoid that gives you that capped, superhero-type look. Remember, this is an isolation movement. Focus on form, not weight.

How to correctly perform the cable lateral raise:

- Set the pulleys of a cable machine to the low setting and select the appropriate weight
- Stand facing away from the machine
- Grab the left handle with your right hand (across your body)
- Keep your elbows high throughout the entire movement
- Keep your arm almost straight, just a few degrees shy of extension
- Abduct your right arm across your body to the right side
- Once you get to shoulder height, pause briefly, and then lower the weight back to starting position

Important note: Lateral raises are one of the most effective medial delt builders. Lateral raises are also one of the most abused exercises. Do a YouTube search and you will see countless videos of bodybuilders recklessly heaving up dumbbells using more momentum than muscle.

The advantage to the cable is the constant tension placed on the muscle so you have to put out maximal effort throughout the entire movement. For a variation, give seated dumbbell lateral raises a try. Remember: form first.

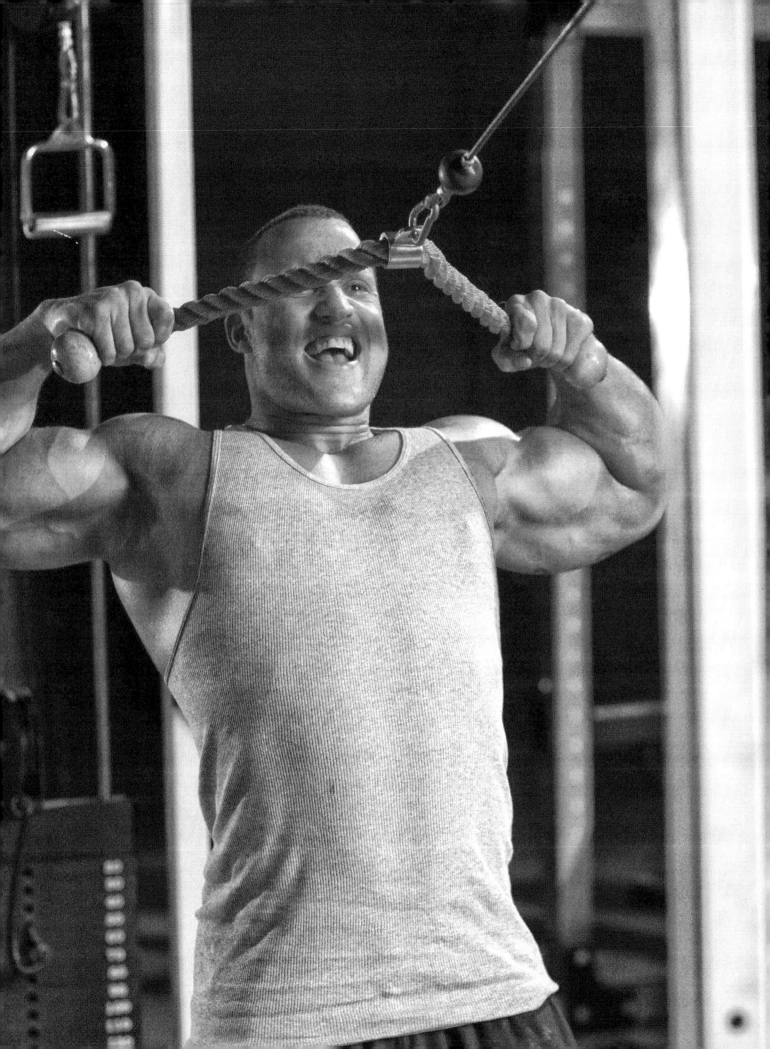

Face Pulls

Face pulls work the posterior deltoid and, surprisingly to most, even put extreme stress on the medial deltoid, according to EMG studies performed by Bret Contreras. They also target your back's weak scapular muscles, which aid in stabilization of your shoulder joints. This is great for shoulder health. Additionally, this movement strengthens your lower traps.

How to correctly perform a face pull:

- Attach a rope to a high pulley station
- Grab the end with each hand, with your palms facing each other
- Back away from the machine until your arms are at extension
- Pull the rope towards your eyes
- Your hands should end up just outside your ears
- Hold for one second and return to the starting position with your arms in full extension

Important note: Keep this exercise strict. It is not an ego exercise.

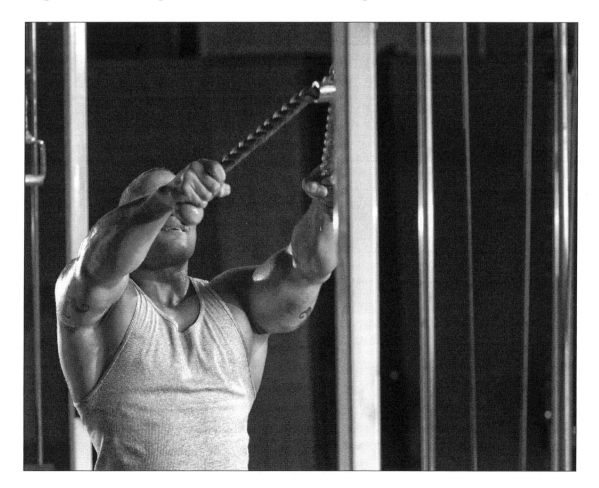

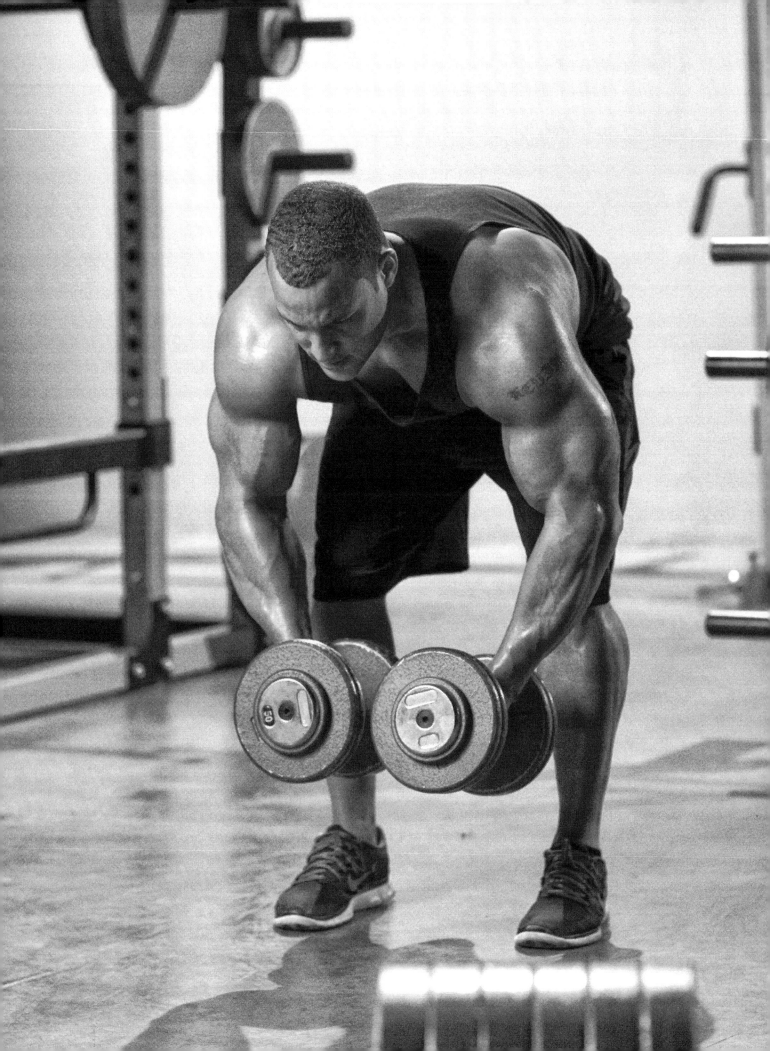

Bent-Over Lateral Raises

Bent-over lateral raises are an isolation exercise for the posterior deltoid. If you want boulders for shoulders, you have to build the back part of the shoulder.

> ***How to correctly perform a bent-over lateral raise:***
> - Lean forward at the waist with your torso at approximately 45 degrees
> - Maintain a strict arch, keeping your back straight
> - Feet should be shoulder width apart with a slight bend in the knees
> - Dumbbells are facing each other
> - With a slight bend in the elbow, raise your arms to your sides (your elbow position does not change)
> - Briefly pause at the top, squeezing your shoulder blades together
> - Return to starting position

Important note: Keep this movement strict. One variation you can do is to make the movement head supported, putting your forehead on the back of an incline bench to make sure your torso position doesn't change.

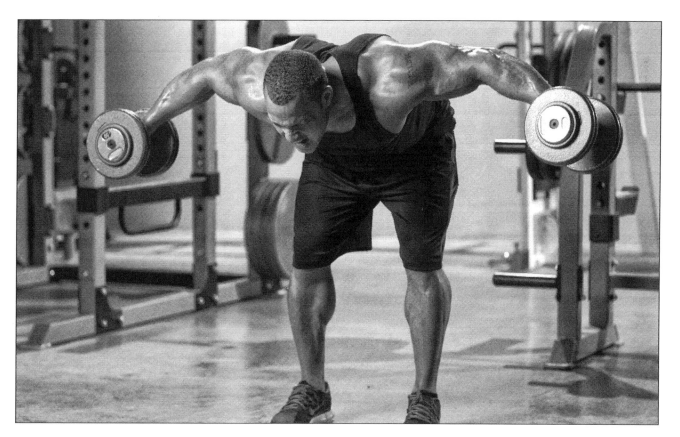

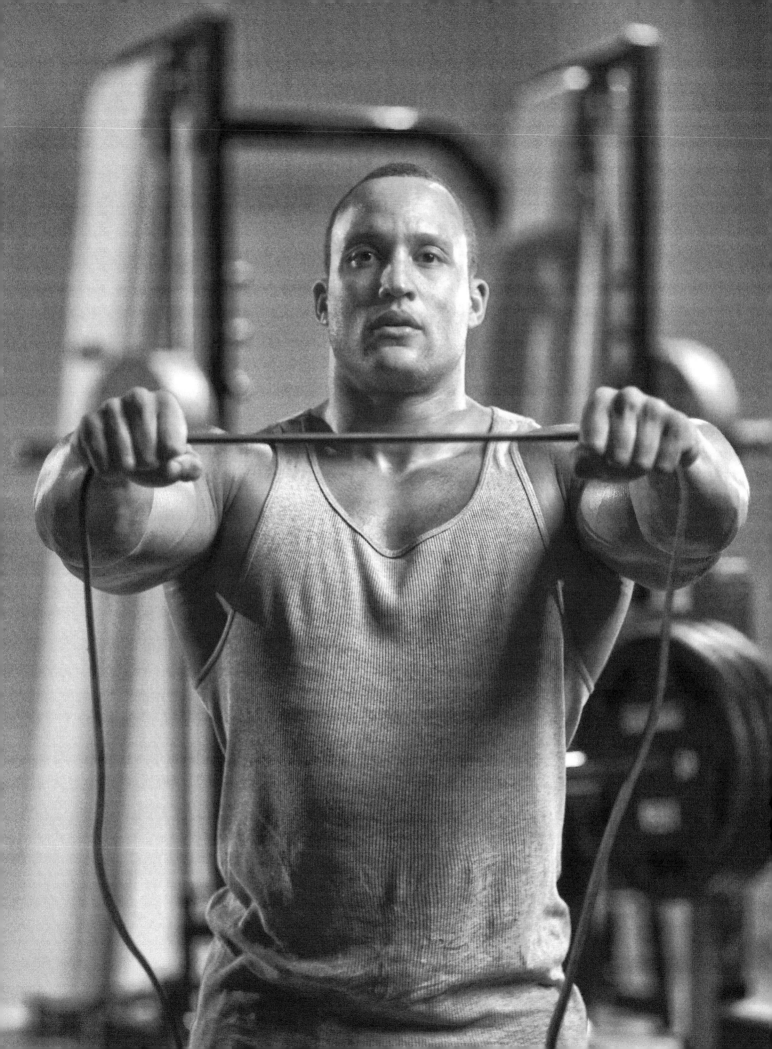

Band Pull Aparts

Poor shoulder health is a problem that plagues the bodybuilding community. Band pull aparts work the rear deltoids, middle back, and traps. These aren't the best muscle builder of all time, but they certainly help maintain optimal shoulder health. That's why exercises like this and the face pull have been included.

How to correctly perform a band pull apart:

- Begin with your arms extended straight out in front of you at chest level
- With a resistance band, which can be purchased from EliteFTS, pull the band apart in a reverse flye motion.
- Keep your arms straight
- Pull the band apart until your arms are at your sides
- Hold this position for a split second
- Return to the starting position

Important note: This is a strict exercise that should be performed for higher reps. The narrower you place your hands at the start of the movement, the more difficult the exercise is because it increases band tension.

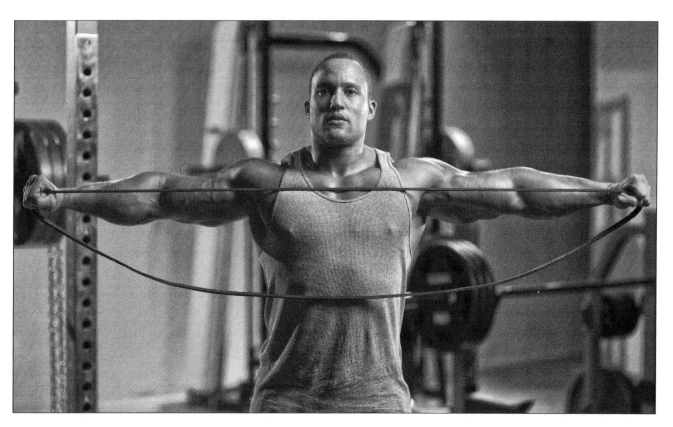

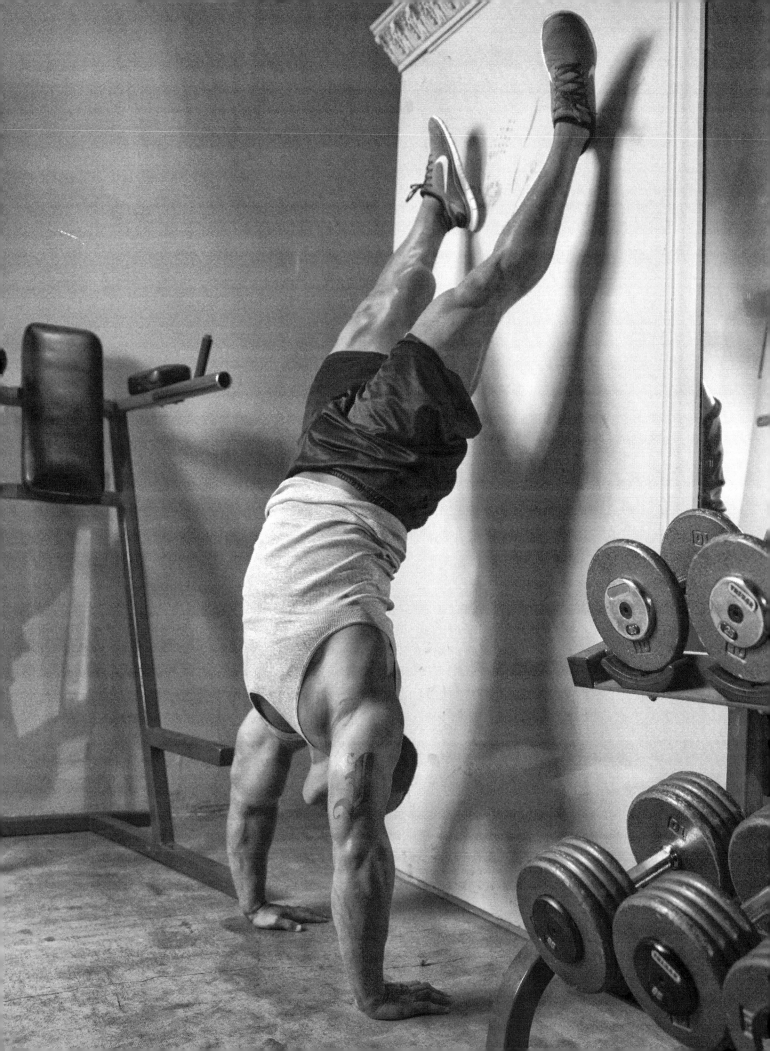

Handstand Push-ups

In 1992, California banned weights from prisons, and much of the nation followed suit. If you take a stroll on the prison tier, it is amazing to look at the shoulder development of inmates with no access to weights.

One reason is the handstand push up, a popular exercise among inmates for decades. This was one of Mike Tyson's favorite exercises to develop large, powerful deltoids.

How to correctly perform a handstand push-up:

- With your back to the wall, bend at the waist and place both your hands on the floor with a shoulder-width or slightly wider stance
- Kick your feet on the wall with your arms straight and walk your body flat against the wall
- Your arms and legs should be fully extended
- From this position, slowly lower yourself to the ground and almost touch your head to the floor
- Push yourself back up to the starting position

Important note: This is a very advanced movement, so proceed with caution.

EXERCISES FOR ABS, CALVES, AND NECK

By performing the aforementioned exercises, you are already working your abs, calves, and neck indirectly.

Here are some helpful exercises that can assist you with reaching your goals:

Leg raises	Standing calf raises
Planks	Seated calf raises
Side planks	Calf raises on the leg press
Landmines	Four-way neck machine
Standing cable crunches	Neck harness

A FEW LAST WORDS

*"Experience without theory is blind, but theory without experience
is mere intellectual play."*
—Immanuel Kant

The gap has been bridged. You now know the what, the why, and the how. But every principle discussed so far goes to hell in a hand basket without proper exercise selection.

_____

SOURCES

Contreras, Bret. "How to Conduct EMG Experiments." *Bret's Blog* (3 February 2010). http://bretcontreras.wordpress.com/2010/02/03/electromyography/.

Contreras, Bret. "Inside the Muscles: Best Back and Biceps Exercises." *T Nation* (1998–2010). http://www.t-nation.com/free_online_article/sports_body_training_ performance/inside_the_muscles_best_back_and_biceps_exercises.

Contreras, Bret. "Inside the Muscles: Best Chest and Triceps Exercises." *T Nation* (1998–2010). http://www.t-nation.com/free_online_article/sports_body_training_ performance/inside_the_muscles_best_chest_and_triceps_exercises.

Contreras, Bret. "Inside the Muscles: Best Leg, Glute, and Calf Exercises." *T Nation* (1998–2010). http://www.t-nation.com/testosterone-magazine-623#inside-the-muscles.

Contreras, Bret. "Inside the Muscles: Best Shoulders and Trap Exercises." *T Nation* (1998–2010). http://www.t-nation.com/free_online_article/sports_body_training_performance/inside_the_muscles_best_shoulders_and_trap_exercises.

Harris, Ron. "Full Deadlifts, Full Results." *Ironman*. N.d. http://bodybuilding.com/articles/full-deadlifts-full-results/.

Kamen, Gary, and David A. Gabriel. *Essentials of Electromyography*. Champaign, IL: Human Kinetics, 2010.

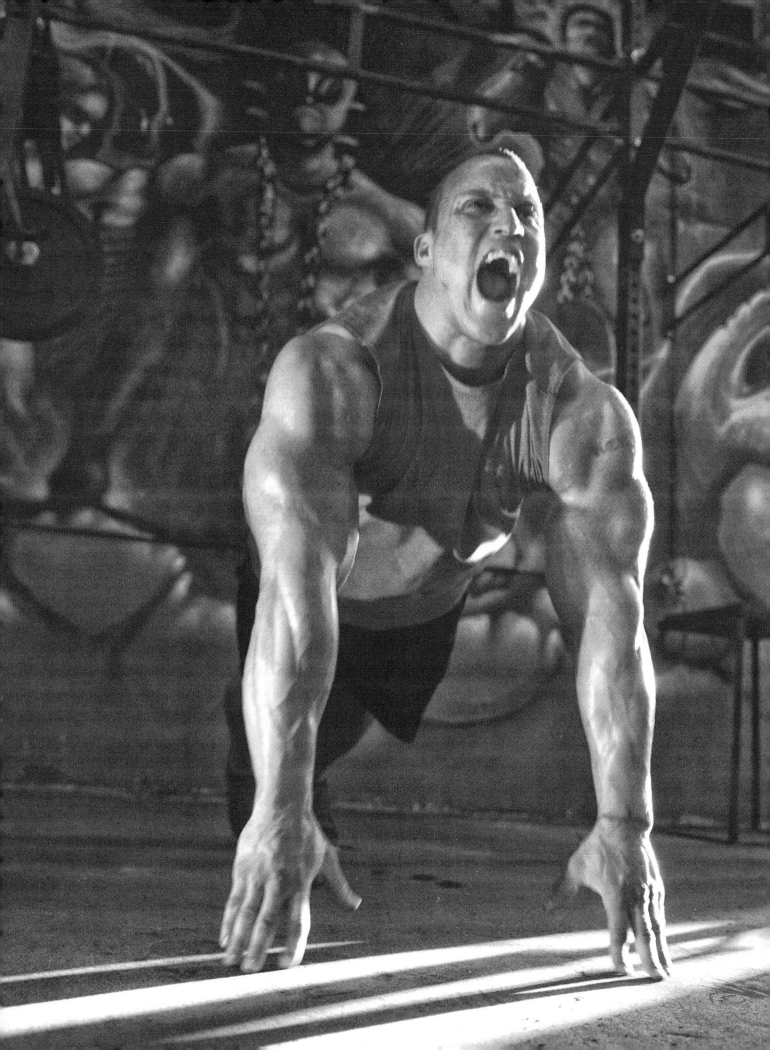

CHAPTER 15.

Bodybuilding Routines

NO-FRILLS, 3-DAY-A-WEEK, FULL-BODY ROUTINE

This routine is basic, simple, and effective for someone who has limited time and is looking to build strength in the compound movements. Give it a shot!

Week 1

Day 1

EXERCISE	REST INTERVAL	INTENSITY	SETS	REPS
Neutral-Grip Chin-ups	120 seconds	Max	4	6–8
Bench Press	120 seconds	75%	4	5
Squats	120 seconds	80%	4	3

Day 2

EXERCISE	REST INTERVAL	INTENSITY	SETS	REPS
Neutral-Grip Chin-ups	120 seconds	Max	4	6–8
Bulgarian Dumbbell Squats	120 seconds	Max	4	6–8
Overhead Press	120 seconds	80%	4	3

Day 3

EXERCISE	REST INTERVAL	INTENSITY	SETS	REPS
Deadlift	120 seconds	80%	4	3
Dips	120 seconds	Max	4	6–10
Squats	120 seconds	Max	4	5-8

Week 2

Day 1

EXERCISE	REST INTERVAL	INTENSITY	SETS	REPS
Neutral-Grip Chin-ups	120 seconds	Max	4	8–10
Bench Press	120 seconds	80%	4	4
Squats	180 seconds	85%	4	3

Day 2

EXERCISE	REST INTERVAL	INTENSITY	SETS	REPS
Narrow-Grip Chin-ups	120 seconds	Max	4	8–10
Bulgarian Dumbbell Squats	120 seconds	Max	4	6–8
Overhead Press	180 seconds	90%	4	2

Day 3

EXERCISE	REST INTERVAL	INTENSITY	SETS	REPS
Deadlift	180 seconds	90%	4	2
Dips	120 seconds	Max	4	6–10
Bent-Over Rows	120 seconds	Max	4	5–8

Week 3

Day 1

EXERCISE	REST INTERVAL	INTENSITY	SETS	REPS
Neutral-Grip Chin-ups	120 seconds	Max	4	4–6
Bench Press	180 seconds	90%	4	2
Squats	180 seconds	90%	4	2

Day 2

EXERCISE	REST INTERVAL	INTENSITY	SETS	REPS
Narrow-Grip Chin-ups	120 seconds	Max	4	8–10
Bulgarian Dumbbell Squats	120 seconds	Max	4	6–8
Overhead Press	120 seconds	75%	4	6

Day 3

EXERCISE	REST INTERVAL	INTENSITY	SETS	REPS
Deadlift	180 seconds	85%	4	3
Dips	120 seconds	Max	4	5–8
Bent-Over Rows	120 seconds	Max	4	5–8

- Day 1 Notes—on last set of bench presses and squats, do as many reps as possible (AMAP). Do not go to failure; stop one rep short of momentary muscular failure (MMF).
- Day 2 Notes—on last set of overhead presses, do AMAP. Do not go to failure; stop one rep short of momentary muscular failure (MMF).
- Day 3 Notes—on last set of deadlifts, do AMAP. Do not go to failure; stop one rep short of momentary muscular failure (MMF).
- Every fourth week is a deload; do three sets per exercise with 65% of the weight used the previous week (not of your one-repetition max). Do not do AMAP on deloads; reps remain the same.
- This cycle can be run three times consecutively; after that, it is advisable to switch exercises. Each time the lifts are recycled after deload, add 5–10 pounds; the key is not to add any more weight than that. If the weight is easy, lift it more explosively and do more reps on the last set.

REST PAUSE TRAINING

These rest pause workouts are plateau busters! You will grow and get stronger. Do not do these workouts more than three weeks in a row without a deload.

Chest: Biggest Hood in the 'Hood, Plateau-Busting Chest Program

EXERCISE	REST INTERVAL	INTENSITY	SETS	REPS
Bench Press	20 seconds	85%	6	2
Incline Press	20 seconds	80%	6	2
Dips	20 seconds	8 rep max	6	2
Incline Cable Flyes	60 seconds	Max	2	15
Dumbbell Pull-over	90 seconds	Max	2	20

- Notes—on bench press, incline press, and dips, do as many reps as possible on the last set; it is to momentary muscular failure. All other sets hit specified reps. Add weight if applicable on dips.

Legs: Take Off the Training "Wheels" Leg Program

EXERCISE	REST INTERVAL	INTENSITY	SETS	REPS
Squats	20 seconds	85%	6	2
Leg Press	20 seconds	12-rep max	6	2
One-Leg Deadlift	60 seconds	Max	2	6
Leg Extension/Leg Curl Superset	60 seconds	Max	2	20…6
Barbell Hip Thrusts	90 seconds	Max	2	12

- Notes—on squats and leg press, do as many reps as possible on the last set.
  Do not go to momentary muscular failure; stop one rep short.

Back: Big Ol' Back Plateau-Busting Program

EXERCISE	REST INTERVAL	INTENSITY	SETS	REPS
Rack Pulls Knee Level	20 seconds	85%	6	2
Snatch Grip Deadlifts	20 seconds	6-rep max	6	2
Bent-Over Rows	20 seconds	10-rep max	6	3
Wide-Grip Chin-ups	120 seconds	Max	2	8
One-Armed Low Cable Rows	60 seconds	Max	2	12
Straight-Arm Pull-downs	60 seconds	Max	2	15

- On rack pulls, snatch grip deadlifts, and bent-over rows, do as many reps as possible.
  On the last set, do not go to momentary muscular failure; stop one rep short.
- Add weight if applicable to chin-ups.

Arms: Fill Your Prison Denim Arms Routine

EXERCISE	REST INTERVAL	INTENSITY	SETS	REPS
Close-Grip Bench Press	20 seconds	85%	6	2
Scott Barbell Curls	20 seconds	10-rep max	6	5
Dicks Press, Close-Grip Push-up, Overhead Rope Extension Giant Set	180 seconds	10-rep max, 15-rep max, 20-rep max	3	Failure
Narrow Grip Chin-up/ Incline Dumbbell Curl Superset (huge stretch)	120 seconds	10-rep max, 15-rep max	3	Failure

- Add weight if applicable to chin-ups.
- Complete the last set on close grip bench press and Scott barbell curls to failure.
- Complete all triceps exercises to failure. For close grip push-ups, additional resistance can be added via bands or a weighted vest.
- Complete narrow-grip chin-ups and incline dumbbell curls both to failure.

Shoulders: Boulders for Shoulders Plateau-Busting Routine

EXERCISE	REST INTERVAL	INTENSITY	SETS	REPS
Overhead Press	20 seconds	85%	6	2
Arnold Press	20 seconds	10-rep max	6	5
Cable Lateral	45 seconds	Max	4	15
Upright Row/Dumbbell Shrug Superset	120 seconds	Max	12/15	3
Face Pulls	60 seconds	Max	3	12
Reverse Pec Deck	60 seconds	Max	2	15

- Overhead presses and Arnold presses are taken to failure.

STAGGERED SET ROUTINE

EXERCISE	REST INTERVAL	INTENSITY	SETS	REPS
Squats	120 seconds	Max	6	4
Cable Lateral Raises		75%	1	15
Lunges	90 seconds	Max	4	12
Upright Rows		75%	1	12
Leg Curl/Leg Extension SupersetPulls	120 seconds	Max	3	6...15
Face Pulls	60 seconds	75%	1	12
One-Leg Deadlift	60 seconds	Max	2	6

- This is an example of a bodybuilder increasing training frequency of shoulders. Legs are the priority, but shoulder work is staggered between exercises.

FORCED REPS: CHEST PLATEAU-BUSTER ROUTINE

Day 1

EXERCISE	REST INTERVAL	INTENSITY	SETS	REPS
Bench Press with Weight Releasers	180 seconds	65%, 75%, 82.5%, 90%–95%	4	10, 8, 6, 4
Face Pulls	60 seconds	Max	2	12
Incline Press	60 seconds	85%, 70%	4 (1 @ 85%, 3 @ 70%)	3, 6
Face Pulls	60 seconds	Max	2	12
Decline Press (against bands)	90 seconds	Max	3	6
Cable Lateral Raises	60 seconds	Max	3	12
Band Resisted Flyes	45 seconds	Max	3	20
Dumbbell Pull Over	90 seconds	Max	3	20

- Weight releasers are 10%–20% over bar weight and not factored to intensity; they release after first rep.
- Last set of bench press will require forced reps; make sure you have a competent spotter.
- Band resistance should be 10%–25% of bar weight for decline presses.

Day 2

EXERCISE	REST INTERVAL	INTENSITY	SETS	REPS
Deadlifts	120 seconds	75%	4	5
Bent-Over Rows	60 seconds	Max	3	6
Cable Lat Pull-downs on Knees	60 seconds	Max	3	12
Incline Dumbbell Curls	60 seconds	Max	3	15
Reverse Fat Bar Curls	60 seconds	Max	3	15

Day 3 off

Day 4

EXERCISE	REST INTERVAL	INTENSITY	SETS	REPS
Close Grip Bench	120 seconds	60%	3	12
Cable Flyes	60 seconds	80%	3	12
Pec Deck	60 seconds	80%	3	12
Dips/Overhead Rope Extension	120 seconds	70%...max	3	15...15
Dumbbell Floor Triceps Extension	60 seconds	Max	3	15

- Chest movements are moderate intensity.
- All-out on triceps movements.

Day 5

EXERCISE	REST INTERVAL	INTENSITY	SETS	REPS
Squats	120 seconds	75%	5	5
Dead Stop Leg Press	60 seconds	Max	2	15
Lunges	60 seconds	Max	2	12
Dead Stop Leg Press	60 seconds	Max	3	15...6

Days 6 and 7 off

- This routine can be used for up to 6 weeks to boost a lagging chest.

ECCENTRIC EMPHASIS TRAINING

Get Negative Chest and Triceps Routine

EXERCISE	REST INTERVAL	INTENSITY	SETS	REPS
Bench Press	180 seconds	65%, 75%, 85%	3	10, 8, 5
Eccentric Bench Press	180 seconds	105%, 115%	2	3
Reverse Grip Bench Press	N/A	Max	1	AMAP
Incline Cable Flyes	60 seconds	Max	3	15
One Armed Overhead Dumbbell Extension Dip Superset	90 seconds	Max	Max	Max

- For dips, you can add weight if applicable.
- On the bench presses with the 5-second eccentric, since they are over your max you will need a reliable spotter to assist you on the positive portion of the lift.
- For the incline press dumbbell mechanical drop set, start with a 45-degree incline with a weight you can do 8–12 times and go to failure. Drop the incline to 30 degrees and go to failure using the same weight. Finally, with the same weight, drop the incline to 15 degrees and lift dumbbells to failure.
- For the triceps bodyweight negative emphasis, grasp a fixed bar and, using a shoulder-width grip, create a 45-degree angle with your body to the floor. Start at bottom position, elbows in flexion and forehead touching the bar. From this position, extend arms to full extension. This is a closed-kinetic-chain version of a triceps extension, a prison yard favorite. From the extended position, lower yourself back down to the starting position but using only one arm, making the negative much more intense. The eccentric contraction should take 4–5 seconds.

Legs

EXERCISE	REST INTERVAL	INTENSITY	SETS	REPS
Squats	120 seconds	90%, 80%, 70%, 60%	4	3, 6, 8, 12
Leg Press (concentric use two legs, eccentric use one leg)	120 seconds	Max	3	6
Leg Extension (concentric use two legs, eccentric use one leg)	90 seconds	Max	3	8
Leg Curl (concentric use two legs, eccentric use one leg)	90 seconds	Max	3	5
Barbell Hip Thrusts	60 seconds	Max	3	12

- Leg curls, presses, and extensions use both legs on the concentric rep and one leg on the eccentric. The eccentric repetition should take 5 seconds.

Back

EXERCISE	REST INTERVAL	INTENSITY	SETS	REPS
Rack Pulls	180 seconds	90%, 85%, 80%, 70%	4	3, 5, 6, 8
Seated Rows (concentric use two legs, eccentric use one leg)	120 seconds	Max	3	6
One-Armed Dumbbell Row/Meadows Rows Superset	90 seconds	Max	3	10/10
T-Bar Row	90 seconds	Max	3	5
Neutral-Grip Chin-ups	90 seconds	Max	3	6

- Rack pulls are performed at knee level.
- Seated rows use neutral grip/narrow handle. Perform the positive portion of the lift with two arms and for the negative use one arm. The negative is for 5 seconds; make sure to get a great stretch on the lats; with a partial stretch you will only get a partial benefit.
- Perform the T-bar row eccentric emphasis on a chest-supported T-bar machine. Have a partner assist you on the positive portion of the rep, then take 5 seconds to lower the negative. Make sure to get a full range of motion and a great stretch at the bottom of the movement.

Shoulders and Biceps

EXERCISE	REST INTERVAL	INTENSITY	SETS	REPS
Overhead Press	60 seconds	70%	6	3
Universal Machine Military Press (concentric use two arms, eccentric use one arm)	120 seconds	Max	3	5
Lateral Raises Seated Machine Negative Emphasis	120 seconds	Max	3	10
Bent-Over Flyes	60 seconds	Max	3	12
One Armed Eccentric Barbell Curls	90 seconds	Max	5	5

- On the universal machine military press, press the weight up with both arms and lower the weight for a 5-second negative using only one arm.
- For lateral raises, perform on a seated machine; have a partner assist you on the positive portion of the reps and lower for a 5-second eccentric.
- For the one armed eccentric barbell curl, lower for an 8-second eccentric and have a partner assist you on the positive, or self-spot with free hand.

Four-Week Arm Specialization Routine

This arm routine I designed was featured in *Muscle & Fitness* magazine. I have made some modifications to make it even more effective from when it was first published in 2010.

Day 1

EXERCISE	REST INTERVAL	SETS	REPS
EZ Curl Decline Bench Press	120 seconds	5	15, 12, 8, 6, 20
Cheat Curl (5-second eccentric)	90 seconds	4	10, 8, 6, 12
One-Armed Eccentric Barbell Curl (8-second eccentric)	60 seconds (after both arms complete)	5	5
One-Armed Cable Push-downs	30 seconds (after both arms complete)	3	15
Close-Grip (full range of motion to 4 Board Mechanical Drop Set)		1	25 (5 reps full ROM, 5 reps 1 board, 5 reps 2 board, 5 reps 3 board, 5 reps 4 board)

Days 2–3 Off

Day 4

EXERCISE	REST INTERVAL	SETS	REPS
Dips/Overhead Rope Extension Superset	120 seconds	4	10/15
Chin-up/Incline Biceps Dumbbell Curl Superset (great stretch on curls)	120 seconds	4	6/15
Fat Bar Reverse Curl to failure, followed by Regular Fat Bar Curls to failure	90 seconds	3	(Start with a weight you can do 12 reverse curls with, keep same weight all 3 sets)
Dicks Press	90 seconds	3	8
One-Arm Overhead Tri Extension	60 seconds	3	15
Forearm Flexion/Extension	60 seconds	3	12

Days 5–7 Off

- Add additional weight to body for chins-ups and dips if possible; use a band for assistance if unable to perform with bodyweight.
- Use as much weight as possible without compromising form.
- If reps descend, add weight; if they ascend, decrease weight.
- Add weight to exercises weekly; the goal is to do more every week, but never at the expense of technique.
- Follow this routine for 4 weeks.

Arm Routine

Once a Week

EXERCISE	REST INTERVAL	SETS	REPS
Close-Grip 2 Board Bench Press With Bands or Chains	120 seconds	4	6
Mechanical Drop Set Dumbbell Curls (Incline Dumbbell Curls to failure, Standing Dumbbell Curls to failure, Hammer Curls to failure)	120 seconds	4	6/15
Overhead Dumbbell Triceps Extension	60 seconds	3	15
Fat Bar 21 Curls	90 seconds	3	7...7...7

- For mechanical drop set curls, start with a weight you can do 8–10 incline curls with. Once you can no longer perform strict curls, switch to standing; and when standing curls with dumbbells can no longer be performed with strict form, switch to hammer curls.
- Do this routine no more than 3 weeks in a row.

Advanced Chest Routine #1

Once a Week

EXERCISE	REST INTERVAL	SETS	REPS
Bench Press with Weight Releasers	120 seconds	4	6
Mechanical Drop Set Incline Press (Steep Incline Dumbbell Press to failure, Medium Incline Dumbbell Press to failure, Low Incline Press to failure)	120 seconds	3	AMAP
Dips	90 seconds	3	Max in 30 seconds

- Weight releasers should contain 20% of bar weight and lower the eccentric for 5 seconds for the first rep with weight releasers. Subsequent reps are performed controlled eccentric, explosive concentric.
- For dips, add weight if applicable; start with a weight you can do for 12 reps.

- For mechanical drop set curls, start with a weight you can do 8–10 steep incline reps with. Once you reach momentary muscular failure, drop to a medium incline and perform repetitions to momentary muscular failure. Finally, drop to a low incline and perform repetitions to momentary muscular failure.
- Do this routine no more than 3 weeks in a row.
- This is a very advanced routine.

Advanced Chest Routine #2

Once a Week

EXERCISE	REST INTERVAL	SETS	REPS
Eccentric Overload Bench Press (lower negatives for 5 seconds)	180 seconds	3	5
Mechanical Drop Set Incline Press (Steep Incline Dumbbell Press to failure, Medium Incline Dumbbell Press to failure, Low Incline Press to failure)	120 seconds	3	AMAP
Decline Flyes	60 seconds	4	15
Dips	120 seconds	3	Max in 30 seconds
Dumbbell Pull-Over	90 seconds	4	20, 20, 15, 15

- For mechanical drop set curls, start with a weight you can do 8–10 steep incline reps with. Once you reach momentary muscular failure, drop to a medium incline and perform repetitions to momentary muscular failure. Finally, drop to a low incline and perform repetitions to momentary muscular failure.
- Do this routine no more than 3 weeks in a row.
- This is a very advanced routine.

"V Is for Victory" V Taper Routine

This routine I designed was Featured in *Muscle & Fitness*. It is a 6-week plan designed to bring up the back and shoulders.

Day 1

EXERCISE	REST INTERVAL	SETS	REPS
Deadlift	180 seconds	4	3, 5, 6, 8
Bent-Over Barbell Row	120 seconds	4	6, 8, 10, 10
Chin-up 21 (7 bottom half, 7 top half, 7 full range of motion)	120 seconds	3	7...7...7
Standing One-Armed Cable Low Row	45 seconds (after both arms complete)	4	15
Straight-Arm Pull-down	60 seconds	5	15
One-Armed Dumbbell Rows	90 seconds	3	8, 10, 15

Day 2–3 Off

Day 4

EXERCISE	REST INTERVAL	SETS	REPS
1/2, 1/2, Full Dumbbell Press	120 seconds	4	6 (1/2, 1/2, full is 1 rep)
Dumbbell Shrugs (right arm 10 reps, left arm 10 reps, both arms 10 reps)	90 seconds	4	10...10...10
Upright Rows	120 seconds	3	12
Cable Lateral Raises	45 seconds (after both arms complete)	3	15
Face Pulls	60 seconds	4	14
Bent-Over Lateral Raises	60 seconds	3	12

Days 5–7 Off

- Add additional weight to body for chin-ups if possible; use a band for assistance if unable to perform with bodyweight.
- Use as much weight as possible without compromising form.
- If reps descend, add weight; if they ascend, decrease weight.

- Add weight to exercises weekly; the goal is to do more every week, but never at the expense of technique.
- Follow this routine for 6 weeks.

Lukenback, Texas, Two-Day-a-Week Back Specialization Routine

Day 1

EXERCISE	REST INTERVAL	SETS	REPS
Deadlifts (against bands)	120 seconds	5	5, 4, 3, 2, 1
Shrugs	90 seconds	4	15
Bent-Over Rows	120 seconds	3	6
One-Armed Dumbbell Rows	45 seconds (after both arms complete)	3	8
Good Mornings	60 seconds	4	8

Rest 3–4 days.

Day 5 or 6

EXERCISE	REST INTERVAL	SETS	REPS
Wide-Grip Lat Pull-downs (chest up face away)	60 seconds	4	15
Neutral-Grip Chin-ups	120 seconds	4	8
Straight-Arm Pull-downs	60 seconds	3	15
One-Armed Standing Cable Rows	45 seconds (after both arms complete)	3	15

Big Ol' Bat Wings, One-Day-a-Week Back Routine

EXERCISE	REST INTERVAL	SETS	REPS
Rack Pulls (knee level)	120 seconds	5	3
Meadows Rows/One-Armed Dumbbell Row Superset	90 seconds	4	10/10
T-Bar Prison Rows	120 seconds	3	12
Cable Lat Pull-downs on Knees	60 seconds	4	6
Seated Rows (one arm eccentric overload)	120 seconds	4	6

- Seated row one-arm eccentric overloads are performed by rowing with two hands on the concentric but on the eccentric releasing the non-working hand; take 5 seconds to return to the start position. You should feel a huge stretch and use much heavier weights than you can use on a concentric only.

TIME UNDER TENSION ROUTINES

Time under tension training is simply performing the maxium amount of reps in the specified time.

Chest, Legs, Shoulders, Arms, and Back

Day 1: Chest

EXERCISE	REST INTERVAL	SETS	REPS
Dumbbell Bench Press	120 seconds	3	Max in 30 seconds
Dumbbell Pull Over	120 seconds	3	Max in 30 seconds
Incline Dumbbell Press	120 seconds	3	Max in 30 seconds
Chain Flyes	120 seconds	3	Max in 30 seconds
Pec Deck	120 seconds	3	Max in 30 seconds

Day 2: Legs

EXERCISE	REST INTERVAL	SETS	REPS
Leg Press	120 seconds	3	Max in 30 seconds
Leg Extensions	120 seconds	3	Max in 30 seconds
Glute Ham Raises	120 seconds	3	Max in 30 seconds
Glute Cable Kickbacks	120 seconds	3	Max in 30 seconds
Seated Calf Raises	120 seconds	3	Max in 30 seconds

Day 3: Shoulders

EXERCISE	REST INTERVAL	SETS	REPS
Dumbbell Military Press	120 seconds	3	Max in 30 seconds
Machine Lateral Raises	120 seconds	3	Max in 30 seconds
Face Pulls	120 seconds	3	Max in 30 seconds
Plate Raises	120 seconds	3	Max in 30 seconds
Reverse Flyes	120 seconds	3	Max in 30 seconds

Day 4: Arms

EXERCISE	REST INTERVAL	SETS	REPS
Dips	120 seconds	3	Max in 30 seconds
Hammer Curls	120 seconds	3	Max in 30 seconds
Rolling Dumbbell Triceps Extension	120 seconds	3	Max in 30 seconds
Incline Dumbbell Curls	120 seconds	3	Max in 30 seconds
Over Rope Triceps Extension	120 seconds	2	Max in 30 seconds

Day 5: Back

EXERCISE	REST INTERVAL	SETS	REPS
Dumbbell Rows	120 seconds	3	Max in 30 seconds
Neutral-Grip Chin-ups	120 seconds	3	Max in 30 seconds
Straight Arm Pull-downs	120 seconds	3	Max in 30 seconds
T-Bar Rows Chest Supported	120 seconds	3	Max in 30 seconds
Seated Rows	120 seconds	2	Max in 30 seconds

- Control on negatives and explode on positives.
- The goal is to keep the weight moving; if you reach momentary muscular failure (MMF), continue with partials. *Do not drop the weight!*
- Start with weights you can do for a true rep max of 8–12 reps; shoot for 10–15, including partial contractions.
- On each set, reduce load by approximately 1/3, so if you start with 90 pounds, set two would be with 60 pounds and set three would be with 40 pounds.
- This technique is very high intensity; do it for a maximum of 3–4 weeks before taking a deload.
- Progression weekly can be to add 5–10 seconds per set, keeping the rest interval the same or keeping the time constant but increasing the weight.
- Use primarily bilateral movements; dumbbell movements need to be with both limbs contracting simultaneously.

Minimal-Time, Maximum-Hypertrophy Three-Day-a-Week Routine

Here is a 3-day-a-week time-under-tension routine designed for someone with minimal time but who is willing to put out maximal effort for training. These routines only work if you put forth an all-out effort.

Day 1

EXERCISE	REST INTERVAL	SETS	REPS
Dumbbell Military Press	120 seconds	3	Max in 30 seconds
Leg Press	120 seconds	3	Max in 30 seconds
Face Pulls	120 seconds	3	Max in 30 seconds
Leg Curls	120 seconds	3	Max in 30 seconds
Machine Lateral Raises	120 seconds	3	Max in 30 seconds
Planks	30 seconds	3	Hold 30 seconds
Seated Calf Raises	60 seconds	3	25

Day 2 Off

Day 3

EXERCISE	REST INTERVAL	SETS	REPS
Incline Dumbbell Press	120 seconds	3	Max in 30 seconds
Incline Dumbbell Biceps Curls	120 seconds	3	Max in 30 seconds
Dumbbell Bench Press	120 seconds	3	Max in 30 seconds
Hammer Curls	120 seconds	3	Max in 30 seconds
Pec Deck	120 seconds	3	Max in 30 seconds
Machine Curls	120 seconds	3	Max in 30 seconds
Leg Raises	30 seconds	3	10-15

Day 4 Off

Day 5

EXERCISE	REST INTERVAL	SETS	REPS
Neutral-Grip Chin-ups	120 seconds	3	Max in 30 seconds
JM Press	120 seconds	3	Max in 30 seconds
Dumbbell Rows	120 seconds	3	Max in 30 seconds
Overhead Rope Triceps Extension	120 seconds	3	Max in 30 seconds
Seated Rows	120 seconds	3	Max in 30 seconds
Rolling Dumbbell Triceps Extension	120 seconds	3	Hold 30 seconds
Weighted Crunches	60 seconds	4	10-15
Standing Calf Raises	60 seconds	4	15-20

Days 6–7 Off

SIZE AND STRENGTH HYBRID PROGRAM

This powerbuilding routine was originally designed by me in the summer of 2012 for *Muscle Mag International*. I have since improved it even more from the great feedback I have received.

Weeks 1–3

Day 1

EXERCISE	REST INTERVAL	SETS	REPS
Bench Press	120 seconds	4	10
Weighted Dip	120 seconds	5	5
Dead Bench Press (from dead stop)	30 seconds	1	8
Flat-Bench Dumbbell Flyes	60 seconds	3	10
Zottman Curl	60 seconds	4	12
Dumbbell Kickback	45 seconds	4	12
Plank	45 seconds	2	60 seconds
Side Plank	30 seconds	2	30 seconds

Day 2

EXERCISE	REST INTERVAL	SETS	REPS
Squat	120 seconds	5	5
Olympic Pause Squat	120 seconds	2	8
Dumbbell Step-up	90 seconds	3	12
Leg Press (with pause)	120 seconds	3	15
Leg Extension	60 seconds	4	12
Single-Leg Deadlift (each side)	60 seconds	3	6
Leg Curl	60 seconds	4	6
Standing Cable Crunch	60 seconds	3	12
Oblique Cable Crunch	60 seconds	3	12

Day 3

EXERCISE	REST INTERVAL	SETS	REPS
Close-Grip Bench Press	120 seconds	4	8
Standing Military Press	120 seconds	3	5
Dumbbell Lateral Raise	60 seconds	3	12
Bent-Over Lateral Raise	60 seconds	3	12
Rope Face Pull	45 seconds	3	12
Lying Triceps Extension	60 seconds	4	12
Triceps Push-down	60 seconds	4	12
Hanging Leg Raise	60 seconds	2	12
Abs Wheel	60 seconds	2	12
Hanging Leg Raise with Twist (each side)	60 seconds	2	12

Day 4

EXERCISE	REST INTERVAL	SETS	REPS
Romanian Deadlift	120 seconds	4	10
Band-Resisted Deadlift	180 seconds	3	5, 3, 2
Deadlift	120 seconds	3	3
High Pull	120 seconds	3	5
Shrug	90 seconds	4	12
Bent-Over Barbell Row	90 seconds	3	5
Weighted Chin-up	120 seconds	3	10
Wide-Grip Lat Pull-down	60 seconds	3	12
Preacher Curl	60 seconds	3	12
Medicine Ball Slam	60 seconds	3	8
Russian Twist	60 seconds	3	10

Week 4

Do all the same exercises but eliminate bands/chains. Do one less set per exercise and use 60% of weights used during week 3; reps remain the same.

Weeks 5–7

Day 1

EXERCISE	REST INTERVAL	SETS	REPS
Bench Press	180 seconds	5	3, 3, 3, 10, 15
Weighted Dip	120 seconds	5	3
Rack Bench Press (from dead stop)	75 seconds	5	1
Flat-Bench Dumbbell Flye (band resisted)	60 seconds	3	12
Zottman Curl	60 seconds	4	15
Dumbbell Kickback	45 seconds	4	15
Plank	30 seconds	2	60 seconds
Side Plank	30 seconds	2	45 seconds

Day 2

EXERCISE	REST INTERVAL	SETS	REPS
Squat	180 seconds	6	3, 3, 4, 4, 4, 4
Olympic Pause Squat	120 seconds	2	10
Dumbbell Step-up	60 seconds	4	12
Hack Squats	60 seconds	2	15
Leg Extension	60 seconds	2	30, 20
Barbell Hip Thrust	120 seconds	3	8
Leg Curl	60 seconds	3	6
Standing Cable Crunch	45 seconds	3	12
Oblique Cable Crunch	45 seconds	3	12

Day 3 Off

Day 4

EXERCISE	REST INTERVAL	SETS	REPS
Close-Grip Bench Press	180 seconds	3	10
Standing Military Press	120 seconds	6	3, 3, 6, 6, 6, 6
Cable Lateral Raise	60 seconds	3	15
Bent-Over Lateral Raise	60 seconds	3	15
Rope Face Pull	60 seconds	3	15
French Press	60 seconds	4	15
Triceps Push-down	45 seconds	3	20
Hanging Leg Raise	45 seconds	3	15
Abs Wheel	45 seconds	4	12

Day 5

EXERCISE	REST INTERVAL	SETS	REPS
Romanian Deadlift	180 seconds	4	8
Band-Resisted Deadlift	180 seconds	4	5
Deadlift	120 seconds	3	3
Shrug	120 seconds	3	20
Meadows Rows	60 seconds	4	10, 8, 6, 15
Weighted Chin-up	120 seconds	3	10, 8, 6
Wide-Grip Lat Pull-down	60 seconds	3	12
Preacher Curl	60 seconds	3	12
V Sit-up	45 seconds	3	12
Medicine Ball Slam	45 seconds	4	12

Days 6–7 Off

Week 8

Do all the same exercises but eliminate bands/chains. Do one less set per exercise and use 60% of weights used during week 3; reps remain the same.

Weeks 9–11

Day 1

EXERCISE	REST INTERVAL	SETS	REPS
Bench Press	180 sec	5	2, 2, 2, 15
Bench Press Against Bands	180 seconds	3	6
Weighted Dips	120 seconds	3	10, 8, 6
Incline-Bench Dumbbell Flyes	60 seconds	3	12
Chin-up/Incline Dumbbell Curl Palms Open Superset	120 seconds	4	6...15
Band Triceps Push-downs	60 seconds	4	30
Plank	45 seconds	2	60 seconds
Side Plank	45 seconds	2	45 seconds

Day 2

EXERCISE	REST INTERVAL	SETS	REPS
Squat	180 seconds	6	2, 2, 3, 3, 3, 3
Front Squats	120 seconds	2	6
Bulgarian Split Squat	60 seconds	2	10
Barbell Hip Thrusts	120 seconds	4	10
Leg Extension	60 seconds	4	12
Single-Leg Deadlift (each side)	60 seconds	3	6
Leg Curl	60 seconds	4	6
Standing Cable Crunch	60 seconds	4	15
Oblique Cable Crunch	60 seconds	4	15

Day 3 Off

Day 4

EXERCISE	REST INTERVAL	SETS	REPS
Close-Grip Bench Press	180 seconds	4	4, 4, 8, 10
Standing Military Press	120 seconds	6	2, 2, 8, 8, 8, 8
Machine Seated Lateral Raise	45 seconds	3	15
Reverse Pec Deck	60 seconds	3	12
Rope Face Pull	60 seconds	3	12
Dicks Press	90 seconds	4	10
Overhead Dumbbell Triceps Extension	60 seconds	2	15
Hanging Leg Raise	60 seconds	3	10
Abs Wheel	60 seconds	4	12

Day 5

EXERCISE	REST INTERVAL	SETS	REPS
Deadlift	180 seconds	5	5, 4, 3, 2, 1
Snatch Grip Deadlift	120 seconds	3	6
Shrug	90 seconds	3	8
Bent-Over Barbell Row	90 seconds	3	8
Weighted Chin-up	120 seconds	3	4
Narrow Grip Lat Pull-down	60 seconds	3	12
Reverse Curls to failure, followed immediately by Barbell Curls to failure	120 seconds	4	As described
Medicine Ball Slam	90 seconds	4	10
Russian Twist	30 seconds	5	12

Week 12

- Do all the same exercises but eliminate bands/chains. Do one less set per exercise, and use 60% of weights used during week 3; reps remain the same.
- Add weight to exercises each week.
- Do not go heavy on light deload weeks.
- Add additional weight to body for chins-ups and dips if possible; use a band for assistance if unable to perform with bodyweight.
- Use as much weight as possible without compromising form.
- If reps descend, add weight; if they ascend, decrease weight.
- Add weight to exercises weekly; the goal is to do more every week, but never at the expense of technique.

POWERBUILDING/STRONGMAN HYBRID ROUTINE

Here is a powerbuilding routine I designed for the "Metroflex Massive Feature." Strongman events are cycled in.

Day 1

EXERCISE	REST INTERVAL	SETS	REPS
Bench Press	120 seconds	5	5
Bench Press	120 seconds	8	1
Bench Press	120 seconds	1	AMAP
Incline Press	120 seconds	3	6
Dumbbell Bench Press	90 seconds	4	8
One-Arm Eccentric Barbell Curl	90 seconds	5	5
Zottman Curl	60 seconds	4	12
Prone Iso Abs	60 seconds	2	60 seconds

Day 2

EXERCISE	REST INTERVAL	SETS	REPS
Back Squat	120 seconds	3	5
Back Squat	240 seconds	1	20
Front Squat	120 seconds	2	6
Sled Drag	60 seconds	5	20 yards
Leg Curls	60 seconds	4	8
One-Leg Squat	90 seconds	3	12
Dumbbell Side Bend	60 seconds	2	8
Landmines	60 seconds	2	10

Day 3

EXERCISE	REST INTERVAL	SETS	REPS
Military Press	120 seconds	5	5
Lateral Raise	60 seconds	4	12
Barbell Front Raise	60 seconds	4	10
Bent-Over Flyes	60 seconds	3	15
Upright Dips	90 seconds	3	AMAP
Skull Crushers	60 seconds	6	15
Leg Raises (knees to chest)	45 seconds	3	12
Leg Raises (straight up)	45 seconds	2	10

Day 4

EXERCISE	REST INTERVAL	SETS	REPS
Deficit Deadlift	120 seconds	5	5
Dumbbell Shrug	60 seconds	5	20
Farmers Walk	120 seconds	4	20 yards
Heavy Tire Flip	120 seconds	3	30 seconds max flips
Chin-ups	120 seconds	5	5
Dumbbell Rows	90 seconds	4	12
Straight-Arm Pull-downs	60 seconds	5	15

PUSH/PULL ROUTINE

Day 1 (Push)

EXERCISE	REST INTERVAL	INTENSITY	SETS	REPS
Squat	120 seconds	75%	5	5
Bench Press	120seconds	75%	5	5
Pause Squats	120 seconds	Max	2	6
Overhead Press	120 seconds	80%	3	3
Weighted Dips	120 seconds	Max	5	5
Seated Calf Raises	60 seconds	Max	5	20

For last set of squats, bench presses and overhead presses, do as many reps as possible.

(Day 2 Combo)

EXERCISE	REST INTERVAL	INTENSITY	SETS	REPS
Lat Pull-downs	60 seconds	Max	4	12
Flyes	60 seconds	Max	3	12
Leg Curls	60 seconds	Max	4	6
Standing Calf Raises	45 seconds	Max	5	15
Abs	60 seconds	Max	5	20

Day 3 (Pull)

EXERCISE	REST INTERVAL	INTENSITY	SETS	REPS
Deadlifts	120 seconds	80%	5	5
Bent Over Rows	60 seconds	Max	5	6–8
Glute Ham Raises	120 seconds	Max	4	6
Chin-ups	120 seconds	Max	3	6
One Armed Dumbbell Rows	120 seconds	Max	5	5
Abs	45 seconds	Max	5	10–15

PROGRAMED OVERREACHING = SUPERCOMPENSATION

Monday/Thursday Morning Workout

EXERCISE	REST INTERVAL	INTENSITY	SETS	REPS
Squats	120 seconds	Max	4	6–8
Leg Curls	60 seconds	Max	3	6
Leg Extensions	60 seconds	Max	3	20
Standing Calf Raises	45 seconds	Max	5	15

Monday/Thursday Evening Workout

EXERCISE	REST INTERVAL	INTENSITY	SETS	REPS
Front Squats	120 seconds	Max	4	4–6
One-Leg Deadlift	60 seconds	Max	3	6
Leg Press	60 seconds	Max	3	20
Abs	45 seconds	Max	5	15–25

Tuesday/Friday Morning Workout

EXERCISE	REST INTERVAL	INTENSITY	SETS	REPS
Bench Press with Band or Chains	120 seconds	Max	4	6–8
Overhead Presses	90 seconds	Max	3	6
Dips/Overhead Rope Triceps Extension Superset	120 seconds	Max	3	10/15

Tuesday/Friday EveningWorkout

EXERCISE	REST INTERVAL	INTENSITY	SETS	REPS
Incline Dumbbell Press	120 seconds	Max	4	6–8
Face Pulls	60 seconds	Max	3	15
Lateral Raises	60 seconds	Max	3	15
Dumbbell Flyes	45 seconds	Max	3	10–15

Wednesday/Saturday Morning Workout

EXERCISE	REST INTERVAL	INTENSITY	SETS	REPS
Snatch Grip Deadlifts	120 seconds	Max	4	3–5
Bent Over Rows	90 seconds	Max	3	6
Incline Dumbbell Curl (huge stretch)	60 seconds	Max	3	15
Leg Raises/Seated Calf Raise Superset	90 seconds	Max	3	12...20

Wednesday/Saturday Evening Workout

EXERCISE	REST INTERVAL	INTENSITY	SETS	REPS
T-Bar Prison Rows	120 seconds	Max	4	6–8
One-Armed Dumbbell Rows	60 seconds	Max	3	15
Weighted Chin-ups	90 seconds	Max	3	6
Hammer Curls	45 seconds	Max	3	10–15

- Do this program for three weeks; then take a full week off from any lifting or intense physical activity.
- This program will beat you down mentally and physically. We are purposefully overreaching to induce supercompensation. You may actually lose muscle during the course of it, but you will gain it back and then some on your week off.
- Supplement with BCAAs (double your normal dosage).
- Eat 500–700 calories daily in addition to what you eat during "normal training."
- Eat 1.5 to 2 grams of protein per pound of body weight daily.
- Do not reduce calories on week off.
- Avoid going to failure; instead, go as hard as you can but stop one rep shy of failure on all exercises.

A FEW LAST WORDS

You know what to do and why to do it. Experiment with the routines as presented, or design your own with variables presented. Most importantly, have fun. Quit reading and hit the pig iron!

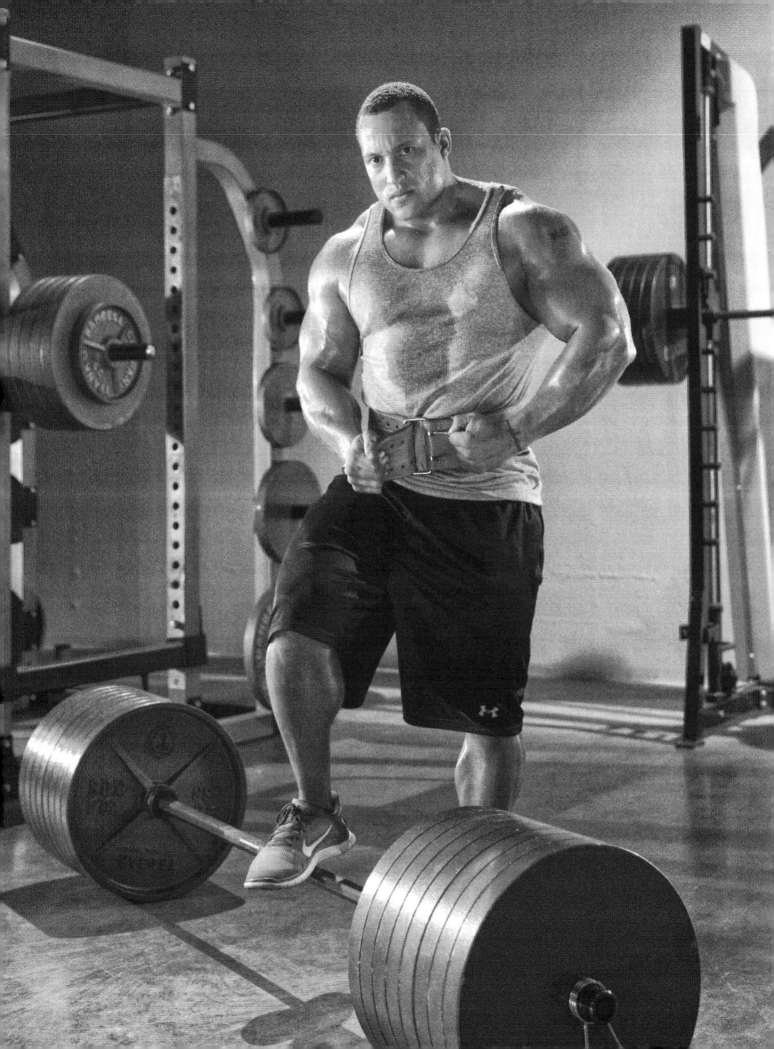

AFTERWORD

Train Your Mind for Success

The straight and narrow path to have a championship physique is initiated by many, but few actually make it.

Why?

A big reason is that they aren't mentally prepared. Mental breakdowns lead to physical mistakes, which can be the beginning of a self-perpetuating, self-sabotaging cycle. You now have the psychological tools to successfully initiate and complete the journey to the physique of your dreams.

No matter how strong your desire, mental toughness, or pain tolerance, you will not get there without a plan. Sure, it takes hard work, but you have to work smart, too. You don't train for pain, you train for gains; pain is part of the process, not the result. The techniques outlined in this book have produced miraculous results for my clients at Metroflex Gym and around the world.

These methods have been proven time and time again in the trenches. Remember, science is the guiding light of the method to the madness, and now you know why!

I really appreciate the opportunity to be a part of your journey. I look forward to hearing about your success. Good luck and God bless you all!

ABOUT THE AUTHOR

Josh Bryant is a speed, strength, and conditioning coach. Josh trains some of the strongest and most muscular athletes in the world in person at Metroflex Gym in Arlington, Texas, and via the Internet. Along with his receiving ISSA certifications in fitness training, nutrition, and conditioning, Josh was recently awarded the prestigious title of Master of Fitness (MFS) by the ISSA. He also has a Master's degree in Exercise Science. Josh has won many national and world titles in powerlifting and strongman and was the youngest person in powerlifting history, at 22, to bench press 600 pounds raw. Josh has squatted 909 in the USPF, officially bench pressed 620 pounds raw, and officially deadlifted 800 pounds raw.

To learn more about Josh Bryant or to sign up for his free training tips newsletter, visit www.JoshStrength.com. You can also follow Josh on Twitter @JoshStrength or on Facebook/TheJoshStrengthMethod.

Josh is available for online training, consultations, and seminars. To learn more, visit www.JoshStrength.com.

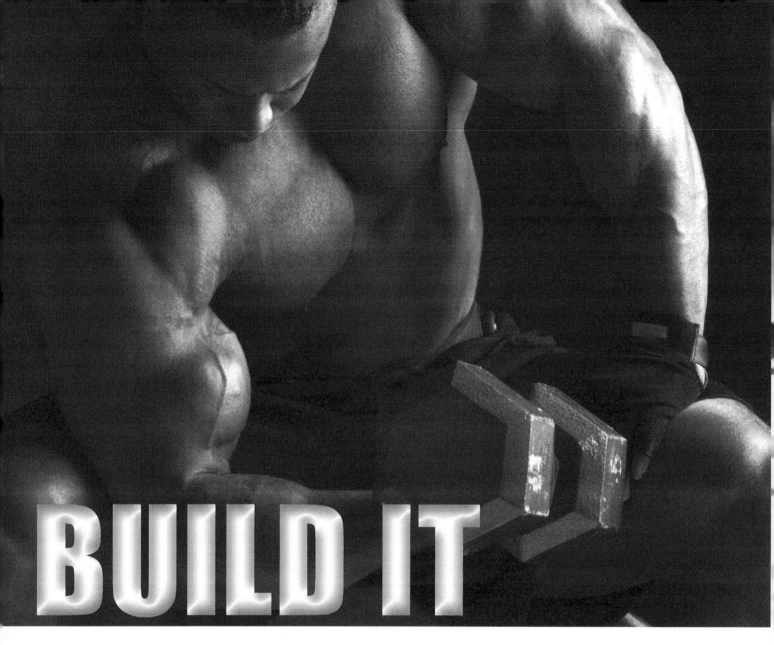

BUILD IT

You're committed to being the best you can be. You train hard, but you train smart. So why not use your passion to help others reach their goals and make great money...doing what you love?

From ISSA's Certified Fitness Trainer program, to our Elite and Master Trainer programs, your education can be the stepping stone to an incredible future.

If you're already certified and looking for a degree, ISSA's nationally accredited Associate's Degree in Exercise Science is the perfect choice because it's entirely online and designed to accommodate your busy schedule!

Since 1988, the ISSA has provided fitness education to nearly 200,000 students in 92 countries. We're nationally accredited by the DETC and Tuition Assistance approved. We support our troops and are honored to help military students and their spouses pursue a career in fitness. Call us and we'll help you every step of the way!

CERTIFICATE & DEGREE PROGRAMS

- *Certified Fitness Trainer*
- *Fitness Nutrition*
- *Exercise Therapy*
- *Youth Fitness Trainer*
- *Senior Fitness*
- *Strength and Conditioning*
- *AS in Exercise Science*

www.ISSAonline.edu

or call (805) 745-8111
1015 Mark Avenue
Carpinteria, CA 93013

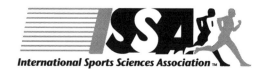

International Sports Sciences Association ™

33906302R00259

Made in the USA
Lexington, KY
15 July 2014